Practical Case Studies in Nephrology

Practical Case Studies in Nephrology

Editor: Percy Cook

AMERICAN
MEDICAL PUBLISHERS
www.americanmedicalpublishers.com

AMERICAN
MEDICAL PUBLISHERS
www.americanmedicalpublishers.com

Cataloging-in-Publication Data

Practical case studies in nephrology / edited by Percy Cook.
p. cm.
Includes bibliographical references and index.
ISBN 979-8-88740-656-5
1. Nephrology. 2. Kidneys--Diseases. I. Cook, Percy.
RC902 .P73 2023
616.61--dc23

American Medical Publishers,
41 Flatbush Avenue,
1st Floor, New York,
NY 11217, USA

ISBN 979-8-88740-656-5 (Hardback)

Contents

Preface

Nephrology is an area of medical science that focuses on the diagnosis, treatment and management of various kidney diseases and disorders. Some common kidney diseases and conditions treated under nephrology include chronic kidney disease, acute kidney injury and kidney stones. Chronic kidney disease is a progressive condition characterized by the gradual loss of kidney function over time. Acute kidney injury refers to the sudden and temporary loss of kidney function, often caused by conditions such as severe infections, dehydration, medications, or reduced blood flow to the kidneys. Kidney stones are hard deposits formed in the kidneys. They can be treated through medications, dietary changes and lifestyle modifications. This book unfolds the innovative aspects of nephrology which will be crucial for the progress of this field in the future. Those in search of information to further their knowledge will be greatly assisted by it.

Significant researches are present in this book. Intensive efforts have been employed by authors to make this book an outstanding discourse. This book contains the enlightening chapters which have been written on the basis of significant researches done by the experts.

Finally, I would also like to thank all the members involved in this book for being a team and meeting all the deadlines for the submission of their respective works. I would also like to thank my friends and family for being supportive in my efforts.

Editor

1

Henoch-Schönlein Nephritis Manifesting with Purpura 15 Years after Diagnosis of IgA Nephropathy

Hideaki Yamabe ,[1,2] Mitsuaki Kaizuka,[1] Satoru Tsunoda,[1] Tasuku Nagasawa,[3] Kazuo Nomura,[4] and Michiko Shimada [2]

[1]*Internal Medicine, EST Clinic, Hirosaki, Japan*
[2]*Department of Nephrology, Hirosaki University Hospital, Hirosaki, Japan*
[3]*Internal Medicine, Japanese Red Cross Ishinomaki Hospital, Ishinomaki, Japan*
[4]*Aoyama Nomura Dermatology Clinic, Hirosaki, Japan*

Correspondence should be addressed to Hideaki Yamabe; h-yamabe@lapis.plala.or.jp

Academic Editor: Kouichi Hirayama

Henoch-Schönlein nephritis or immunoglobulin A (IgA) vasculitis is characterized by purpura, arthralgia, abdominal pain, and glomerulonephritis with glomerular IgA deposition. Notably, the presence of purpura is essential to diagnose this disease. We report the case of a patient in whom proteinuria and haematuria were detected during screening tests and he was diagnosed with IgA nephropathy at 20 years of age. Corticosteroids were administered for 7 years and were subsequently tapered. At 35 years of age, he noticed purpura on his lower extremities and was diagnosed with anaphylactoid purpura. Following the appearance of purpura, urinalysis revealed an increase in urinary protein levels from 0.7 g/g creatinine (Cr) to 1.4 g/gCr, and his serum Cr levels increased from 1.1 mg/dL to 1.35 mg/dL. Two months later purpura subsided, and his urinary protein level and serum Cr level were restored to the former levels. Although the cause remains unknown, an interval may occasionally be observed between the appearance of purpura and urinary abnormalities. However, to our knowledge to date, a 15-year interval is the longest interval, in such cases, reported in the literature.

1. Introduction

Henoch-Schönlein nephritis or immunoglobulin A (IgA) vasculitis (IgAV) is characterized by purpura, arthralgia, abdominal pain, and glomerulonephritis with glomerular IgA deposition. Notably, the presence of purpura is essential to establish the diagnosis in these patients [1]. Usually, patients show urinary abnormalities with a purpuric rash concomitantly or within a month. We report a patient of Henoch-Schönlein nephritis who developed purpura 15 years after the diagnosis of IgA nephropathy (IgAN). To our knowledge to date, 15 years is the longest interval between the detection of urinary abnormalities and the development of purpura.

2. Case Report

A 35-year-old Japanese man with a history of renal disease presented to a dermatology clinic with sudden onset of a purpuric rash on his lower extremities (Figure 1) and was diagnosed with anaphylactoid purpura. Although he was asymptomatic, proteinuria, and haematuria were detected during a screening test when he was 20 years old, and he was diagnosed with IgAN based on renal biopsy. Histopathological examination of renal biopsy specimens revealed mild mesangial proliferation (Figure 2). Immunohistochemical examination revealed mesangial IgA (Figure 3), IgG and C3 (Figure 4) depositions, and he was treated with corticosteroids. Thereafter, he moved to our city and continued to be treated here. Corticosteroids treatment was continued for 7 years and was subsequently tapered.

Physical examination following the appearance of purpura revealed purpuric rash without any pitting oedema on his legs. Blood pressure was 147/78 mmHg. Urinalysis showed (+++) urinary protein, no urinary glucose, 6–10 red blood cells/high power field, urinary protein was 1.4 g/g creatinine (Cr). A peripheral blood smear showed a white blood cell (WBC)

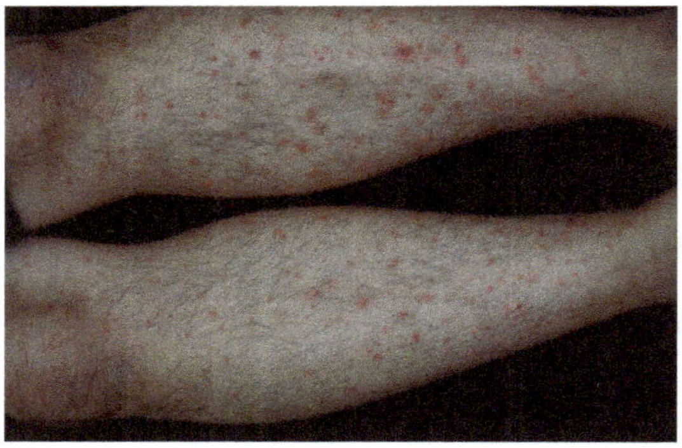

FIGURE 1: Purpuric rash on the patient's lower extremities.

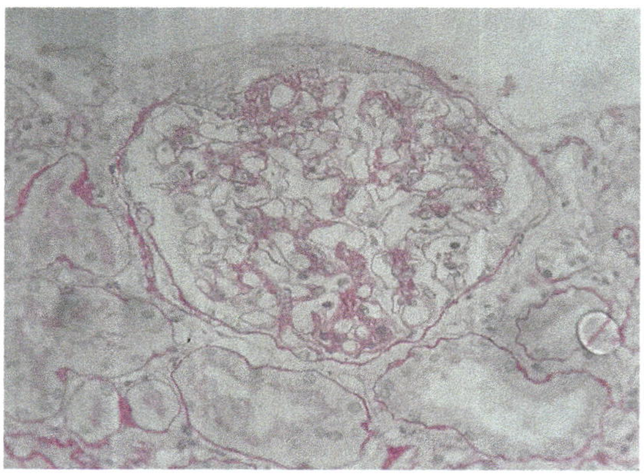

FIGURE 2: Mesangial proliferative glomerulonephritis was demonstrated (PAS stain).

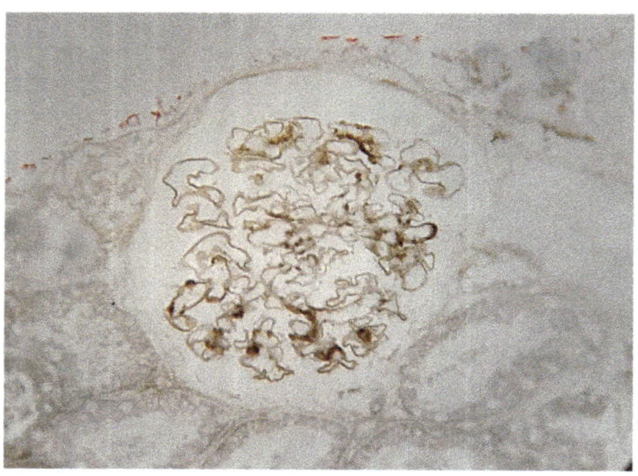

FIGURE 3: Mesangial IgA deposition was observed by immunohistochemistry.

count of 12,100 cells/mm3, red blood cell of 5.16 million cells/mm3, and platelets 192,000 cells/mm3. Serum haemoglobin was 16.6 g/dL and haematocrit 45.4%. Blood chemistry showed total serum protein 7.2 g/dL, serum albumin 4.2 g/dL, serum sodium 141 mEq/L, potassium 4.3 mEq/L, chloride 105 mEq/L, serum Cr 1.35 mg/dL, serum aspartate aminotransferase 21 IU/L, serum alanine aminotransferase 28 IU/L, blood glucose 96 mg/dL, glycosylated haemoglobin 4.8%, and serum C-reactive protein (CRP) 1.57 mg/dL. Immunological

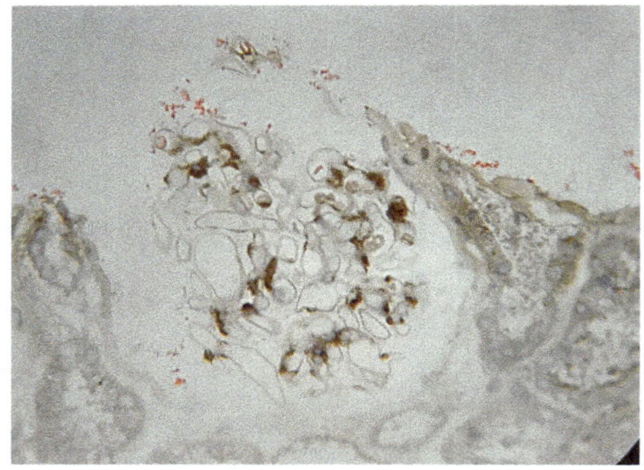

FIGURE 4: Mesangial C3 deposition was observed.

examination showed an antistreptolysin O (ASO) titer 24 IU/mL, IgG 1095 mg/dL, IgA 315 mg/dL, IgM 133 mg/dL, C3 164 mg/dL, C4 35 mg/dL, and CH50 67.0 U/mL. A month before the appearance of purpura urinalysis revealed (++) protein, absence of haematuria, urinary protein level of 0.73 g/gCr, and serum Cr level of 1.10 mg/dL. Two months thereafter, purpura subsided, and his urinary protein level and serum Cr level were restored to the former levels. Skin biopsy was not performed because his purpura was typical for anaphylactoid purpura.

3. Discussion

We report a patient who developed anaphylactoid purpura 15 years after the diagnosis of IgAN. Schönlein first described a child with purpura and arthritis in 1837. Subsequently in 1874, Henoch described a patient who showed purpura, arthralgia, and abdominal pain. Therefore, this condition is referred to Henoch-Schönlein purpura. These patients often present with proteinuria and haematuria. Histopathological examination of renal biopsy specimen shows focal segmental mesangial proliferative glomerulonephritis, and mesangial deposition of IgA is a consistent finding. C3 deposition occurs in 90% and IgG deposition in 70% of the cases. The eponym Henoch-Schönlein purpura was replaced with IgAV at the 2012 Chapel Hill Consensus Conference. Based on the revised nomenclature IgAV was defined as vasculitis with IgA1-dominant immune deposits affecting small vessels in the skin and gastrointestinal tract commonly associated with arthritis. IgAV is also associated with glomerulonephritis indistinguishable from IgAN [2]. Currently, it is being recognized that IgAV and IgAN share pathogenic mechanisms. In patients with systemic IgAV or renal-limited IgAN, IgA1 in serum and in tissues deposits shows reduced terminal glycosylation in the hinge regions [3]. Emerging data suggest that patients with IgAV and IgAN have circulating immune complexes containing abnormally glycosylated IgA1 and passively glycan-specific IgG antibodies that form IgA1-IgG and anti-IgA1 immune complexes [4]. IgG antibodies directed against abnormal glycosylation reportedly bind to IgA1 molecules and localize in vessel walls, causing inflammation. Our patient showed increased urinary protein and serum Cr levels coinciding with the appearance of purpura, which indicates a close association between IgAV and IgAN. Notably, the presence of purpura is the only distinguishing feature between IgAV and IgAN. Glomerulonephritis in patients with IgAV is diagnosed on the basis of proteinuria and haematuria and occurs concomitantly with purpura or within a month of onset of purpura. A long interval between the appearance of purpura and the detection of urinary abnormalities is rare [5]. To our knowledge to date, 15 years is the longest interval between the detection of urinary abnormalities and the development of purpura in patients diagnosed with this condition.

The cause of the long interval in our patient remains unknown and could be attributed to the following possibilities: (a) mild purpura could have been present at the time of detection of proteinuria and haematuria. However, considering that the urinary abnormalities were identified during screening, purpura, arthralgia, or abdominal pain was not recognized. Thus, this possibility can be excluded. (b) Previous studies have reported that corticosteroids may effectively treat the extrarenal manifestations in these patients [6] and may inhibit the appearance of purpura. A previous report has described a patient who developed purpura 13 years after being diagnosed with IgAN. Notably, he did not receive corticosteroids [7]. Our patient received corticosteroids for 7 years. Based on these observations, the effect of corticosteroids remains unclear. (c) It is possible that our patient developed an infection at the time of appearance of purpura. Reportedly, 30–50% of patients with IgAV were shown to have streptococcal infection [8]. Although the patient was asymptomatic, his peripheral blood smear showed elevation of the WBC count, and he also showed elevated serum CRP levels suggesting an infection. Infection is a known trigger for vasculitis. However, his ASO titer was within normal limits, and the elevated WBC count and positive results with CRP testing may only represent vasculitis. Diagnosis of IgAV is based on the existence of purpura and is challenging in patients with a long interval between the occurrence of purpura and the diagnosis of IgAN.

4. Conclusion

In summary, we describe a rare patient of IgAV who showed purpura 15 years after the diagnosis of IgAN. Therefore, patients with IgAN require close and prolonged follow-up.

References

[1] C. E. Gota, "Vasculitis," in *The Merck Manual*, R. S. Porter, J. L. Kaplan, R. B. Lynn, and M. T. Reddy, Eds., pp. 353–354, Merck Sharp & Dohme Corp. A Subsidiary of Merck & CO., INC, Kenilworth, NJ, 20th edition, 2018.

[2] J. C. Jennette, R. J. Falk, P. A. Bacon et al., "2012 revised international Chape Hill consensus conference nomenclature of vasculitides," *Arthritis & Rheumatism*, vol. 65, no. 1, pp. 1–11, 2013.

[3] H. Suzuki, K. Kiryluk, J. Novak et al., "The pathophysiology of IgA nephropathy," *Journal of American Society of Nephrology*, vol. 22, no. 10, pp. 1795–1803, 2011.

[4] H. Suzuki, R. Fan, Z. Zhang et al., "Aberrantly glycolsylated IgA1 in IgA nephropathy patients is recognized by IgG antibodies with restricted heterogeneity," *The Journal of Clinical Investigation*, vol. 119, no. 6, pp. 1668–1677, 2009.

[5] K. Kamei, "Purpura nephritis and IgA nephropathy. Jin to Touseki," vol. 82, no. 4, pp. 589–594, 2017, Japanese.

[6] J. Feehally and J. Floege, "IgA nephronpathy and Henoch-Schönlein nephritis," in *Comprehensive Clinical Nephrology*, J. Floege, R. J. Johnson, and J. Feehally, Eds., pp. 270–281, Elsevier Saunders, St Louis, 4th edition, 2010.

[7] D. M. Siverstein, I. Greifer, V. Folkeert, B. Bennett, H. E. Corey, and A. Spitzer, "Sequential occurrence of IgA nephropathy and Henoch-Schönlein purpura: support for common pathogenesis," *Pediatric Nephrology*, vol. 8, no. 6, pp. 752–753, 1994.

[8] D. M. Kraft, D. Mckee, and C. Scott, "Henoch-Schönlein nephritis: a review," *American Family Physician*, vol. 58, no. 2, pp. 405–408, 1998.

2

Peritoneal Dialysis with Marked Pneumoperitoneum

Norio Nakamura[1] **Masamichi Nakata,**[2] **Daiki Nagawa,**[2] **Ikuyo Narita,**[2] **Takeshi Fujita,**[2] **Reiichi Murakami,**[2] **Michiko Shimada,**[2] **and Hirofumi Tomita**[2]

[1]*Community Medicine, Hirosaki University Graduate School of Medicine, Aomori, Japan*
[2]*Department of Cardiology and Nephrology, Hirosaki Graduate School of Medicine, Aomori, Japan*

Correspondence should be addressed to Norio Nakamura; nnakamur@r2.dion.ne.jp

Academic Editor: Ze'ev Korzets

Pneumoperitoneum, the presence of free air within the peritoneal cavity, is often caused by the perforation of gas-containing viscus and commonly requires surgical treatment. However, in patients with peritoneal dialysis, free air is commonly seen on X-ray. We present the case of a patient with peritoneal dialysis with marked pneumoperitoneum. A 75-year-old Japanese male with end-stage renal disease due to antineutrophil cytoplasmic antigen-associated vasculitis had been receiving continuous ambulatory peritoneal dialysis for 9 years. He had a poor appetite and general malaise without abdominal pain or fever. These symptoms gradually worsened, and he was hospitalized. At the time of admission, chest X-ray revealed bilateral free air in the abdomen. Subsequent computed tomography of the abdomen revealed marked pneumoperitoneum. Peritonitis due to perforation of the digestive tract was considered; however, the absence of abdominal pain, fever, and turbidity of dialysis drainage indicated that peritonitis was unlikely. Insufficient air venting during continuous ambulatory peritoneal dialysis bag replacement was suspected. The bag was carefully changed, resulting in a gradual decrease in the free air. We encountered a patient with continuous ambulatory peritoneal dialysis who had significant free air in the abdominal cavity in the absence of peritonitis. The source of the air was determined to be the dialysis bag due to insufficient venting during replacement. This case underscores the importance of instructing patients with continuous ambulatory peritoneal dialysis on the thorough removal of air from the bag during replacement.

1. Introduction

Pneumoperitoneum (PP) is the presence of free air within the peritoneal cavity. This condition is often caused by perforation of gas-containing viscus and commonly requires surgical treatment [1]. However, in patients with peritoneal dialysis (PD), free air is commonly seen on X-ray [2]. We present the case of a patient with PD with marked PP.

2. Case Presentation

A 75-year-old Japanese male with end-stage renal disease due to antineutrophil cytoplasmic antigen (ANCA)-associated vasculitis had been receiving continuous ambulatory peritoneal dialysis (CAPD) for 9 years. He also had an implanted defibrillator (cardio-resynchronized therapy with defibrillator) to treat chronic heart failure resulting from a myocardial infarction. He had a poor appetite and general malaise without abdominal pain or fever. These symptoms gradually worsened, and he was hospitalized. At the time of admission, his blood pressure was 94/52 mmHg, his height was 165 cm, and his weight was 53 kg. At auscultation, no gallop rhythm was heard, and his extremities were not edematous. The laboratory parameters at the time of admission were as follows: white blood cells, 8080/μL; hemoglobin, 13.5 g/dL; platelets, $121 \times 10^3/\mu$L; total protein, 5.2 g/dL; albumin, 1.8 g/dL; lactate dehydrogenase, 309 U/L; glutamate oxaloacetate transaminase, 25 U/L; glutamate pyruvate transaminase, 19 U/L; blood urea nitrogen, 28 mg/dL; creatinine, 4.97 mg/dL; sodium, 125 mmol/L; potassium, 2.7 mmol/L; chlorine, 91 mmol/L; calcium, 6.8 mg/dL; phosphorus, 4.1 mg/dL; C-reactive protein, 0.092 mg/dL; procalcitonin, 0.21 ng/mL; BNP, 319 pg/mL; intact parathyroid hormone, 149 pg/mL; and β_2-microglobulin,

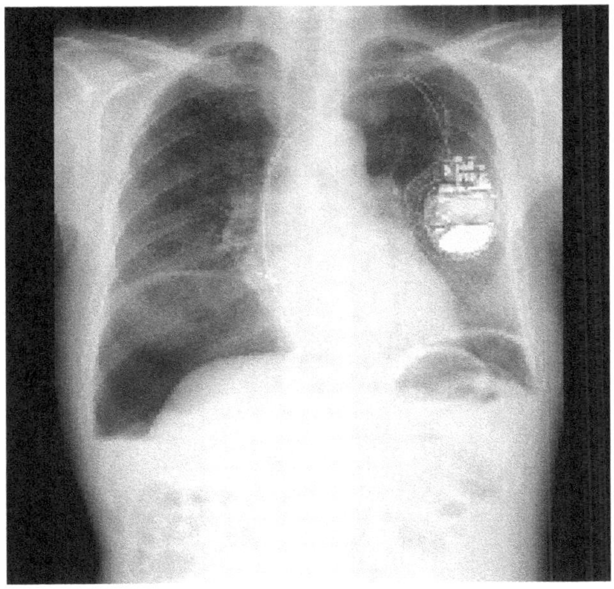

FIGURE 1: Chest X-ray upon admission. Bilateral free air in the abdomen was observed.

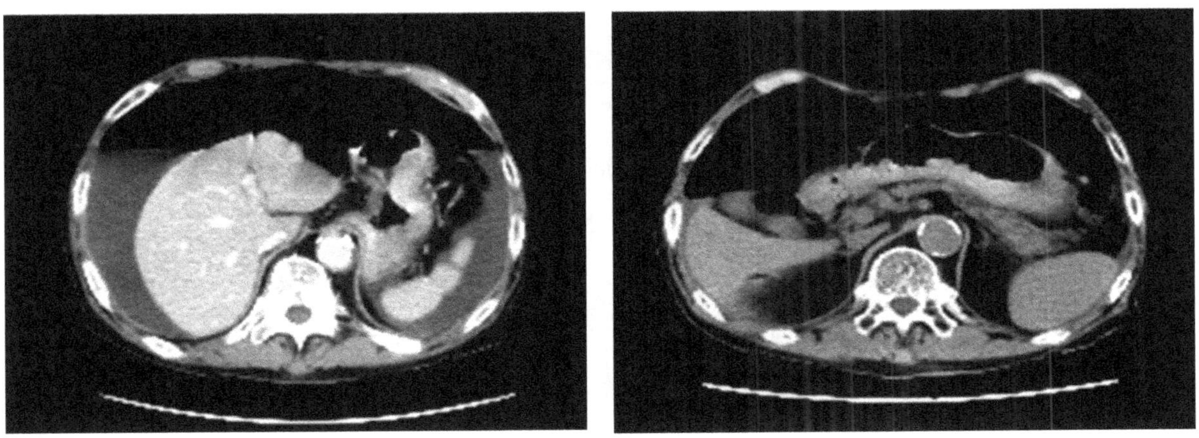

(a) (b)

FIGURE 2: (a), (b) Computed tomography of the abdomen one day after admission. Marked pneumoperitoneum was observed.

23.4 μg/mL. Chest X-ray revealed bilateral free air in the abdomen (Figure 1). Subsequent computed tomography of the abdomen revealed marked PP (Figures 2(a) and 2(b)).

Peritonitis due to perforation of the digestive tract was suspected, but the possibility of perforation was considered very low because of the absence of abdominal pain, fever, and turbidity of dialysis drainage. Insufficient priming (air removal) at the time of peritoneal dialysis bag replacement was suspected, and the patient was instructed on how to perform sufficient priming. As a result, the free air in his abdominal cavity gradually disappeared (Figure 3).

3. Discussion

We encountered a patient with marked abdominal free air during CAPD. The patient exhibited no pain, fever, or drainage opacification, eliminating peritonitis due to gastrointestinal perforation as the cause. Insufficient air venting during CAPD bag replacement was suspected. The bag was carefully changed, resulting in a gradual decrease in the free air.

In general, free air in the abdominal cavity is a strong indicator of peritonitis due to gastrointestinal perforation [3]. However, this condition has been observed in the absence of gastrointestinal perforation in 20%–23% of patients with PD [2, 4, 5]. Idiopathic PP has been reported, sometimes resulting from iatrogenic causes, including PD [6].

Intraperitoneal free air is an independent risk factor for peritonitis in patients with PD [7] and is thought to be caused by inadequate PD procedures. The most likely cause of intraperitoneal free air in patients with PD is aeration due to insufficient air removal during bag replacement. In the present case, complete air removal during bag replacement led to a gradual decrease in intraperitoneal free air. This case

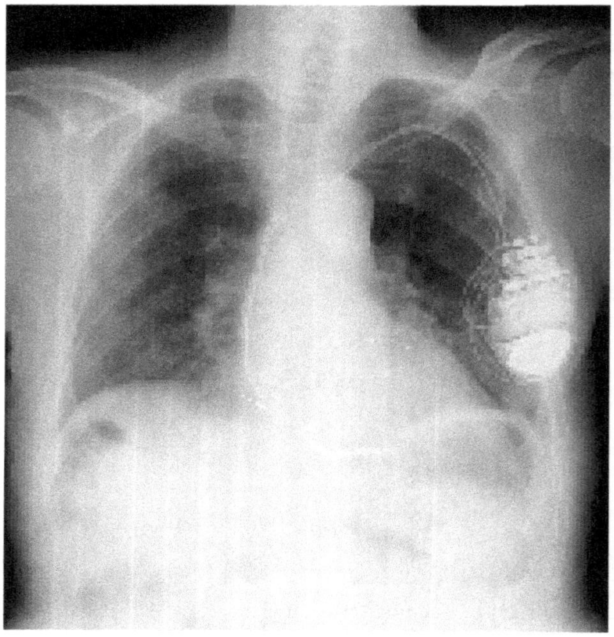

FIGURE 3: Chest X-ray one day after admission. The free air in the abdomen had disappeared.

underscores the importance of providing sufficient instructions to patients with CAPD regarding thorough air removal during bag replacement.

Consent

Written informed consent was obtained from the patient for publication of the case report and any accompanying images.

Acknowledgments

The authors would like to thank Enago (http://www.enago.jp) for the English language review.

References

[1] J. J. Roth, J. S. Thompson, R. K. Harned, and P. E. Hodgson, "Value of pneumoperitoneum in the diagnosis of visceral perforation," *American Journal of Surgery*, vol. 146, no. 6, pp. 830–833, 1983.

[2] T. Kiefer, U. Schenk, J. Weber, E. Hiubel, and U. Kuhlmann, "Incidence and significance of pneumoperitoneum in continuous ambulatory peritoneal dialysis," *American Journal of Kidney Diseases*, vol. 22, no. 1, pp. 30–35, 1993.

[3] T. G. Winek, H. S. Mosely, G. Grout, and D. Luallin, "Pneumoperitoneum and its association with ruptured abdominal viscus," *Archives of Surgery*, vol. 123, no. 6, pp. 709–712, 1988.

[4] J. J. Chang, J. Y. Yeun, and J. A. Hasbargen, "Pneumoperitoneum in peritoneal dialysis patients," *American Journal of Kidney Diseases*, vol. 25, no. 2, pp. 297–301, 1995.

[5] G. C. Cancarini, O. Carli, M. R. Cristinelli, L. Manili, and R. Maiorca, "Pneumoperitoneum in peritoneal dialysis patients," *Journal of Nephrology*, vol. 12, no. 2, pp. 95–99, 1999.

[6] R. A. Mularski, M. L. Ciccolo, and W. D. Rappaport, "Nonsurgical causes of pneumoperitoneum," *Western Journal of Medicine*, vol. 170, no. 1, pp. 41–46, 1999.

[7] T. Okamoto, T. Ikenoue, K. Matsui et al., "Free air on CT and the risk of peritonitis in peritoneal dialysis patients: a retrospective study," *Renal Failure*, vol. 36, no. 10, pp. 1492–1496, 2014.

3

Anaphylactic Reactions Caused by Nafamostat Mesylate during Hemodialysis before Surgery for Carpal Tunnel Syndrome

Yuta Nakamura, Kaoru Tada, Masashi Matsuta, Atsuro Murai, and Hiroyuki Tsuchiya

Department of Orthopaedic Surgery, Graduate School of Medical Sciences, Kanazawa University, 13-1 Takara-machi, Kanazawa 920-8641, Japan

Correspondence should be addressed to Kaoru Tada; tdkr@med.kanazawa-u.ac.jp

Academic Editor: Yoshihide Fujigaki

Nafamostat mesylate (NM) has been used to treat pancreatitis and disseminated intravascular coagulation during hemodialysis (HD). However, there have been some reports of adverse effects related to anaphylactic reactions. We present a case in which anaphylactic reactions caused by NM during preoperative HD caused repeated postponement of surgery for carpal tunnel syndrome. Symptoms including fever, shivering, chills, low blood pressure, tachycardia, nausea, and vomiting appeared during preoperative HD, and surgery was postponed thrice. Initially, the patient was misdiagnosed with sepsis because of elevated C-reactive protein and procalcitonin levels. However, since the symptoms appeared only when NM was administered and disappeared quickly after the administration of NM was terminated, the condition was diagnosed as anaphylactic reactions caused by NM. Therefore, it is essential to consider anaphylactic reactions caused by NM as differential diagnoses, when symptoms, such as fever, are observed during perioperative HD.

1. Introduction

Nafamostat mesylate (NM) was developed in Japan as a serine protease inhibitor to inhibit various proteases in the coagulation system, fibrinolytic system, complement system, and trypsin [1]. In Japan, in 1986, it was approved as a therapeutic agent for pancreatitis, and in 1989 as a therapeutic agent for disseminated intravascular coagulation (DIC) and an anticoagulant drug during hemodialysis (HD). However, there are reports of adverse effects related to allergic reactions, including anaphylactic reactions [2–5], apart from other side effects [6,7]. Here, we report a case in which anaphylactic reactions caused by NM occurred during preoperative HD, and surgery for carpal tunnel syndrome was postponed thrice.

2. Case Report

A 66-year-old man started HD 20 years ago with end-stage renal disease due to diabetic nephropathy. Numbness of the left thumb, index, and middle fingers appeared a year ago. Numbness of the fingers worsened at night, and Tinel's sign and Phalen's test were both positive. On electrophysiological examination, the right median distal motor latency from the wrist to the abductor pollicis brevis muscle was 10.86 ms, and the right sensory conduction velocity between the index finger and the wrist was undetectable. Based on the symptoms and physical and laboratory findings, the patient was diagnosed with carpal tunnel syndrome on the right side. Surgery was planned as conservative treatment was ineffective. The preoperative blood test results are presented in Table 1. HD was performed 3 times a week for 4 hours each using ABH-21F (Asahi Kasei Medical, Tokyo, Japan) as a hemodiafilter, and heparin as an anticoagulant before admission. The blood flow rate was 200 ml/min, and the dialysate flow rate was 500 ml/min. NM had never been used previously for this patient. The patient was scheduled to be operated upon immediately following HD.

However, surgery was postponed because a fever of approximately 38°C suddenly appeared during HD before surgery. Surgery was postponed for a week. Once again, a

Table 1: Blood test on hospital admission.

WBC	7480/μL
RBC	$378 \times 10^4/\mu l$
Hb	11.8 g/dL
Ht	36.8%
Plt	$12.4 \times 10^4/\mu L$
TP	5.7 g/dL
Alb	3.5 g/dL
AST	11 IU/L
ALT	7 IU/L
LDH	197 IU/L
T-Bil	0.4 mg/dL
AMY	79 IU/L
CK	65 IU/L
BUN	50 mg/dL
Cr	7.87 mg/dL
UA	6.1 mg/dL
Na	142 mEq/L
K	3.2 mEq/L
Cl	106 mEq/L
CRP	0.33 mg/dL
HbA1c	6.7%
PT	12.5 sec
PT ratio	1.05
APTT	29.5 sec
Fbg	356 mg/dL

fever of approximately 38°C appeared during HD before the second surgery. Surgery was postponed for a second time, as the patient presented with fever, shivering, chills, low blood pressure, and tachycardia (Figure 1). Physical findings were as follows: height, 168.4 cm; weight, 72.2 kg; systolic blood pressure, 80–90 mmHg; pulse, 108 beats/min. The blood test results are shown in Table 2. DIC was diagnosed based on the DIC diagnostic criteria established by the Japanese Association for Acute Medicine [8], which consists of 8 points (systemic inflammatory response syndrome, 1 point; platelet, 3 points; prothrombin time ratio, 1 point; fibrin degradation product, 3 points). Whole-body computed tomography scan and echocardiography findings were normal, and blood culture was negative; however, sepsis was suspected at first because blood tests indicated an inflammatory response, and procalcitonin levels were high. Meropenem (0.5 g/day) and vancomycin (0.5 g/each HD) were administered. Symptoms, including fever, disappeared a few hours after HD. Although the patient's condition had improved clinically, blood tests performed several days later showed elevated levels of C-reactive protein (CRP) of 4.97 mg/dL and procalcitonin (PCT) of 162 mg/dL, still indicative of sepsis. However, there was no recurrence of symptoms. Subsequently, CRP and PCT levels improved gradually and became negative 17 days after antibiotic treatment; therefore, antibiotic treatment was completed.

One month after antibiotic treatment, surgery for carpal tunnel syndrome was rescheduled. Once again, fever (approximately 38°C), nausea, and vomiting appeared during HD before surgery, and surgery had to be postponed. Symptoms, including fever, disappeared a few hours after HD, as on the previous two occasions. At this point, it was found that the anticoagulant during HD had been changed

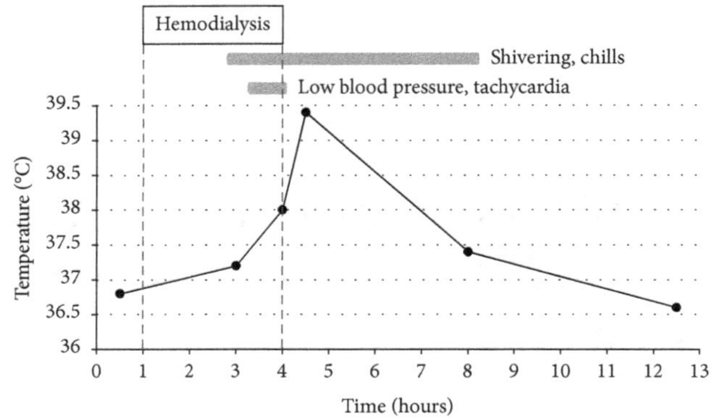

Figure 1: The clinical course of the anaphylactic episode leading to postponement of surgery for a second time.

Table 2: Blood test when a fever appeared for the second time.

WBC	2240/μL
RBC	$337 \times 10^4/\mu l$
Hb	10.3 g/dL
Ht	32.3%
Plt	$6.4 \times 10^4/\mu L$
TP	5.5 g/dL
Alb	3.2 g/dL
AST	21 IU/L
ALT	12 IU/L
LDH	517 IU/L
T-Bil	0.6 mg/dL
AMY	33 IU/L
CK	36 IU/L
BUN	23 mg/dL
Cr	4.45 mg/dL
UA	3.7 mg/dL
Na	144 mEq/L
K	3.1 mEq/L
Cl	108 mEq/L
CRP	0.66 mg/dL
PT	14.6 sec
PT ratio	1.24
APTT	32.1 sec
Fbg	100.8 mg/dL
D-Dimer	36.9 μg/dL
FDP	75.3 g/dL
PCT	2.9 ng/mL
βD-Glucan	<6.0 pg/mL
T-SPOT	–

from heparin to NM only during the perioperative period to control bleeding. The symptoms appeared only when NM was used and disappeared quickly after administration of NM was stopped, leading to the diagnosis of anaphylactic reactions caused by NM. The drug-induced lymphocyte stimulation test (DLST) for NM was negative.

3. Discussion

HD requires anticoagulants to prevent coagulation during extracorporeal circulation. Heparin is the most frequently used anticoagulant, but preoperative administration carries a risk of bleeding. In such cases, changing to NM, which has a shorter half-life, is one of the options for controlling bleeding. NM exhibits an anticoagulant effect by inhibiting proteases associated with thrombin and activated coagulation factors (XIIa, Xa, and VIIa). NM has a low molecular weight of approximately 540 Da and is efficiently removed by HD with a half-life of 8 min. Therefore, the anticoagulant effect does not work inside the body but only during extracorporeal circulation [9]; thus, it is used during HD for the perioperative period and bleeding tendencies, such as gastric ulcers and certain conditions such as aortic dissection and heparin-induced thrombocytopenia.

However, side effects must be carefully considered while administering NM. According to the database provided by the Pharmaceuticals and Medical Devices Agency in Japan, there were 2008 cases of side effects caused by NM during the 16 years from 2004 to 2019; of these, 1072 cases (53.4%) were anaphylactic reactions, 45 cases (2.2%) were leukocytosis/leukopenia or thrombocytosis/thrombocytopenia, 43 cases (2.1%) were fever, 29 cases (1.4%) were nausea and vomiting, and 10 cases (0.5%) were shivering and chills. It has also been reported that anaphylactic reactions occur in 0.16% of patients. These reports indicate that side effects related to anaphylactic reactions are among the most common side effects of NM. In the case of anaphylactic reactions caused by NM, it is necessary to note that symptoms may not occur or may be mild at the first use of NM, but may worsen after multiple uses [2, 3].

In this case, CRP and PCT levels were elevated in addition to fever, shivering, chills, and low blood pressure. Since patients on HD are 26 times more likely to suffer from bacteremia than the general population [10], sepsis was strongly suspected at first. However, all culture tests were negative, and imaging tests showed no other lesions that could cause infection or fever. It was also atypical for the course of sepsis as fever and other symptoms disappeared promptly after HD on all occasions. In this case, the DLST for NM was negative. However, although DLST for the drug is widely used for diagnosis, when anaphylactic reactions are suspected, the test has low sensitivity [11]. Another blood test for antigen-specific IgE antibodies also has similar low sensitivity. Therefore, the diagnosis of anaphylactic reactions requires a comprehensive judgment based on clinical symptoms, clinical course, and laboratory findings. Therefore, this patient's condition was diagnosed as anaphylactic reactions caused by NM based on a comprehensive judgment, since DLST for NM was negative, but his condition was stable during HD, except during the perioperative period; symptoms appeared only during HD using NM and disappeared promptly after.

There are several reasons why the diagnosis was delayed in this case. First, despite anaphylactic reactions, PCT, which is known to be specifically elevated in sepsis, was observed. However, it has been reported that 21% of patients with allergy have elevated PCT levels, and PCT levels correlate with the severity of allergic reactions [12]. Therefore, there is a need to pay attention to anaphylactic reactions that mimic bacterial infections. Secondly, the change in anticoagulant during HD was known after a long delay, slowing the diagnosis. This underlines the need for surgeons/physicians to keep in close contact with the dialysis unit.

4. Conclusion

We encountered a case of a patient whose surgery for carpal tunnel syndrome was postponed thrice due to acute symptoms, including fever, chills, and tachycardia, during perioperative HD. If such symptoms are observed during perioperative HD, it is necessary to consider anaphylactic reactions to NM as a differential diagnosis.

Acknowledgments

The authors would like to thank Editage (https://www.editage.com) for English language editing.

References

[1] S. Fujii and Y. Hitomi, "New synthetic inhibitors of C1r̄, C1 esterase, thrombin, plasmin, kallikrein and trypsin," *Biochimica et Biophysica Acta (BBA) - Enzymology*, vol. 661, no. 2, pp. 342–345, 1981.

[2] N. Higuchi, H. Yamazaki, H. Kikuchi, and F. Gejyo, "Anaphylactoid reaction induced by a protease inhibitor, nafamostat mesilate, following nine administrations in a hemodialysis patient," *Nephron*, vol. 86, no. 3, pp. 400-401, 2000.

[3] M. Yamazato, R. Mano, S. Oshiro-Chinen et al., "Severe abdominal pain associated with allergic reaction to nafamostat mesilate in a chronic hemodialysis patient," *Internal Medicine*, vol. 41, no. 10, pp. 864–866, 2002.

[4] S. Ookawara, K. Ito, and Y. Morishita, "Sustained deterioration of hepatic oxygenation after nafamostat mesilate-induced anaphylactic shock during hemodiafiltration," *Artificial Organs*, vol. 42, no. 6, pp. 674-675, 2018.

[5] H. S. Kim, K. E. Lee, J. H. Oh et al., "Cardiac arrest caused by nafamostat mesilate," *Kidney Research and Clinical Practice*, vol. 35, no. 3, pp. 187–189, 2016.

[6] H. Okada, H. Suzuki, N. Deguchi, and T. Saruta, "Agranulocytosis in a haemodialysed patient induced by a proteinase inhibitor, nafamostat mesilate," *Nephrology Dialysis Transplantation*, vol. 7, no. 9, p. 980, 1992.

[7] S. Muto, M. Imai, and Y. Asano, "Mechanisms of hyperkalemia caused by nafamostat mesilate," *General Pharmacology: The Vascular System*, vol. 26, no. 8, pp. 1627–1632, 1995.

[8] S. Gando, T. Iba, Y. Eguchi et al., "A multicenter, prospective validation of disseminated intravascular coagulation diagnostic criteria for critically ill patients: comparing current criteria," *Critical Care Medicine*, vol. 34, no. 3, pp. 625–631, 2006.

[9] J.-Y. Choi, Y.-J. Kang, H. M. Jang et al., "Nafamostat mesilate as an anticoagulant during continuous renal replacement therapy in patients with high bleeding risk," *Medicine*, vol. 94, no. 52, Article ID e2392, 2015.

[10] L. S. Dalgaard, M. Nørgaard, J. V. Povlsen et al., "Risk and prognosis of bacteremia and fungemia among peritoneal dialysis patients: a population-based cohort study," *Peritoneal Dialysis International: Journal of the International Society for Peritoneal Dialysis*, vol. 36, no. 6, pp. 647–654, 2016.

[11] M. Aiso, H. Takikawa, K. Tsuji, and N. Sakamoto, "Analysis of 307 cases with drug-induced Liver Injury between 2010 and

2018 in Japan," *Hepatology Research*, vol. 49, no. 1, pp. 105–110, 2019.

[12] S.-Y. Yoon, S. H. Baek, S. Kim et al., "Serum procalcitonin as a biomarker differentiating delayed-type drug hypersensitivity from systemic bacterial infection," *The Journal of Allergy and Clinical Immunology*, vol. 132, no. 4, pp. 981–983, 2013.

4

Lanthanum-Induced Radiopaque Intestinal Precipitates: A Potential Cause of Intestinal Foreign Bodies

Jason Galo, Bianca Madrid, and Warren Kupin

Jackson Memorial Hospital/University of Miami Hospital, Miami, FL, USA

Correspondence should be addressed to Jason Galo; jasongalo92@gmail.com

Academic Editor: Salih Kavukcu

Lanthanum carbonate is a commonly prescribed oral phosphate binder for use in patients with acute or chronic kidney disease. The elemental form of lanthanum is a soft metal, which will appear radiopaque on a standard X-ray radiograph. This case report illustrates the potential for Lanthanum to masquerade as multiple radiopaque intestinal foreign bodies, leading to the extensive mobilization of medical resources and consultations including serial X-ray monitoring, multiple consultants including acute care and colorectal surgery. Given the few published reports describing this finding in the literature, it is essential to consider Lanthanum precipitates in the differential diagnosis of radiopaque intestinal foreign bodies in patients with chronic kidney disease to avoid unnecessary utilization of medical resources for this predominantly benign condition.

1. Case Presentation

Lanthanum carbonate is a commonly prescribed oral phosphate binder used exclusively in patients with acute or chronic kidney disease to prevent secondary hyperparathyroidism. Lanthanum, a rare earth metal, is minimally absorbed systemically after oral ingestion. Dietary phosphorus in the gastrointestinal tract is avidly bound to lanthanum and excreted in the stool in a soluble state. However, failure to properly chew and dissolve the lanthanum carbonate pills may result in the appearance of multiple radiopaque objects on the abdomen since lanthanum carbonate appears radiopaque on X-rays.

We report the rare finding of lanthanum induced multiple radiopaque intestinal foreign bodies in a patient with acute kidney injury as a consequence of kidney transplant rejection.

This patient is a 21-year-old male with a medical history significant for end stage renal disease secondary to brachio-oto-renal syndrome and born with a solitary small kidney, who underwent a successful deceased donor kidney transplant in 2013. After 5 years, he was admitted with acute kidney failure due to biopsy proven T-cell and antibody-mediated rejection. At the time of his presentation, he was complaining of worsening nausea and vomiting for the last five days prior to presentation. His previously normal serum creatinine had risen to 27 mg/dL, and his phosphate level on presentation was 6.9 mg/dL. He was treated with the institutional protocol for antibody-mediated rejection, which included thymoglobulin, rituximab, bortezomib, and plasmapharesis. As a result of his acute renal failure, he developed hyperphosphatemia with levels up to 8.9 mg/dL (range: 6.4 mg/dL–8.9 mg/dL) and was started on oral lanthanum carbonate tablets with each meal, with the doses titrated up to 1000 mg three times daily. During his hospitalization a renal ultrasound detected the presence of a "foreign body" localized within or adjacent to the transplant. An abdominal radiograph was obtained that revealed multiple radiopacities scattered throughout the entire abdomen (Figure 1). A computed tomography scan of the abdomen was obtained to better characterize the opacities, which also revealed radiopaque material within the colon consistent with some form of ingested material. Repeat abdominal radiography (Figure 2) showed the same foreign bodies in the bowel, which appeared to be moving along the gastrointestinal tract en route towards the rectum. Gastroenterology and Colorectal Surgery were consulted for further evaluation of the suspected foreign bodies seen on abdominal imaging. Close monitoring was recommended

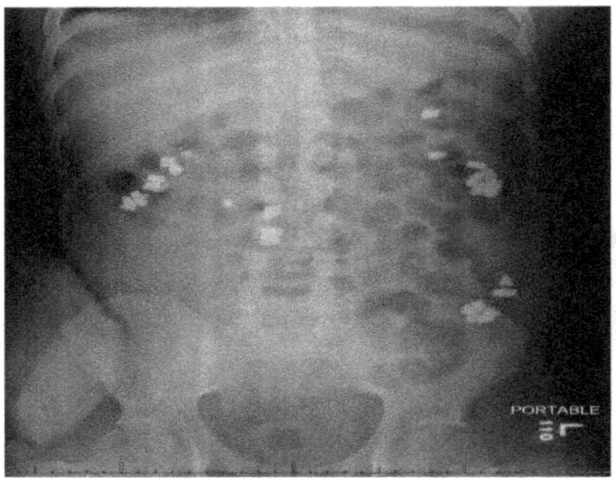

Figure 1: An abdominal radiograph from 6/26/18 showing multiple radiopaque objects in the bowel.

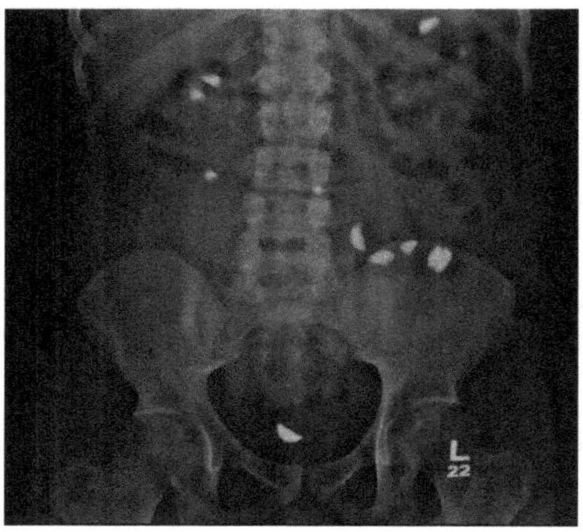

Figure 2: Repeat abdominal radiograph from 6/28/18 shows radiopaque objects moving towards rectum.

with serial abdominal imaging since the patient was asymptomatic with no immediate risk of perforation. The patient's stool was also collected in an attempt to identify any passed foreign objects, but no foreign material in the stool was found. A psychiatrist was consulted to determine if the patient was ingesting any foreign objects.

Serial abdominal radiography revealed an increase in quantity of the radiopaque densities scattered about the abdomen (Figures 2 and 3). The patient's medications were subsequently reviewed, and it was determined that lanthanum carbonate was the likely etiology of the radiography findings. Discontinuation of the Lanthanum Carbonate led to complete resolution of the findings.

2. Discussion

Oral ingestion of foreign objects both intentional and unintentional is common among children and adults. Many of these foreign bodies are radiopaque such as metal-based products, glass, certain plastics, and animal bones. Intestinal foreign bodies can cause perforation, obstruction, intussusception, fistula formation, abdominal abscess formation, and death, and their discovery should be considered a medically urgent situation [1].

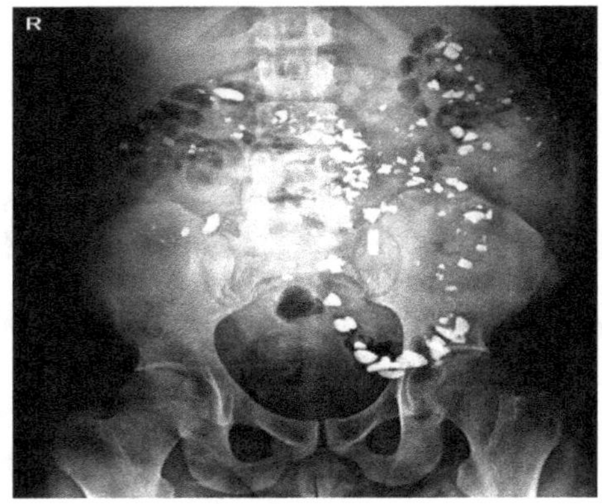

Figure 3: KUB from 7/4/18 shows new radiopaque foreign material in bowel concerning for foreign ingestion.

Alternatively, many medications can be radiopaque and would represent benign findings that do not require additional investigation. Drugs that typically cause radiopaque appearance can be grouped according the mneumonic CHIPES (chloral hydrate, heavy metals, iodides, phenothiazines, enteric-coated pills, and solvents) [2].

Hyperphosphatemia is associated with increased mortality in chronic kidney disease, and the American Kidney Foundation recommends treating dialysis patients who are hyperphosphatemic (serum phosphorus >5.5 mg/dL) with calcium based phosphate binders such as calcium acetate or noncalcium-containing binders such as lanthanum carbonate or sevelamer [3]. In the setting of acute kidney injury, hyperphosphatemia is a common electrolyte abnormality that should be treated with medical therapy and dietary phosphorus restriction [4]. Acute hyperphosphatemia may cause massive phosphate overload and severe acute kidney injury [5]. In the case of Acute Phosphate Nephropathy, acute kidney injury accompanied by severe hyperphosphatemia may cause life-threatening hypocalcemia, with complications such as cardiovascular collapse, tetany, and mental status changes [6]. Our patient presented with acute kidney injury secondary to renal allograft rejection and hyperphosphatemia. Fortunately, his calcium was within normal limits during the hospitalization. Given his already existing severe acute kidney injury, persistent hyperphosphatemia could potentially have made the already existing kidney damage worse. Due to the patient's young age, short length of having the kidney transplant, and relatively few comorbidities, an attempt was made to treat the acute allograft rejection with steroids, immunotherapy, and plasmapharesis. Persistent and untreated hyperphosphatemia could have cause worsening kidney damage, and treatment was indicated.

Lanthanum carbonate is a natural earth metal used as an oral phosphate binder prescribed to patients with advanced renal insufficiency for control of hyperphosphatemia [7]. Formulations available include chewable tablets or powder packets. The chewable tablets should be fully chewed or crushed prior to ingestion. The drug then dissociates in the gastrointestinal tract into its elemental form to bind dietary phosphorus. The elemental form of lanthanum is a soft metal, hence appears radiopaque on radiography [7–11]. The most common adverse effects reported are gastrointestinal symptoms such as nausea, diarrhea, and abdominal pain; rarely with ileus or bowel obstruction [12–14]. Because of the possibility of gastrointestinal side effects, one should first rule out abdominal diseases before prescribing lanthanum carbonate. Overall, the medication is overall tolerated well. The patient presented in this case had not completely chewed the lanthanum carbonate tablets as prescribed. Therefore, the tablets did not fully dissociate in the gut, and was passed in the stool essentially unchanged. Previously published case reports have reported lanthanum carbonate on radiographic imagining being confused to be barium, with a "starry sky appearance" on CT imagining [9]. In a different case report, an elderly man developed cough, dysphagia, and hoarseness, and a chest X-ray determined there was a radiopaque coin-shaped foreign body in the aero digestive tract. Further intervention included an upper endoscopy, where it was determined that the culprit was lanthanum carbonate, which was being taken for treatment of hyperphosphatemia [11]. Some authors of similar case reports have suggested as far as to temporarily switching from lanthanum carbonate to a different phosphate-lowering medication prior to radiologic examination, despite the drug's effectiveness [15]. On the other hand, lanthanum carbonate's characteristic radiopaque appearance may be used as an advantage to assess the patient's drug adherence [8, 9, 16].

Lanthanum carbonate should now be considered in the differential diagnosis of radiopaque foreign bodies in patients with acute or chronic kidney disease. Recognition of this association can avoid extensive and costly use of medical resources for this benign condition.

Additional Points

Learning Objective 1. Define the use and radiographic appearance of lanthanum carbonate. *Learning Objective 2.* Analyze and adapt to uncommon presentations of radiopaque objects on X-ray imaging. *Learning Objective 3.* Formulate a plan to assess possible causes of radiopaque foreign objects on imaging, including iatrogenic causes such as medications.

Disclosure

This manuscript was presented at the National Kidney Foundation Meeting Abstracts from May 8-12, 2019, in Boston, MA and was one of five winning posters out of >500 presentations.

References

[1] T. B. Hunter and M. S. Taljanovic, "Foreign bodies," *RadioGraphics*, vol. 23, no. 3, pp. 731–757, 2003.

[2] S. M. Spiegel and B. B. Hyams, "Radiographic demonstration of a toxic agent," *Journal of the Canadian Association of Radiologists*, vol. 35, no. 2, pp. 204–205, 1984.

[3] National Kidney Foundation, "K/DOQI clinical practice guidelines for bone metabolism and disease in chronic kidney disease," *American Journal of Kidney Diseases*, vol. 42, no. 4 Suppl 3, pp. S1–S201, 2003.

[4] G. Kumar and A. Vasudevan, "Management of acute kidney injury," *The Indian Journal of Pediatrics*, vol. 79, no. 8, pp. 1069–1075, 2012.

[5] N. Hamano and M. Fukagawa, "Pathogenesis and clinical condition of hyperphosphatemic diseases," *Clinical Calcium*, vol. 26, no. 2, pp. 207–213, 2016.

[6] A. Monfared, S.M. Habibzadeh, S.A. Mesbah, "Acute phosphate nephropathy," *Iranian Journal of Kidney Diseases*, vol. 8, no. 3, pp. 246–249, 2009.

[7] G. J. Behets, S. C. Verberckmoes, P. C. D'Haese, and M. E. De Broe, "Lanthanum carbonate: a new phosphate binder," *Current Opinion in Nephrology and Hypertension*, vol. 13, no. 4, pp. 403–409, 2004.

[8] F. Aucella, T. Marinelli, D. Paoletti, M. Vigilante, and V. Vocino, "Why does a patient on hemodialysis have radiopaque material in his abdomen?," *Giornale Italiano di Nefrologia*, vol. 26, no. 2, pp. 246–249, 2009.

[9] F.-M. Chang, D.-C. Tarng, and C.-Y. Yang, "Starry-sky bowels," *International Journal of Colorectal Disease*, vol. 33, no. 12, pp. 1807–1808, 2018.

[10] Y. Nishinaga, S. Miyazaki, R. Yamashita, and T. Ikeda, "Airway foreign body manifested as a coin lesion," *Clinical Case Reports*, vol. 6, no. 9, pp. 1913–1914, 2018.

[11] S. Paranji, N. Paranji, and A. S. Weltz, "All that glitters is not gold: a case of lanthanum carbonate aspiration," *SAGE Open Medical Case Reports*, vol. 5, p. 2050313X1771264, 2017.

[12] V. Camarero-Temino, V. Mercado-Valdivia, B. Hijazi-Prieto, and P. Abaigar-Luquin, "Intestinal pseudo-obstruction secondary to persistent constipation due to lanthanum carbonate," *Nefrologia*, vol. 32, no. 1, p. 129, 2012.

[13] A. Martinez Pobes de Salinas, I. Blanco Rodríguez, L. Quiñones Ortiz, and A. Suárez Laurés, "Intestinal pseudo-occlusion due to lanthanum carbonate," *Nefrologia*, vol. 30, no. 3, p. 376, 2010.

[14] T. Black, G. Philips, and R. Burbridge, "Pharmacobezoar in a patient on an oral phosphate binder," *Gastrointestinal Endoscopy*, vol. 77, no. 3, pp. 511–512, 2013.

[15] J. Pafcugova, M. Horackova, M. Hraskova, J. Forejt, M. Szabo, and R. Padr, "Radio-opaque appearance of lanthanum carbonate in a patient with chronic renal failure," *Nephrology Dialysis Transplantation*, vol. 23, no. 5, pp. 1776–1777, 2008, author reply 1777-8.

[16] J. P. Walsh and A. A. Lteif, "Lanthanum carbonate interference with lumbar spine DXA," *Journal of Clinical Densitometry*, vol. 14, no. 4, pp. 499–501, 2011.

5

Hypercalcemia, Acute Kidney Injury and Metabolic Alkalosis

Faten Aqeel[1] **Jennifer Del Castillo,**[2] **Bernard G. Jaar**[1,3,4,5] **and Mohamad Hanouneh**[1,3]

[1]*Johns Hopkins University School of Medicine, Department of Medicine, Division of Nephrology, Baltimore, MD, USA*
[2]*Department of Internal Medicine, MedStar Health, Baltimore, MD, USA*
[3]*Nephrology Center of Maryland, Baltimore, MD, USA*
[4]*The Johns Hopkins Bloomberg School of Public Health, Department of Epidemiology, Baltimore, MD, USA*
[5]*The Welch Center for Prevention, Epidemiology, and Clinical Research, Baltimore, MD, USA*

Correspondence should be addressed to Faten Aqeel; faqeel1@jh.edu

Academic Editor: David Mudge

Calcium regulation is tightly controlled in the body. Multiple causes of hypercalcemia have been studied including primary hyperparathyroidism, hypercalcemia of malignancy, and chronic granulomatous disorders. Among the less studied causes is calcium-alkali syndrome. Here, we discuss a case of hypercalcemia secondary to calcium-alkali syndrome, presenting with hypercalcemia, metabolic alkalosis, and acute kidney injury as a result of ingestion of a large amount of calcium supplements. Hypercalcemia can result in impaired collecting duct system sensitivity to antidiuretic hormone, afferent arteriole constriction, and activation of calcium sensor receptors in multiple tissues. The net effect is an increase in calcium reabsorption with a salt and water diuresis which leads to volume depletion, acute kidney injury, and metabolic alkalosis.

1. Introduction

Calcium-alkali syndrome is one of the leading causes of hypercalcemia. It is caused by the ingestion of large amounts of calcium and alkali. The classic triad of calcium-alkali syndrome includes hypercalcemia, metabolic alkalosis, and acute kidney injury (AKI). Here, we report a case of calcium-alkali syndrome secondary to ingestion of calcium carbonate and we review the pathophysiology of this syndrome.

2. Case Presentation

A 54-year-old woman with a past medical history of bipolar disorder and gastroesophageal reflux disease (GERD) presented to the emergency room with altered mental status and epigastric pain. Her symptoms were associated with nausea and vomiting for 3 days. Home medications included lithium 300 mg three times a day and quetiapine 100 mg daily. On physical examination, her vital signs revealed a temperature of 99.2°F, heart rate 95 beats per minute, blood pressure 127/72 mm Hg, respiration rate 26 breaths per minute, and oxygen saturation 97% on room air. Pertinent physical findings included soft abdomen with mild epigastric tenderness. She was alert but oriented to person only. Initial laboratory values are listed in Table 1. Electrocardiogram showed a short QT interval (270 ms, QTc 327 ms). Cardiac enzymes were unremarkable. Chest X-ray was normal. CT brain and abdomen without contrast were also unremarkable. Her age-appropriate cancer screening was up to date. Intact parathyroid hormone (i-PTH) level was 13 pg/mL (normal 18–80 pg/mL) which indicated PTH-independent hypercalcemia. Further workup demonstrated a thyroid stimulating hormone (TSH) level of 2.5 μU/mL (normal 0.5–5 μU/mL) and total 25-hydroxy vitamin D level of 11 ng/mL (normal 30–100 ng/mL), excluding hyperthyroidism and vitamin D intoxication, respectively. Parathyroid hormone-related peptide (PTH-rp) was 14 pg/mL (normal 18–80 pg/mL) and total 1,25 dihydroxy vitamin D < 5.0 pg/mL (normal 18–72 pg/mL), making hypercalcemia of malignancy and chronic granulomatous disorder unlikely. In addition, monoclonal gammopathy workup was negative including normal serum and urine electrophoresis with normal serum free light chains ratio. Our patient had the classic triad of calcium-alkali syndrome including hypercalcemia, metabolic

Table 1: Initial laboratory data.

Labs	Results	Normal values
White blood count	17.9 K/uL	4–10.8
Neutrophils	80%	
Lymphocytes	8%	
Monocytes	10%	
Hemoglobin	12.8 g/dL	12.5–16.5
Platelet count	327 K/uL	140–400
Sodium	134 mmol/L	135–145
Potassium	3.2 mmol/L	3.5–5.1
Chloride	86 mmol/L	98–107
Sodium bicarbonate	34 mmol/L	22–31
Blood urea nitrogen	50 mg/dL	7–20
Creatinine	4.05 mg/dL (baseline 0.6 mg/dL)	0.7–1.3
Calcium	>20 mg/dL	8.4–10.2
Ionized calcium	3.2 mmol/L	1.17–1.38 mmol/L
Phosphorus	2.6 mg/dL	2.5–4.5
Total protein	7.3 g/dL	6.1–8.2
Albumin	4.7 g/dL	3.5–5.0
Total bilirubin	0.5 mg/dL	0.2–1.2
Aspartate aminotransferase	23 U/L	17–59
Alanine aminotransferase	12 U/L	21–72
Alkaline phosphatase	63 U/L	35–104 U/L
Arterial blood gas		
pH	7.52	7.35–7.45
PCO2	35	35–45 mmHg
PO2	90	75–100 mmHg
HCO3-	32	18–23 mmHg
Urine calcium (mg/dL):urine creatinine (mg/dL) ratio	0.41	<0.14

alkalosis, and acute kidney injury (AKI). The patient was started emergently on normal saline 300 cc/hour and received IV zoledronic acid 4 mg × 1 dose and calcitonin 4 units/Kg × 1 dose with plans to initiate hemodialysis. However, she responded promptly following the medical therapy (IV fluids, zoledronic acid, and calcitonin) with urine output 200 cc/hour and significant drop in her serum calcium level to 18.3 mg/dL in 1 hour and 15.9 mg/dL in 4 hours. Denosumab was not used due to its lack of availability. Serum calcium level and mental status returned to normal in 24 hours. AKI and metabolic alkalosis resolved in 48 hours. She later reported taking up to 20 tablets of calcium carbonate 500 mg daily for 3 weeks to control her severe GERD symptoms. Given her history of bipolar disorder, her excessive calcium carbonate intake was thought to be related to Münchausen syndrome, prompting a psychiatric evaluation.

3. Discussion

The causes of PTH-independent hypercalcemia are summarized in Table 2 [1]. Chronic lithium use can be associated with mild hypercalcemia; however, it is usually PTH dependent (normal to high PTH) [2]. Calcium-alkali syndrome is usually caused by ingestion of large amount of calcium supplements, and it is one of the leading causes of hypercalcemia [3–5]. The classic triad of calcium-alkali syndrome includes hypercalcemia, metabolic alkalosis, and acute kidney injury (AKI). Serum vitamin D is usually suppressed in patients with calcium-alkali syndrome. However, it could be elevated in the case of concomitant excessive intake of vitamin D supplements.

Table 2: Causes of PTH-independent hypercalcemia.

Hypercalcemia mediated by elevated levels of 1,25-dihydroxy vitamin D
Granulomatous disorders
Foreign material (e.g., silicone)
Pneumocystis jirovecii pneumonia
Hypercalcemia from excess calcium intake
Calcium-alkali syndrome
Calcium sulfate beads
Calcium alginate
Hypercalcemia medicated by PTH-related protein
Malignancy
Benign tumors
Sarcoidosis
Systemic lupus erythematous
Pregnancy/lactation related
Medications
Vitamin D and A
Thiazides
Foscarnet
Parenteral nutrition
Omeprazole in interstitial nephritis

Ingestion of large amounts of calcium leads to an increase in intestinal reabsorption of calcium causing hypercalcemia. Hypercalcemia can result in impaired collecting duct sensitivity to antidiuretic hormone and vasoconstriction of mainly the afferent arteriole in the

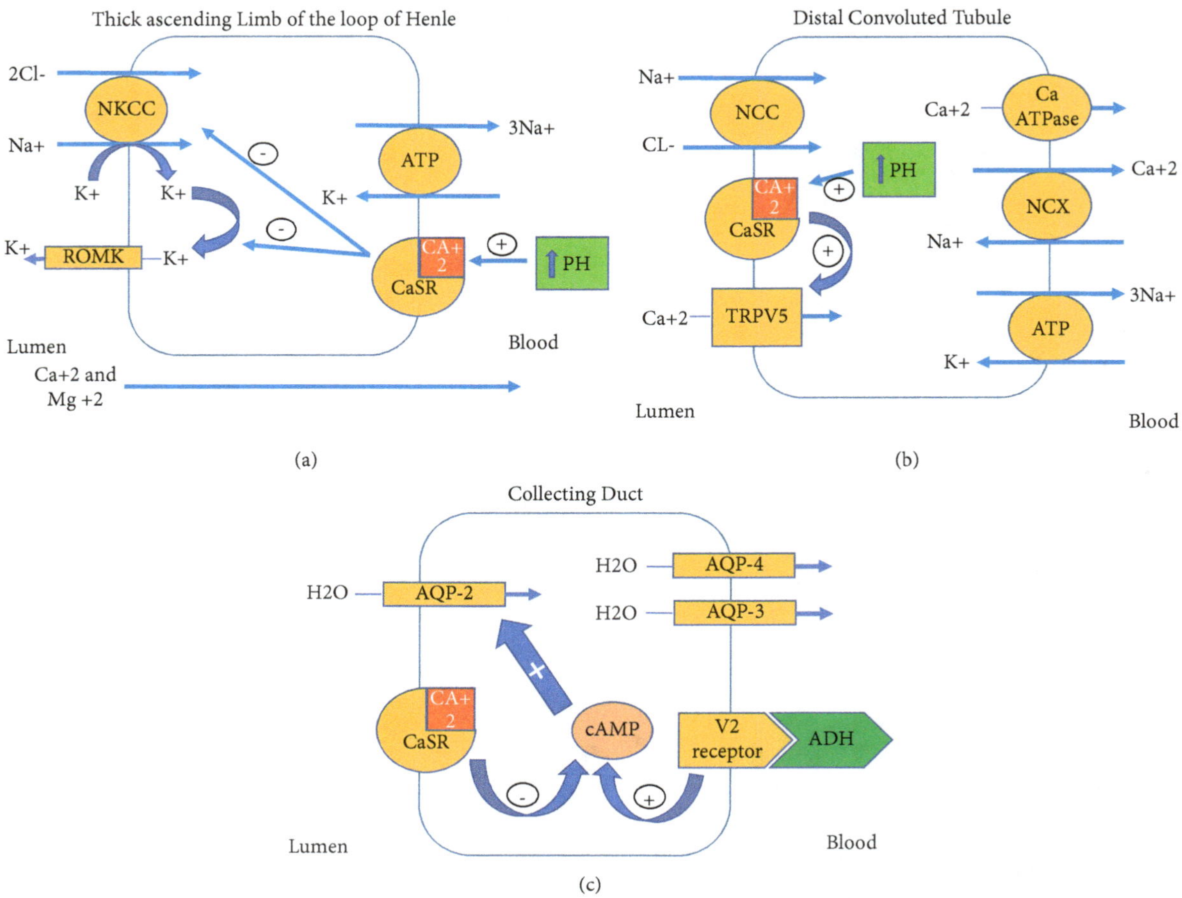

FIGURE 1: (a) Thick ascending limb of the loop of Henle. (b) Distal convoluted tubule. (c) Collecting duct.

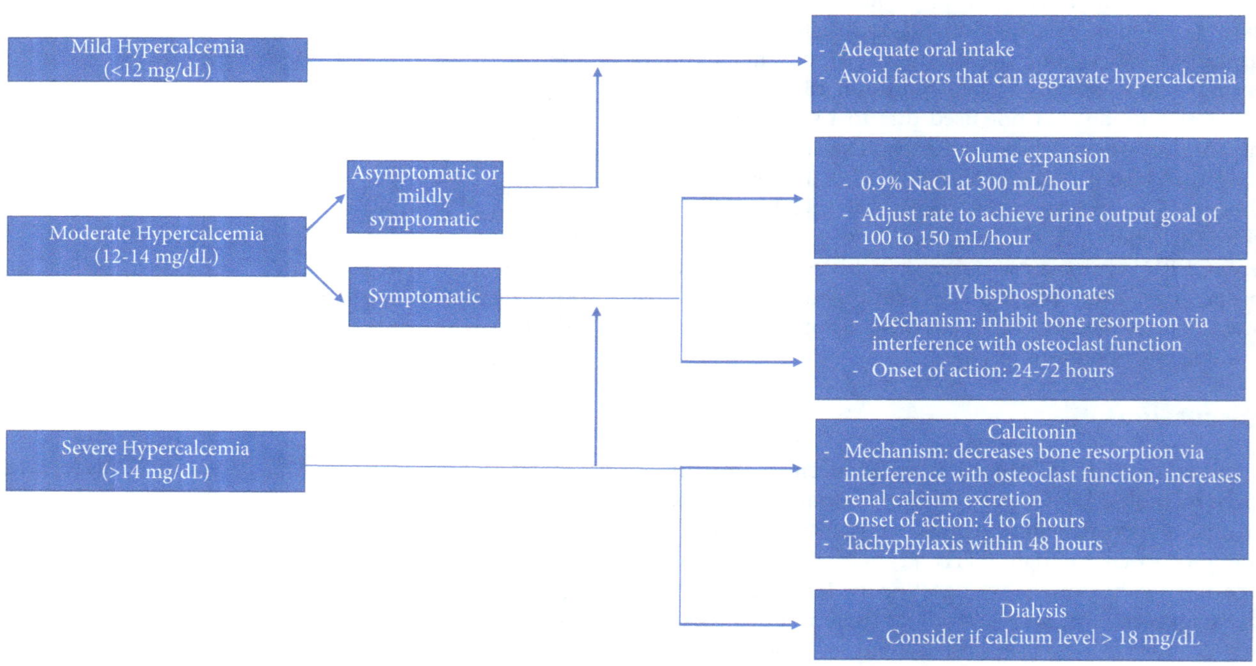

FIGURE 2: Treatment of hypercalcemia.

glomerulus, leading to AKI [5]. Hypercalcemia activates calcium sensor receptors (CaSRs) in multiple tissues. Activation of CaSR in parathyroid gland causes suppression of the parathyroid hormone. Activation of CaSRs on the basolateral membrane of the thick ascending limb of the loop of Henle results in the inhibition of sodium chloride reabsorption and leads to a loop diuretic-like effect and an increase in urinary calcium excretion (Figure 1(a)) [6]. The increase in urinary calcium concentration activates the CaSRs on the luminal membrane of the distal convoluted tubule and the collecting duct cells. Activation of CaSRs on the luminal membrane of the distal convoluted tubules leads to an increase in calcium reabsorption via TRPV5 transporter and worsening hypercalcemia (Figure 1(b)) [6]. Activation of CaSRs on the luminal membrane of the collecting duct reduces the expression of aquaporin 2 water channels, resulting in a decrease in water reabsorption (Figure 1(c)) [6].

The net effect is an increase in calcium reabsorption along with a salt and water diuresis which leads to worsening volume depletion and metabolic alkalosis. Additionally, elevated serum pH perpetuates this cycle by increasing the affinity of CaSRs to calcium. Hypercalcemia causes nausea and vomiting which can also lead to volume depletion and metabolic alkalosis [5].

The treatment of hypercalcemia is focused on lowering the serum calcium level, while investigating and possibly treating the underlying disease. Figure 2 summarizes the treatment options of hypercalcemia.

Data Availability

Previously reported data were used to support this study and are available at [doi:10.1007/s00268-017-4328-5]. These data are cited at relevant places within the text as references [1]. Previously reported data were used to support this study and are available at [doi:10.1681/ASN.2010030255]. These data are cited at relevant places within the text as references [2]. Previously reported data were used to support this study and are available at [doi: 10.1097/00005792-199503000-00004]. These data are cited at relevant places within the text as references [3]. Previously reported data were used to support this study and are available at [doi:10.2215/CJN.01451005]. These data are cited at relevant places within the text as references [4]. Previously reported data were used to support this study and are available at [doi: 10.1152/ajprenal.00608.2009]. These data are cited at relevant places within the text as references [5].

References

[1] Y. Motlaghzadeh, J. P. Bilezikian, and D. E. Sellmeyer, "Rare causes of hypercalcemia: 2021 update," *The Journal of Clinical Endocrinology & Metabolism*, vol. 106, no. 11, pp. 3113–3128, 2021.

[2] A. D. Meehan, R. Udumyan, M. Kardell, M. Landén, J. Järhult, and G. Wallin, "Lithium-associated hypercalcemia: pathophysiology, prevalence, management," *World Journal of Surgery*, vol. 42, no. 2, pp. 415–424, 2018.

[3] A. M. Patel and S. Goldfarb, "Got calcium? Welcome to the calcium-alkali syndrome," *Journal of the American Society of Nephrology*, vol. 21, no. 9, pp. 1440–1443, 2010.

[4] D. P. Beall and H. R. Scofield, "Milk-alkali syndrome associated with calcium carbonate consumption: report of 7 patients with parathyroid hormone levels and an estimate of prevalence among patients hospitalized with hypercalcemia," *Medicine*, vol. 74, no. 2, pp. 89–96, 1995.

[5] A. J. Felsenfeld and B. S. Levine, "Milk alkali syndrome and the dynamics of calcium homeostasis," *Clinical Journal of the American Society of Nephrology*, vol. 1, no. 4, pp. 641–654, 2006.

[6] D. Riccardi and E. M. Brown, "Physiology and pathophysiology of the calcium-sensing receptor in the kidney," *American Journal of Physiology-Renal Physiology*, vol. 298, no. 3, pp. F485–F499, 2010.

6

Temporal Arteritis and Vision Loss in Microscopic Polyangiitis: A Case Report and Literature Review

Alexander G. Goglia,[1] Michael Makar,[2,3] Craig Vanuitert,[4] and Vadim Finkelstein[5]

[1]*Rutgers Robert Wood Johnson Medical School, 675 Hoes Ln W, Piscataway, NJ 08854, USA*
[2]*Rutgers Robert Wood Johnson Medical School, Department of Internal Medicine, 125 Paterson Street, New Brunswick, NJ 08901, USA*
[3]*Penn Medicine Princeton Medical Center, Department of Internal Medicine, 1 Plainsboro Rd, Plainsboro Township, NJ 08536, USA*
[4]*Penn Medicine Princeton Medical Center, Department of Pathology, 1 Plainsboro Rd, Plainsboro Township, NJ 08536, USA*
[5]*Penn Medicine Princeton Medical Center, Princeton Hypertension and Nephrology, 1 Plainsboro Rd, Plainsboro Township, NJ 08536, USA*

Correspondence should be addressed to Michael Makar; michaelmakar5@gmail.com

Academic Editor: Ze'ev Korzets

Microscopic polyangiitis (MPA) is an idiopathic autoimmune disease characterized by systemic vasculitis. While the lungs and kidneys are the major organs affected by MPA, it is known to involve multiple organ systems throughout the body. Temporal artery involvement is a very rare finding in MPA. This report presents a patient whose initial presentation was consistent with giant cell arteritis but was ultimately found to have microscopic polyangiitis. It highlights the importance of considering alternative types of vasculitis in the differential diagnosis for patients with atypical temporal artery biopsy findings.

1. Introduction

Primary vasculitides are a diverse group of disorders characterized by an autoimmune response against host blood vessels that often leads to multisystem disease [1]. These conditions have traditionally been classified into one of three categories based on the size of the vessels they affect: either large, medium, or small vessel vasculitides [2]. However, in rare cases, a primary vasculitis can involve vessels of various sizes, leading to heterogeneous and widely overlapping clinical features that require careful investigation.

Microscopic polyangiitis (MPA) is an idiopathic autoimmune disease characterized by systemic vasculitis [3]. It is a predominantly small vessel disease associated with anti-neutrophil cytoplasmic antibodies (ANCA), which are thought to play a causative role in its pathophysiology. While the lungs and kidneys are the major organs affected by MPA, it is known to involve multiple organ systems throughout the body. Notably, temporal artery involvement is a very rare manifestation of ANCA-associated vasculitides and is a finding more consistent with the large/medium vessel predominant vasculitis giant cell arteritis (GCA).

Here we report the case of a patient whose clinical picture was consistent with giant cell arteritis but was ultimately found to have microscopic polyangiitis. This case highlights the importance of identifying the proper diagnosis in these mixed vasculitides and provides the most up-to-date literature review in patients with temporal artery findings in MPA.

2. Case Description

An 81-year-old Caucasian male with hypertension and hyperlipidemia presented with one day of complete unilateral loss of vision in his right eye, along with jaw claudication, and bitemporal headaches. He reported 1 to 2 months of weight loss, worsening fatigue, decreased oral intake, and severe bilateral lower extremity pain and edema.

On physical exam, the patient was cachectic and ill-appearing with severe anasarca. He exhibited bilateral tenderness to gentle temporomandibular joint palpation, and visual exam revealed complete unilateral right-sided vision loss. Initial labs showed elevated ESR (64 mm/hr) and serum creatinine (11.9 mg/dL) levels, while urinalysis revealed moderate hematuria (10–20 RBCs/hpf) and proteinuria (urine protein/creatinine ratio of 1.15). Further testing revealed high-titer p-ANCA anti-myeloperoxidase IgG (79 AU/mL; normal, <19 AU/mL) antibodies and weakly positive antinuclear antibody titers (1 : 80). C-ANCA anti-proteinase-3 (PR3) and complement levels (c3, c4) were within normal limits.

Given these findings, the patient was started on pulsed steroids and began to exhibit signs of clinical improvement. A subsequent right temporal artery biopsy (Figure 1) identified vasculitis with fibrinoid necrosis and leukocytoclasis in an arteriolar branch of the temporal artery (Figure 2). Furthermore, a chest CT scan identified multiple areas of ground-glass opacities involving the right upper and middle lobes and within the lingula, consistent with interstitial lung disease from a systemic vasculitis.

Based on these findings, the patient was diagnosed with microscopic polyangiitis with systemic involvement of the temporal and ophthalmic arteries. He was treated with three days of pulsed steroids and intermittent hemodialysis and was then transitioned to maintenance steroids. He received one dose of rituximab induction therapy in the hospital. Given his respiratory, cardiac, and hemodynamic instability, a renal biopsy was not obtained.

During his hospitalization, the patient developed acute hypoxic respiratory failure requiring BiPAP ventilation, likely secondary to his interstitial lung disease. In addition, he experienced repeated episodes of supraventricular tachyarrhythmia that required treatment with a chronotropic therapy (diltiazem drip). As his condition worsened, he was transferred to the ICU and ultimately developed an acute right-sided cerebral infarct with left hemiparesis. Given his multiorgan failure (respiratory failure and kidney failure) and stroke, his family chose to transition him to comfort care and he passed away in the hospital.

3. Discussion

The size of affected vessels has long been used to classify the various types of systemic vasculitis [2]. While these distinctions are informative for understanding the underlying pathophysiology, it is important to recognize that vessel involvement and thus clinical presentations can vary widely. Giant cell arteritis (GCA) is the most common systemic vasculitis in adults. Typical presentation includes involvement of temporal, vertebral, and ophthalmic arteries [4]. Involvement of the large arteries, such as the aorta, is less common. Clinical features are often vague, consisting of constitutional symptoms (e.g., fever, malaise, and weight loss) along with localized headache, temporal artery tenderness, and elevated ESR [4]. By comparison, microscopic polyangiitis (MPA) is a systemic small vessel vasculitis that often presents with renal and pulmonary manifestations and can, in rare cases, also involve medium and large caliber vessels such as the aorta [3].

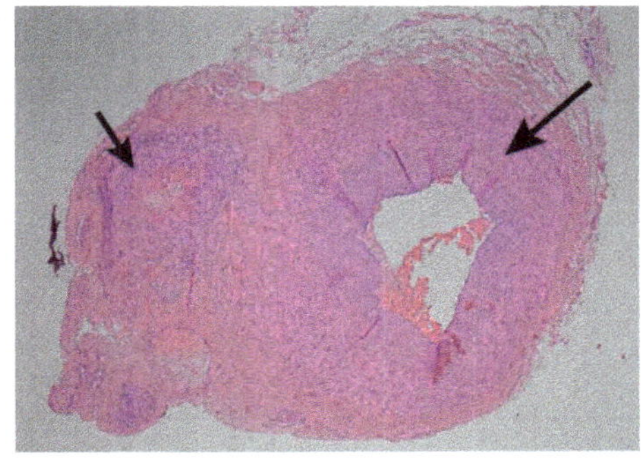

Figure 1: Temporal artery biopsy. The larger unaffected temporal artery can be seen on the right (large arrow) while the smaller arteriole involved by vasculitis (small arrow) extends to the left of the temporal artery.

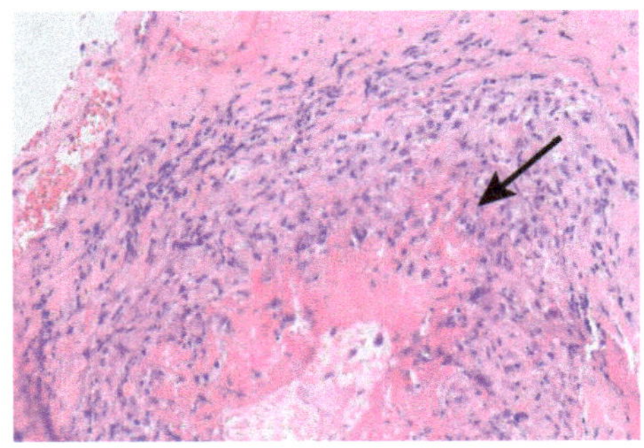

Figure 2: Vasculitis in arteriolar branch of the temporal artery. Extensive fibrinoid necrosis (arrow) and leukocytoclasis with vascular dilatation, destruction of the vascular wall, fibrin deposition, and inflammatory infiltrate in and around the vascular wall.

Notably, it is exceedingly rare for MPA to present with temporal artery involvement, as only a small handful of such cases have been reported to date [5–13]. In our review of the literature, we identified only 14 cases of MPA reported to involve the temporal artery (Table 1). The true frequency of temporal artery involvement has been difficult to establish, but a recently published case series reported that ANCA-associated vasculitis occurred in <1% of patients with temporal artery biopsies (TAB) [5]. Cavazza et al. examined 871 patients with TAB and only identified three cases of MPA in 317 patients diagnosed with GCA. When considering a possible diagnosis of GCA, fibrinoid necrosis is a rare finding in the temporal artery and its presence should prompt the clinician to consider a broad differential diagnosis including MPA. While the patient's initial symptoms reflected temporal artery involvement, our findings demonstrate that it is important for clinicians to consider MPA as well as GCA. Given the inherent severity of MPA and other pauci-immune vasculitides, temporal artery biopsy findings may be used to help guide the treatment and management of patients with an unclear diagnosis.

Table 1: Literature review of temporal artery involvement in patients with MPA.

	Patients	Presenting symptoms	Organ systems involved	Biopsy findings
Cavazza et al. [5]	3/322	NA	NA	TAB: small-vessel vasculitis; no fibrinoid necrosis or leukocytoclasis
Chirinos et al. [6]	1	Constitutional symptoms (e.g., weight loss, weakness, fever, night sweats, myalgias), recurrent pulmonary infiltrates, no temporal arteritis	Renal, pulmonary, cutaneous, aorta	Palmar lesion: leukocytoclastic vasculitis Renal: pauci-immune necrotizing crescentic glomerulonephritis
Genereau et al. [7]	3/27	Headache (temporal), vision loss, jaw claudication, constitutional symptoms	Pulmonary, renal, URT, cutaneous, cardiovascular, PNS	TAB: fibrinoid necrosis in 3/3
Hamidou et al. [9]	3/120	Headache, jaw claudication, mononeuritis, scleritis, constitutional symptoms	Renal, middle ear, ocular, URT	TAB: fibrinoid necrosis in 2/3
Morinaga et al. [10]	1	Headache (temporal), dysphagia, hoarseness, dysgeusia, gait instability, cranial neuropathies	Renal, CNA	Renal: necrotizing glomerulonephritis with fibrinoid necrosis TAB: temporal arteritis, no giant cells
Planté-Bordeneuve et al. [11]	1	Upper extremity hemiparesis, jaw claudication, bitemporal headache with tenderness	Pulmonary, renal, muscular	TAB: transmural inflammation, focal zones of fibrinoid necrosis
Tanaka et al. [12]	1	Bitemporal pain/tenderness, fever	Renal, pulmonary (on relapse)	TAB: fibrinoid necrosis and luminal stenosis in surrounding SV Renal: pauci-immune necrotizing crescentic glomerulonephritis
Zuckerman et al. [13]	1*	Headache, bitemporal tenderness, jaw claudication, visual disturbances	Renal (on follow-up presentation)	TAB: chronic inflammation. Within arterial wall, giant cells present Renal: pauci-immune necrotizing crescentic glomerulonephritis

TAB, temporal artery biopsy; URT, upper respiratory tract; PNS, peripheral nervous system; CNS, central nervous system; SV, small vessels. *GCA diagnosed, followed by diagnosis of renal-limited MPA 4 years later.

Further research studies are needed in this unique patient population.

4. Conclusion

Here, we describe a patient whose clinical presentation appeared to be entirely consistent with GCA (e.g., constitutional symptoms, bitemporal headaches with localized tenderness to palpation and jaw claudication, and elevated inflammatory markers), but whose biopsy results and further diagnostic workup revealed the presence of ANCA-positive MPA. This case is an important example of a difficult clinical presentation of small vessel vasculitis with temporal artery involvement in an older adult with unilateral vision loss and acute renal failure. It highlights the importance of considering alternative types of vasculitis in the differential diagnosis for patients with atypical temporal artery biopsy findings.

Consent

Informed consent was obtained for this case report.

References

[1] W. L. Gross, A. Trabandt, and E. Reinhold-Keller, "Diagnosis and evaluation of vasculitis," *Rheumatology*, vol. 39, no. 3, pp. 245–252, 2000.

[2] J. C. Jennette, R. J. Falk, K. Andrassy et al., "Nomenclature of systemic vasculitides," *Arthritis & Rheumatism*, vol. 37, no. 2, pp. 187–192, 1994.

[3] G. G. Hunder, D. A. Bloch, B. A. Michel et al., "The American College of Rheumatology 1990 criteria for the classification of giant cell arteritis," *Arthritis and Rheumatism*, vol. 33, no. 8, pp. 1122–1128, 1990.

[4] C. G. M. Kallenberg, "The diagnosis and classification of microscopic polyangiitis," *Journal of Autoimmunity*, vol. 48-49, pp. 90–93, 2014.

[5] A. Cavazza, F. Muratore, L. Boiardi et al., "Inflamed temporal artery," *The American Journal of Surgical Pathology*, vol. 38, no. 10, pp. 1360–1370, 2014.

[6] J. A. Chirinos, L. J. Tamariz, G. Lopes et al., "Large vessel involvement in ANCA-associated vasculitides: report of a case and review of the literature," *Clinical Rheumatology*, vol. 23, no. 2, pp. 152–159, 2004.

[7] T. Genereau, O. Lortholary, M. A. Pottier et al., "Temporal artery biopsy: a diagnostic tool for systemic necrotizing vasculitis: French Vasculitis Study Group," *Arthritis and Rheumatism*, vol. 42, no. 12, pp. 2674–2681, 1999.

[8] E. Guerin, P. Alexander, P. Lanyon, K. Robinson, and A. Foss, "A reminder that temporal arteritis is not necessarily giant cell arteritis," *Eye*, vol. 23, no. 7, pp. 1608-1609, 2009.

[9] M. A. Hamidou, A. Moreau, C. Toquet, D. El Kouri, P. de Faucal, and J. Y. Grolleau, "Temporal arteritis associated with systemic necrotizing vasculitis," *The Journal of Rheumatology*, vol. 30, no. 10, pp. 2165–2169, 2003.

[10] A. Morinaga, K. Ono, K. Komai, and M. Yamada, "Microscopic polyangitis presenting with temporal arteritis and multiple cranial neuropathies," *Journal of the Neurological Sciences*, vol. 256, no. 1-2, pp. 81–83, 2007.

[11] T. Planté-Bordeneuve, L. Henckaerts, E. Lerut, E. Verbeken, and D. Blockmans, "Not every case of temporal arteritis is giant cell arteritis. Microscopic polyangiitis involving the temporal artery," *JCR: Journal of Clinical Rheumatology*, vol. 24, no. 8, pp. 440–442, 2018.

[12] A. Tanaka, I. Tsujimoto, Y. Ito, Y. Sugiura, N. Ujihira, and R. Sezaki, "Temporal artery involvement in microscopic polyangitis," *Internal Medicine*, vol. 50, no. 9, pp. 1033–1037, 2011.

[13] R. Zuckerman, M. Patel, and D. R. Alpert, "A tale of two vasculitides: biopsy-proven giant cell arteritis followed by the independent development of renal-limited microscopic polyangiitis," *BMJ Case Reports*, vol. 2017, 2017.

Clinicopathological Implications of Proteinuria after Long-Term Isolated Hematuria due to Thin Basement Membrane Nephropathy and Focal Segmental Glomerulosclerosis

Ryo Togashi,[1] Yoshikazu Nemoto,[1] Kaito Waki,[1] Michito Nagura,[1] Shigeyuki Arai,[1] Yoshifuru Tamura,[1] Yasutoshi Oshima,[2] Fukuo Kondo,[2] Ryuji Ohashi,[3] Shunya Uchida,[1] Shigeru Shibata,[1] and Yoshihide Fujigaki[1]

[1]*Department of Internal Medicine, Teikyo University School of Medicine, Itabashi-ku, Tokyo, Japan*
[2]*Department of Pathology, Teikyo University Hospital, Itabashi-ku, Tokyo, Japan*
[3]*Department of Diagnostic Pathology, Nippon Medical School Musashikosugi Hospital, Kasasaki-City, Kanagawa, Japan*

Correspondence should be addressed to Yoshihide Fujigaki; fujigaki@med.teikyo-u.ac.jp

Academic Editor: Władysław Sułowicz

A 45-year-old obese man presented with persistent hematuria for 21 years. At the age of 37, he developed hypertension and proteinuria which later increased up to 1.6 g/g creatinine. Kidney biopsy revealed thin basement membrane nephropathy (TBMN) and focal segmental glomerulosclerosis (FSGS), which explained his urinary abnormalities. Although a subgroup of TBMN can be complicated by FSGS, his FSGS was associated with obesity because of its histological features. Reduction of body weight and increasing a dose of angiotensin-receptor blocker could transiently reduce the amount of proteinuria. Clinicopathological implications of proteinuria after long-term hematuria by TBMN and FSGS were further discussed.

1. Introduction

The common causes of isolated microscopic hematuria among children and young adults are IgA nephropathy, thin basement membrane nephropathy (TBMN) and Alport syndrome (AS) [1, 2]. It is well recognized that both IgA nephropathy and AS could develop proteinuria, hypertension and renal dysfunction, resulting in end-stage kidney disease (ESKD). Although the renal outcome was believed to be generally good in TBMN, recent studies showed that a subgroup of TBMN is at increased risk of ESKD due to the late onset of focal segmental glomerulosclerosis (FSGS) [3]. Therefore, patients with persistent isolated microscopic hematuria, whatever the cause among children and young adults, need long-term follow-up to monitor proteinuria, renal function and blood pressure to provide patients with proper treatment at an appropriate timing.

We herein report a 45-year-old obese man who presented with proteinuria after long-term persistent hematuria. Kidney biopsy revealed TBMN and FSGS. We judged that his FSGS was caused by obesity because of its histological features. Differential diagnoses of clinical situations involving co-occurrence of TBMN and FSGS were also discussed.

2. Case Report

A 45-year-old man presented with occult blood in urine since 24 years old. He began to treat hypertension at the age of 37, when he had microscopic hematuria and proteinuria of 0.4 g/g creatinine. Since proteinuria was gradually increased to 1.16 g/g creatinine, he was admitted to our hospital to evaluate urinary abnormalities. He did not experience macroscopic hematuria. He was full-term birth, but birth weight information could not be obtained. He had no family history of renal diseases. On admission, height and body weight were 177 cm and 98.7 kg, respectively. Body mass index (BMI) was 31.5 kg/m^2. He had over 80 kg (BMI >25.5 kg/m^2) since 15 years old. Blood pressure was 140/78 mmHg. He was treated with the dosage of 25 mg/day of losartan potassium, 5 mg/day of amlodipine OD and 20 mg/day of febuxostat. Physical examination was not

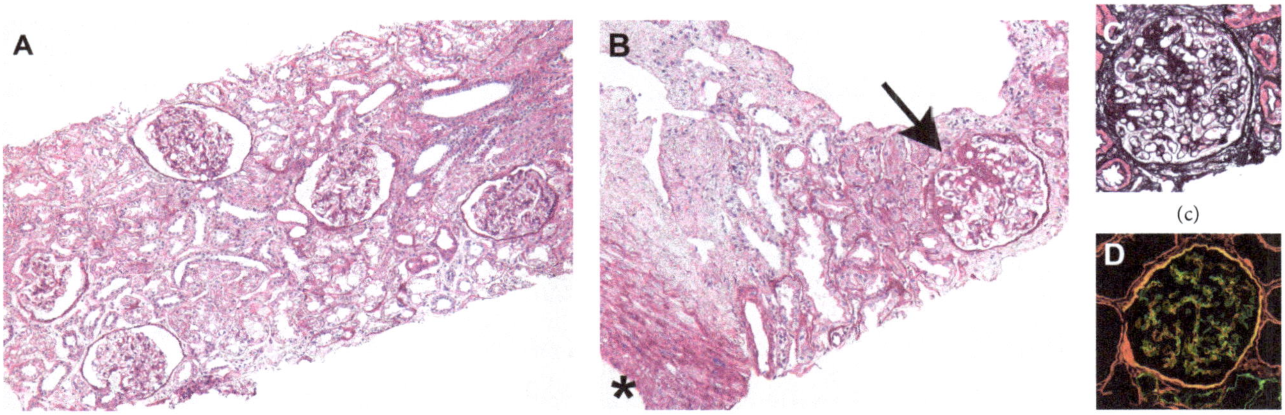

(a) (b) (c) (d)

FIGURE 1: Kidney biopsy findings. (a): Light microscopic observation reveals glomeruli with slight enlargement. Periodic acid-Schiff staining. Original magnification ×200. (b) One glomerulus with focal segmental sclerosis is found at a corticomedullary junction area (arrow). *; arcuate artery. Periodic acid-Schiff staining. Original magnification ×200. (c) This glomerulus shows perihilar type of segmental sclerosis. Periodic acid-methenamine-silver staining. Original magnification ×200. (d) Immunofluorescent finding shows linear alpha-2 (red) and alpha-5 (green) of type IV collagen staining along the glomerular basement membrane. Yellow stain indicates merged image of co-localization of alpha-2 (red) and alpha-5 (green) of type IV collagen.

remarkable. Urinary examination showed proteinuria of 0.7 g/g creatinine, red blood cell of 10-19/high power filed and positive red cell casts. Blood chemistry showed serum creatinine of 0.69 mg/dL, cystatin C of 0.74 mg/L, albumin of 4.1 g/dL, uric acid of 6.3 mg/dL, LDL-cholesterol of 144 mg/dL and HbA1c of 5.5%. The estimated glomerular filtration rate calculated by the revised serum creatinine–based Japanese equation [4] was 97.6 mL/min/1.73 m^2. Immunological examination indicated no abnormal results including C-reactive protein, IgG, IgA, complement and anti-nuclear antibody. The electrocardiogram and chest X-ray were normal. Abdominal ultrasound detected normal shape and size in the kidneys.

With a clinical suspicion of IgA nephropathy, kidney biopsy was performed. Kidney biopsy revealed 1 global sclerosis out of 16 obtained glomeruli. Nonsclerotic glomeruli exhibited slight enlargement (glomerular diameter from 180 μm to 200 μm) without significant proliferative changes. One glomerulus showed segmental sclerosis at the perihilar region, diagnostic of FSGS (Figures 1(a)–1(c)). There were mild degree of tubular atrophy and interstitial fibrosis accompanied by mononuclear cell infiltration. Mild intimal thickening in small arteries and arteriolar hyalinosis were found. Immunofluorescent study showed no deposition of immnoreactants and a preserved linear alpha-5 of type IV collagen staining (Figure 1(d)), supportive for TBMN rather than AS [5]. Electron microscopy showed thinning of the glomerular basement membrane (GBM) (GBM width between 140 nm and 250 nm) without splitting or lamellation, fulfilling the diagnostic criteria of TBMN (Figure 2) [5]. Foot process effacement was partial, and glomerular epithelial detachment was not seen (Figure 2). Hypertension can be a cause of FSGS [6]. However, it is less likely that FSGS lesion in our patient was caused by hypertension because that his hypertension was less severe degree and that kidney biopsy did not include ischemic glomerular lesions, which are a common feature in hypertensive nephrosclerosis [7]. As our patient has significant obesity, the presence of glomerulomegaly and perihilar segmental glomerulosclerosis, and the absence of diffuse foot process effacement collectively supported the diagnosis of obesity-associated FSGS [8].

We further examined possible additional lesions consistent with obesity-related glomerulopathy (ORG). The glomerular density (the number of nonsclerotic glomeruli per renal cortical area) measured using an image analysis program (Aperio ImageScope, Leica, Buffalo Grove, IL, USA) was 1.7 mm^2, which was low compared with that in nonobese kidney donors and comparable to the reported glomerular density in patients with ORG [9]. GBM width of the nonsclerotic area of the glomerulus with perihilar sclerosis was expected to be thick or normal in ORG [10], however, electron microscopic specimen including the glomerulus was not obtained. Since there was no detachment of podocytes from GBM, the expected reduction of the coating area of podocyte on the glomerular surface in ORG was not evident [8]. Other characteristics of ORG, such as tubular hypertrophy and the presence of the lipid droplets in the mesangial cells, podocytes and proximal tubular cells were not found [11].

Reduction of body weight by diet therapy from 98.7 kg to 92.0 kg, and increasing a dose of angiotensin-receptor blocker, losartan potassium to 100 mg/day successfully reduced blood pressure to 125/75 mmHg and proteinuria from 1.16 to 0.16 g/g creatinine 9 months after the kidney biopsy. However, subsequently re-increase in body weight brought about increasing proteinuria up to 1.2 g/g creatinine. Microscopic hematuria persisted, and renal function was stable during the clinical course.

3. Discussion

IgA nephropathy, TBMN and AS, all of three conditions can present with the manifestations of proteinuria after short or long-term isolated hematuria [1, 2]. Our patient with

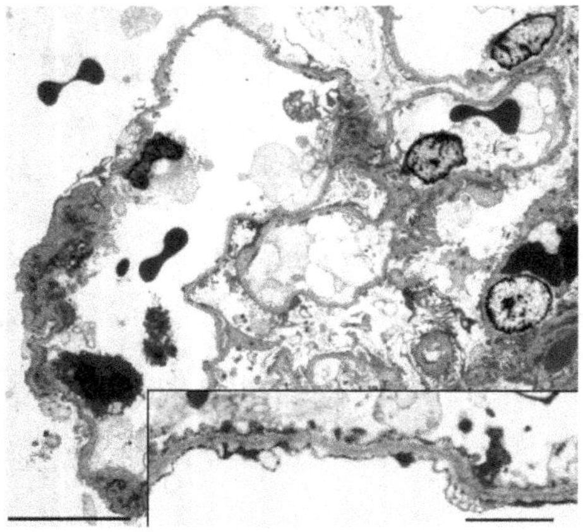

FIGURE 2: Electron micrograph of a glomerulus. Glomerular basement membranes are diffusely thinned without lamellation or reticular formation. Overlying podocytes are fairly preserved with focal foot process effacement. There are no electron dense deposits within glomerular capillary walls and a mesangial region. A red blood cell is seen in Bowman's space. Bar =10.0 μm. Inset; Peripheral glomerular capillary wall. Bar =1.0 μm.

proteinuria after long-term hematuria had no family history of renal diseases and no visual or auditory deficits, thus IgA nephropathy was initially suspected. However, kidney biopsy revealed a dual diagnosis of TBMN and FSGS. The cause of FSGS needs to be clarified carefully in patients with such manifestations.

First, we postulated that FSGS might be a result of a co-inherited glomerulopathy with TBMN. TBMN is characterized by persistent isolated hematuria often in childhood or young adults. TBMN is usually autosomal dominant and caused by mutations in the genes encoding type IV collagen and heterozygous *COL4A3/COL4A4* mutations may explain about 40% of familial microscopic hematuria due to TBMN [12]. Although the renal outcome was believed to be generally good, it is now recognized that up to 20–30% of patients of familial and sporadic TBMN cases with carriers of heterozygous *COL4A3/COL4A4* mutations may progress to the ESKD due to late-onset FSGS often with nonnephrotic proteinuria [3, 12–14] or due to possible subset of AS [15]. Interestingly certain hypomorphic podocin variants may act as adverse genetic modifiers predisposing to FSGS when co-inherited with *COL4A3 or COL4A4* mutations [16, 17]. No genotype-phenotype correlation was observed [18]. AS and TBMN have a common molecular basis. These conditions arise as a result of mutations in genes *COL4A3, COL4A4* and *COL4A5* that affect the synthesis, assembly, deposition or function of the collagen IV α345 molecules. Recently, the Alport Syndrome Classification Working Group proposed the classification of all disorders arising from abnormalities of the collagen IV α345 molecules as forms of AS with the goal of improving renal outcomes through regular monitoring and early treatment [19]. As our patient did not undergo genetic analysis, we were unable to determine if FSGS was caused by genetic abnormalities. Histopathologically, however, we believe that our FSGS was a secondary lesion because strong evidence of podocytopathy, such as diffuse process effacement and glomerular epithelial detachment, was absent by electron microscopic analysis.

Next, out of various factors leading to secondary FSGS, obesity was more likely to be the main cause because of our patient's morbid obesity. ORG is usually defined as glomerulomegaly with or without perihilar segmental glomerular sclerosis and partial foot process effacement in patients with BMI $\geq$30 kg/m^2 [8]. Typically ORG presents with either subnephrotic or less commonly nephrotic range proteinuria [8]. A glomerulomegaly with perihilar FSGS and relatively mild foot process effacement with moderate proteinuria can help to diagnose obesity-associated FSGS in our patient. However, it may not be easy to distinguish secondary FSGS from primary one from morphological aspects especially in the early phase of disease without any risk factors for secondary FSGS. As reported [8], reduction of body weight and reinforcement of renin angiotensin system inhibition were effective on reduction of proteinuria in our patient. This also supported a dual diagnose of TBMN and obesity-associated FSGS.

TBMN is not a rare disease since about 1% of the population is affected [20]. However, there is no evidence that TBMN alters the prognosis of another glomerulopathy [21]. On the other hand, obesity seems to worsen the renopathological state in chronic kidney disease [8, 22]. It is largely unknown whether obesity-associated FSGS or hypertension-associated FSGS is easy to develop in patients with TBMN. Given that the incidence of obesity and ORG has been increasing worldwide, we predict that more cases with a dual diagnose of TBMN and obesity-associated FSGS might be reported in the future [8, 23].

In summary, we experienced a patient with proteinuria after long-term isolated hematuria, diagnosed as TBMN complicated by secondary FSGS associated with obesity. Analysis of *COL4A3* or *COL4A4* mutations might be helpful to know the underlying risk not only for FSGS but also for AS in patients with long-term isolated hematuria [3, 15]. However, genetic diagnosis that can predict a progression of FSGS in patients with TBMN has not been established, therefore careful evaluation of clinicopathological findings is essential for a proper diagnosis and an appropriate treatment.

Additional Points

This article does not contain any studies with human participants performed by any of the authors.

Consent

Written informed consent was obtained from the patient.

Acknowledgments

We would like to thank Ms. Hiromi Yamaguchi for her technical assistance.

References

[1] C. Nieuwhof, C. Doorenbos, W. Grave et al., "A prospective study of the natural history of idiopathic nonproteinuric hematuria," *Kidney International*, vol. 49, pp. 222–225, 1996.

[2] K. M. Chow, B. C. Kwan, P. K. Li, and C. C. Szeto, "Asymptomatic isolated microscopic haematuria: long-term follow-up," *Quarterly Journal of Medicine*, vol. 97, pp. 739–745, 2004.

[3] C. Gast, R. J. Pengelly, M. Lyon et al., "Collagen, *(COL4A)* mutations are the most frequent mutations underlying adult focal segmental glomerulosclerosis," *Nephrology Dialysis Transplantation*, vol. 31, no. 6, pp. 961–970, 2016.

[4] S. Matsuo, E. Imai, M. Horio et al., "Revised equations for estimated GFR from serum creatinine in Japan," *American Journal of Kidney Diseases*, vol. 53, no. 6, pp. 982–992, 2009.

[5] K. Tryggvason and J. Patrakka, "Thin basement membrane nephropathy," *Journal of the American Society of Nephrology*, vol. 17, no. 3, pp. 813–822, 2006.

[6] V. D. D'Agati, A. B. Fogo, J. A. Bruijn, and J. C. Jennette, "Pathologic classification of focal segmental glomerulosclerosis: a working proposal," *American Journal of Kidney Diseases*, vol. 43, pp. 368–382, 2004.

[7] S. Liang, W. Le, D. Liang et al., "Clinico-pathological characteristics and outcomes of patients with biopsy-proven hypertensive nephrosclerosis: a retrospective cohort study," *BMC Nephrology*, vol. 11, no. 17, 42 pages, 2016.

[8] V. D. D'Agati, A. Chagnac, A. P. de Vries et al., "Obesity-related glomerulopathy: clinical and pathologic characteristics and pathogenesis," *Nature Reviews Nephrology*, vol. 12, no. 8, pp. 453–471, 2016.

[9] Y. Okabayashi, N. Tsuboi, T. Sasaki et al., "Glomerulopathy associated with moderate obesity," *Kidney International Reports*, vol. 1, no. 4, pp. 250–255, 2016.

[10] D. S. Goumenos, B. Kawar, M. El Nahas et al., "Early histological changes in the kidney of people with morbid obesity," *Nephrology Dialysis Transplantation*, vol. 24, no. 12, pp. 3732–3738, 2009.

[11] I. A. Bobulescu, Y. Lotan, J. Zhang et al., "Triglycerides in the human kidney cortex: relationship with body size," *PLoS One*, vol. 9, no. 8, e101285 pages, 2014.

[12] L. Papazachariou, P. Demosthenous, M. Pieri et al., "Frequency of *COL4A3/COL4A4* mutations amongst families segregating glomerular microscopic hematuria and evidence for activation of the unfolded protein response. Focal and segmental glomerulosclerosis is a frequent development during ageing," *PLoS One*, vol. 9, no. 12, e115015 pages, 2014.

[13] K. Voskarides, L. Damianou, V. Neocleous et al., "*COL4A3/COL4A4* mutations producing focal segmental glomerulosclerosis and renal failure in thin basement membrane nephropathy," *Journal of the American Society of Nephrology*, vol. 18, no. 11, pp. 3004–3016, 2007.

[14] E. Marcocci, V. Uliana, M. Bruttini et al., "Autosomal dominant Alport syndrome: molecular analysis of the *COL4A4* gene and clinical outcome," *Nephrology Dialysis Transplantation*, vol. 24, no. 5, pp. 1464–1471, 2009.

[15] J. Savige, "Should we diagnose autosomal dominant Alport syndrome when there is a pathogenic heterozygous *COL4A3* or *COL4A4* variant?," *Kidney International Reports*, vol. 3, no. 6, pp. 1239–1241, 2018.

[16] K. Voskarides, M. Arsali, Y. Athanasiou, A. Elia, A. Pierides, and C. Deltas, "Evidence that NPHS2-R229Q predisposes to proteinuria and renal failure in familial hematuria," *Pediatric Nephrology*, vol. 27, no. 4, pp. 675–679, 2012.

[17] C. Stefanou, M. Pieri, I. Savva et al., "Co-inheritance of functional podocin variants with heterozygous collagen IV mutations predisposes to renal failure," *Nephron*, vol. 130, pp. 200–212, 2015.

[18] P. Plevová, J. Gut, and J. Janda, "Familial hematuria: a review," *Medicine (Kaunas)*, vol. 53, no. 1, pp. 1–10, 2017.

[19] C. E. Kashtan, J. Ding, G. Garosi et al., "Alport syndrome: a unified classification of genetic disorders of collagen IV α345: a position paper of the Alport syndrome classification working group," *Kidney International*, vol. 93, no. 5, pp. 1045–1051, 2018.

[20] M. C. Gregory, "The clinical features of thin basement membrane nephropathy," *Seminars in Nephrology*, vol. 25, no. 3, pp. 140–145, 2005.

[21] S. M. Norby and F. G. Cosio, "Thin basement membrane nephropathy associated with other glomerular diseases," *Seminars in Nephrology*, vol. 25, no. 3, pp. 176–179, 2005.

[22] S. Kato, A. Nazneen, Y. Nakashima et al., "Pathological influence of obesity on renal structural changes in chronic kidney disease," *Clinical and Experimental Nephrology*, vol. 13, no. 4, pp. 332–340, 2009.

[23] N. Kambham, G. S. Markowitz, A. M. Valeri, J. Lin, and V. D. D'Agati, "Obesity-related glomerulopathy: an emerging epidemic," *Kidney International*, vol. 59, no. 4, pp. 1498–509, 2001.

Calciphylaxis: Successful Management of a Rare Complication of Chronic Kidney Disease in Two Patients

Ibtissam Fares, [1,2] **Tarik Bouattar**, [1,2] **Hadja Moussokoro Kone**, [1,2] **Hajar Benzouina**, [1,2] **Meryem Benbella**, [1,2] **Naima Ouzeddoun**, [1,2] **Rabia Bayahia**, [1,2] **and Loubna Benamar** [1,2]

[1] *Nephrology Dialysis and Transplantation Department, Ibn Sina Teaching Hospital, Rabat, Morocco*
[2] *Faculty of Medicine and Pharmacy of Rabat, Morocco*

Correspondence should be addressed to Ibtissam Fares; nephro.fares@gmail.com

Academic Editor: Phuong Chi Pham

Calciphylaxis, or calcification uremic arteriolopathy, is a rare disease thought to occur due to arteriolar calcifications of the dermis and is responsible for ischemia with cutaneous necrosis and painful panniculitis. Its mechanism remains poorly understood which makes its management challenging and difficult to standardize. We report our management of two patients diagnosed with calciphylaxis. In one patient, calciphylaxis was mentioned upon admission given the context of preexisting secondary hyperparathyroidism and the existence of multiple risk factors. In both patients, the diagnosis was confirmed histologically. Our two observations highlight the difficulty of the diagnosis and the complexity of the therapeutic management that has been personalized according to patient characteristics and clinical evolution. Several therapeutic means can be implemented once the diagnosis is made; nevertheless, its prognosis remains pejorative despite the therapeutic advances. Broad debridement, good phosphocalcic balance control, and the correction of the risk factors top the list of any therapeutic strategy. One of the major challenges of the therapy is normalizing the calcium-phosphate balance. Thus, Cinacalcet and sodium thiosulfate appear to be promising treatments.

1. Background

Calciphylaxis, or calcific uremic arteriolopathy, is a rare disease with a poor prognosis. The mechanism involves arteriolar calcifications of the dermis, responsible for ischemia, with cutaneous necrosis and painful panniculitis [1].

Risk factors are multiple: female sex, dialysis, advanced age, diabetes, obesity, undernutrition, antivitamin K, and poor phosphocalcic balance control [2, 3].

The treatment is primarily based on managing the wounds, eliminating all the possible precipitating factors of ectopic calcification, administering agents capable of inhibiting the process of calcification, and controlling risk factors to avoid recurrences.

This disease is associated with high mortality ranging between 30% and 80% depending on the comorbidities and the configuration of cutaneous involvement. In recent years, mortality seems to have improved; especially, since the pathology is better known, the action is taken more quickly and some treatment alternatives are available [4].

We report a successful evolution of two patients with calciphylaxis managed in our department.

2. Cases Presentation

2.1. Patient 1. A 56-year-old woman with a 27-year history of type 2 diabetes mellitus being poorly controlled the last 3 years and high blood pressure under angiotensin-converting enzyme inhibitor (ACEI) for 4 years was diagnosed with end-stage kidney disease presumably due to diabetic nephropathy. After three years of thrice-weekly hemodialysis treatment (with a single-pool Kt / V at 1.27 and dialysate Ca at 1.5 mmol/L), our patient presented with necrotic and painful extremities skin lesions (Figure 1). The clinical examination found a patient in good general health with present

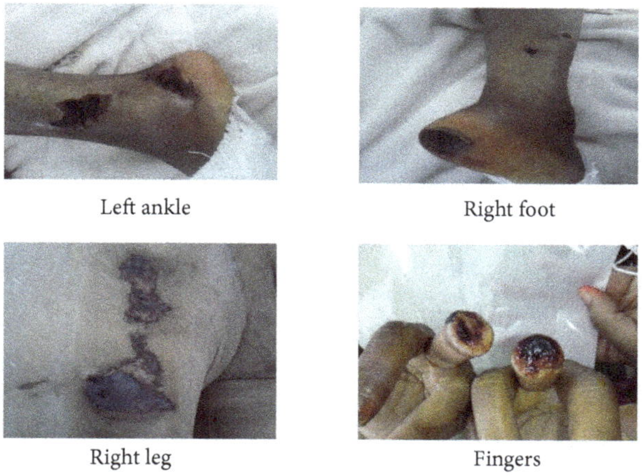

FIGURE 1: Topography and aspect of Calciphylaxis lesions of patient 1.

and symmetrical peripheral pulses. Its biological assessment revealed phosphocalcic balance disorders with an elevated parathormone (PTH) and alkaline phosphatase (PAL) at 919 pg /ml and 348 UI /l, respectively, a calcium level at 2.2 mmol / l under calcium carbonate, a normal serum phosphorus at 1.03 mmol / l, a vitamin D deficiency at 14.2 ng / ml, and normocytic normochromic anemia. Dosage of prothrombotic factors (C and S proteins, antiphospholipid antibodies, anticardiolipin antibody, anti-b2 glycoprotein 1 antibody, circulating anticoagulant, and cryoglobulinemia) was normal. Cervical ultrasound has found bilateral parathyroid nodules. X-rays of the skeleton showed bone demineralization with extensive calcification of the vessels. The patient initially received symptomatic treatment with an opioid analgesic (Tramadol sometimes associated with Nefopam), blood transfusion, and erythropoietin to correct anemia.

She underwent a wide debridement of the necrotic cutaneous lesions whose anatomopathological examination returned in favor of a calciphylaxis. Once the diagnosis was established, the patient first benefited from a parathyroidectomy in order to correct the phosphocalcic balance. One week after parathyroidectomy, the patient had asymptomatic hypocalcemia at 1.74 mmol/l, following which she was dialyzed with a dialysate rich in calcium 1.75 mmol/l and given calcium supplementation based on calcium carbonate. 3 weeks later, its balance sheet improved significantly with a PTH at 432 pg/ml, a serum calcium level at 2.29 mmol/l, and a hypophosphatemia at 0.64 mmol / l. In addition, the patient received several hyperbaric oxygen therapy sessions that started from the second week of her admission and had been maintained until the fourth month with a total of 36 sessions. Sodium thiosulfate perfusions (25g three times a week at the end of each hemodialysis session) were also administered to our patient that started from the fourth week to the sixteenth week with a total of 36 bottles. No adverse effects have been reported. Local care was performed daily until complete healing of the lesions (Figure 2).

2.2. Patient 2. A 69-year-old woman with a long history of arterial hypertension under ACEI, complicated by end-stage kidney disease was placed on automated peritoneal dialysis (APD) for 21 months with a KT/V urea at 1,69. The patient was also under calcium carbonate for secondary hyperparathyroidism diagnosed during her follow-up (a PTH at 780 pg/ml). The patient was consulted for erythematous, necrotic, and painful skin lesions of her right leg (Figure 3.1). The clinical examination found inflammatory signs with redness and pain around these lesions. Peripheral pulses were present and symmetrical. Her body mass index was at 28,3 kg/m^2. The lesions worsened and spread to the contralateral leg within 5 days (Figure 3.2). CT angiography did not indicate stenosis of the vascular axes but showed diffuse calcifications that extended to the lower limbs. Calciphylaxis was mentioned in view of the different risk factors present in our patient, as well as the quite telling clinical presentation occurring in a known context of secondary hyperparathyroidism. The initial treatment consisted of the correction of anemia with erythropoietin to optimize the tissue perfusion as well as analgesics to manage the pain. Parathyroidectomy was performed as soon to control the disturbances of the phosphocalcic balance and the PTH levels decreased to 417 pg/ml the 2nd day after parathyroidectomy. A concomitant biopsy of skin lesions confirmed the already mentioned diagnosis of calciphylaxis (Figure 4). Necrosectomy with local care and optimization of dialysis parameters were also implemented. A treatment based on sodium thiosulfate and hyperbaric oxygen was proposed to our patient but was not performed due to a lack of her financial resources. Fortunately, the complete healing of the lesions was obtained by 4 months (Figure 5).

3. Discussion

Calciphylaxis was described in 1968 by Anderson et al. in a context of secondary hyperparathyroidism with hypercalcemia [9]. Since then, it has been more frequently observed in patients with chronic kidney disease with a frequency ranging from 1 to 4% according to the studies [1, 10].

The average age of onset is between 50 and 60 years with a clear female predominance. The risk factors for calciphylaxis commonly cited in the literature are as follows: the number of years of dialysis, the presence of phosphocalcic balance abnormalities (including hypercalcemia, hyperphosphatemia, and secondary hyperparathyroidism, favoured by calcium supplementation and vitamin D deficiency), the use of antivitamin K or corticosteroids, the presence of diabetes, obesity, female sex, hypoalbuminemia, and liver diseases. Thrombophilia also appears to be one of the predisposing factors for calciphylaxis [7, 9, 10].

Both of our patients had an obvious predisposing ground. Besides the female sex, dialysis, and secondary hyperparathyroidism risk factors were diabetes in the first patient and the overweight in the second.

The pathogenesis of calciphylaxis remains incompletely understood. It has been advanced that these lesions are secondary to calcification of the small vessel's wall, with fibrosis and endovascular thrombosis, leading to tissue ischemia and necrosis of the dermis and hypodermis.

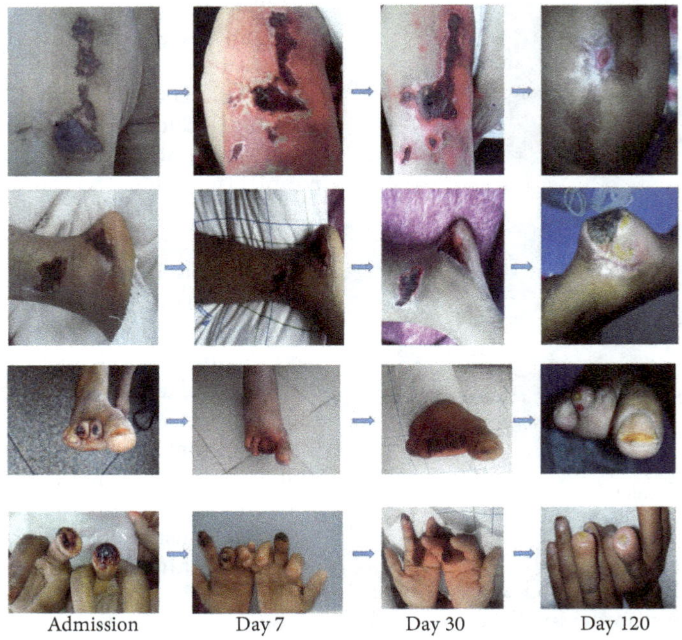

FIGURE 2: Evolution of Calciphylaxis lesions over 4 months of treatment in patient 1. Necrosectomy could not be performed at the heels because of the risk of injury to the Achilles tendon.

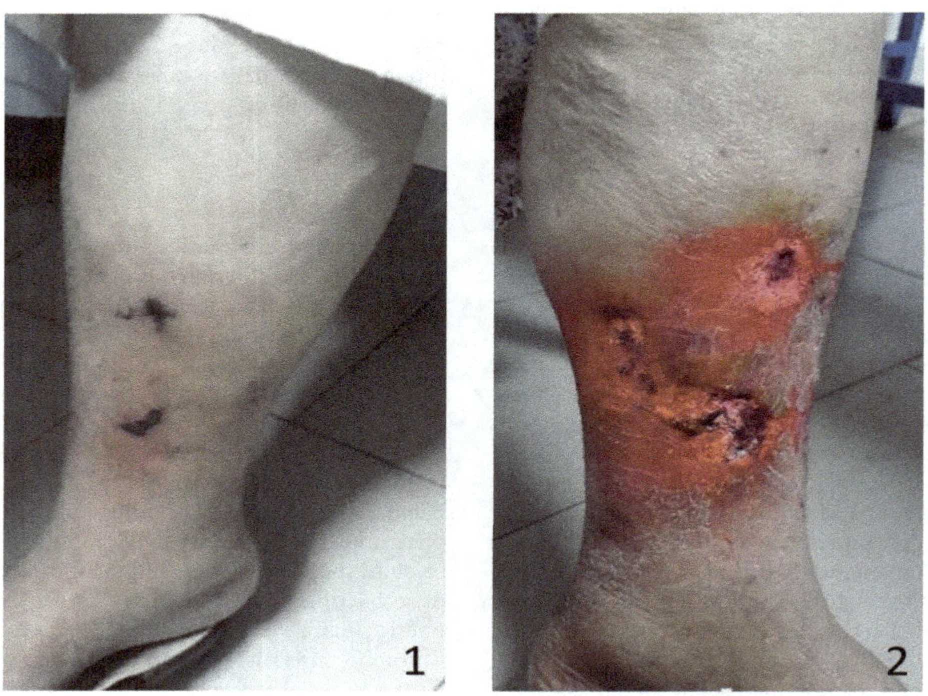

FIGURE 3: Calciphylaxis lesions at the admission of patient 2 (A: right leg, B: left leg).

The development of calciphylaxis goes through two phases: a silent phase where vascular calcifications are formed in the media with intimal hyperplasia of dermal and hypodermic arterioles, and then a phase of microcirculatory decompensation, which corresponds to thrombosis ischemia most often [8].

The diagnosis of calciphylaxis is based on a set of arguments essentially clinical [3, 8].

Clinical signs include skin lesions which start as subcutaneous indurated nodules or plaques extremely painful (a pain disproportionate to the cutaneous lesion) accompanied by livedo reticularis, often initially labeled dermis-hypodermis.

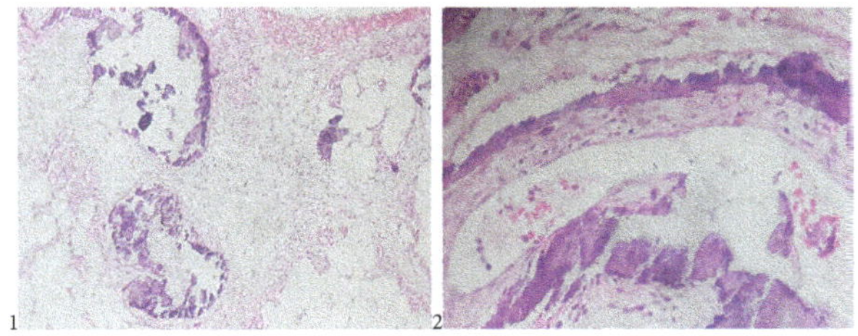

FIGURE 4: (1) A skin biopsy and adipose tissue in patient 2 with foci of necrosis, calcification of arteriolar walls, and necrotizing panniculitis in the context of a uremic calcifying arteriopathy. (2) Intimal thickening and fibrin thrombi in patient 2 skin biopsy.

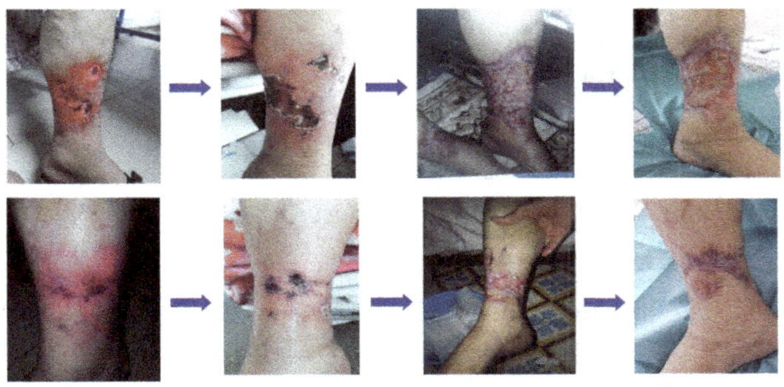

FIGURE 5: Evolution of Calciphylaxis lesions over 3 months of treatment in patient 2.

The evolution is done in a few days towards the formation of superficial and then deep ulcerations leading to the constitution of a blackish eschar, always strongly painful with centrifugal extension [11].

This suggestive clinical presentation associated with risk factors should rapidly evoke the diagnosis and initiate early therapeutic management to avoid serious infectious and ischemic complications, which can lead to death [1–3, 8, 10]

Indeed, in patients presenting with plaques only, the mortality rate was 33% at six months. Once ulceration develops, the mortality rate increased to above 80% [12].

Two strong arguments in favor of a diagnosis of calciphylaxis are the presence of pulse distal and lack of neuropathy [13].

Imaging tests may contribute to the diagnosis of calciphylaxis. A simple X-ray of the affected area can demonstrate the presence of calcifications of the vessels of medium-small caliber.

The biological context is very particular. In the vast majority of cases, there are secondary hyperparathyroidism and profound disorders of phosphocalcic metabolism with hypercalcemia and hyperphosphatemia. The thrombophilia assessment is useful and must be performed according to antecedents [8, 11].

Although in the context of the clinical signs biological and radiological features guide the diagnosis, the biopsy of skin lesions would confirm the diagnosis of calciphylaxis [4, 8].

Pathologically, this entity is characterized by the existence of calcifications of the media of deep and hypodermic dermal arterioles, hypertrophy of the intima, vascular thrombi formation, adipose tissue calcification, and infiltration by inflammatory cells [1, 8, 10].

Given the low level of evidence and the lack of randomized studies in this field, optimal treatment is far from being standardized. It involves a medical and surgical approach.

Management will, therefore, aim at the restoration of phosphocalcic balance, effective detoxification of affected areas, and the elimination of various risk factors [3, 8, 10].

Surgical wound cleaning is the first step in the management of this disease. McCarthy et al. reported in their retrospective monocentric study that a lack of surgical debridement was associated with a lower 6-month survival and significantly poorer survival for the entire duration of follow-up [6].

Other measures would be essential, notably the management of ulcerations (debridement, directed cicatrization, and broad-spectrum antibiotherapy depending on the evolution) and the optimization of healing (nutritional management, pressure ulcer prevention, and physiotherapy) [3].

Some authors advocate hyperbaric oxygen therapy in addition to previous treatments to accelerate wound healing [5].

The effective treatment of pain with analgesics using opioids is often appropriate. In our cases, opioids were used essentially during local care and dressing changes where the pain was at its peak.

The correction of anemia (by erythropoietin or transfusion of red blood cells) and the optimization of dialysis parameters (daily dialysis for patients on hemodialysis) allow better tissue oxygenation, essential for good healing of lesions [3].

Table 1: Therapies that have been suggested to improve calciphylaxis and their mechanism of action.

Therapies	Mechanism of action
Hyperbaric oxygen therapy	Promote tissue oxygenation [5]
Correction of anemia	Promote tissue oxygenation [3]
Stopping alpha-hydroxylated vitamin D derivatives	Slow down calcification phenomena [1, 3]
Dialysate calcium 1.5 mmol / L	Slow down calcification phenomena [3]
Parathyroidectomy	Slow down calcification phenomena [1, 3, 6]
Sodium thiosulfate	Slow down calcification phenomena [1–3, 6–8]
Debridement	Ulcerations treatment [1, 6]

It is accepted by several authors that the normalization of calcium phosphate balance is the primary variable for the treatment of calciphylaxis lesions [6].

Optimal dialysate poor in calcium and stopping the intake of calcium and alpha hydroxylated derivatives of vitamin D help to fight against the phenomena of calcification [3].

The control of hypoprothrombinemia by calcimimetics is strongly recommended or, more radically, parathyroidectomy in case of secondary hyperparathyroidism. McCarthy et al. found that, in patients with stage 5 / 5D chronic kidney disease (CKD), subtotal parathyroidectomy (performed only in patients with secondary hyperparathyroidism) was associated with better 6-month survival and overall survival [6].

Cinacalcet represents an interesting alternative for controlling hyperparathyroidism and decreasing the phosphocalcic product especially for patients with surgical contraindications [14].

In our patients, we used parathyroidectomy for the rapid treatment of secondary hyperparathyroidism and better control of the calcium phosphate balance. However, we have used a calcium carbonate substitution given the hypocalcemia threatening after parathyroidectomy. In addition, we did not correct the hypovitaminosis D during the 4 months of evolution.

Sodium thiosulfate, a calcium ion chelator, is a specific treatment that proved its worth in slowing calcification phenomena. Its mechanism of action is based on its ability to form soluble complexes with many metals and minerals, as well as being a possible effect as a vasodilator, antioxidant, and direct inhibitor of the calcification process [1–3, 6–8].

Bisphosphonates are the drugs of choice in the management of bone disorders including osteoporosis, Paget's disease, multiple myeloma, bone cancer, and cancer-induced hypocalcemia. It has shown response mainly in dystrophic calcifications of dermatomyositis and systemic sclerosis by reducing calcium turnover and resorption [15]. Furthermore, because of an additional property of inhibiting calcium phosphate crystal formation, bisphosphonates were used as inhibitors of ectopic calcification in two different types of vascular disease, atherosclerosis, and calciphylaxis [16, 17]. We do not have the experience of the use of bisphosphonates in our cases.

The calciphylaxis is one of the most feared complications of patients with CKD and dialysis. Its prognosis is very poor with mortality that reached 100% at 12 months as reported by Jean et al. [3]

Despite being improved in recent years by a better understanding of the pathology, the mortality remains high ranging between 33% and 80% mainly related to sepsis in most than half of the cases [8, 18].

The severity of calciphylaxis is related to the underlying condition of the patient (obesity, diabetes, and arteritis), diagnosis delay, the extent of the lesions, and the topography of the affected area with a better prognosis for distal forms [1, 3, 8, 18].

Our little experience in the management of calciphylaxis made us more optimistic toward this feared disease. We believe that the creation of a national registry for calciphylaxis and referral of patients to centers with experience in the management of calciphylaxis may help to carry out studies on a larger number of patients and then may help in improving the knowledge of calciphylaxis and therefore the survival of patients facing this disease.

Table 1 includes the nonexhaustive list of different therapies suggested to improve calciphylaxis in our patients and their mechanism of action.

Consent

Written informed consent for publication of clinical details and clinical images were obtained from the two patients. A copy of the consent form is available for review by the Editor of this journal.

References

[1] M. Chettati, A. Adnouni, W. Fadili, and I. Laouad, "Calcific uremic arteriolopathy in hemodialysis patient, review of literature through five cases reports," *Néphrologie & Thérapeutique*, vol. 14, no. 6, pp. 439–445, 2018.

[2] S. Devey, A. Valois, G. Cazajous et al., "Calciphylaxis in hemodialysis patients: 8 cases treated with sodium thiosulfate," *Annales de Dermatologie et de Venereologie*, vol. 145, no. 4, pp. 288–292, 2018.

[3] G. Jean, J.-C. Terrat, T. Vanel et al., "Calciphylaxis in dialysis patients: To recognize and treat it as soon as possible," *Néphrologie & Thérapeutique*, vol. 6, no. 6, pp. 499–504, 2010.

[4] D. Cucchiari and J.-V. Torregrosa, "Calciphylaxis in patients with chronic kidney disease: A disease which is still bewildering and potentially fatal," *Nefrología*, vol. 38, no. 6, pp. 579–586, 2018.

[5] T. Podymow, C. Wherrett, and K. D. Burns, "Hyperbaric oxygen in the treatment of calciphylaxis: A case series," *Nephrology Dialysis Transplantation* , vol. 16, no. 11, pp. 2176–2180, 2001.

[6] J. T. McCarthy, R. A. el-Azhary, M. T. Patzelt et al., "Survival, risk factors, and effect of treatment in 101 patients with calciphylaxis," *Mayo Clinic Proceedings*, vol. 91, no. 10, pp. 1384–1394, 2016.

[7] S. U. Nigwekar, D. Kroshinsky, R. M. Nazarian et al., "Calciphylaxis: risk factors, diagnosis, and treatment," *American Journal of Kidney Diseases*, vol. 66, no. 1, pp. 133–146, 2015.

[8] G. Perceau, "Uraemic and non-uraemic calcific arteriopathy: The need for rapid diagnosis and therapy," *Annales de Dermatologie et de Venereologie*, vol. 142, no. 8-9, pp. 506–512, 2015.

[9] D. C. Anderson, W. K. Stewart, and D. M. Piercy, "Calcifying panniculitis with fat and skin necrosis in a case of uraemia with autonomous hyperparathyroidism.," *The Lancet*, vol. 2, no. 7563, pp. 323–325, 1968.

[10] V. Esteve Simó, J. Almirall, J. Luelmo, A. Sáez, X. Andreu, and M. García, "Calcific uraemic ateriolopathy (calciphylaxis): Incidence, clinical features and long term outcomes," *Nefrología*, vol. 27, no. 5, pp. 599–604, 2007.

[11] O. Trost, N. Kadlub, P. Trouilloud, G. Malka, and A. Danino, "Calciphylaxis: A severe but unrecognized complication in end-stage renal disease patients. A review of 2 cases," *Annales de Chirurgie Plastique Esthétique*, vol. 50, no. 6, pp. 746–750, 2005.

[12] A. Fine and J. Zacharias, "Calciphylaxis is usually non-ulcerating: risk factors, outcome and therapy," *Kidney International*, vol. 61, no. 6, pp. 2210–2217, 2002.

[13] M. Angelis, L. L. Wong, S. A. Myers, and L. M. Wong, "Calciphylaxis in patients on hemodialysis: a prevalence study," *Surgery*, vol. 122, no. 6, pp. 1083–1090, 1997.

[14] S. Prey, A. Sparsa, H. Durox et al., "Calciphylaxis treated by cinacalcet: A medical alternative to parathyroidectomy," *La Revue de Médecine Interne*, vol. 30, no. 2, pp. 186–189, 2009.

[15] D. Jiménez-Gallo, L. Ossorio-García, and M. Linares-Barrios, "Calcinosis Cutis and Calciphylaxis," *Actas Dermo-Sifiliográficas*, vol. 106, no. 10, pp. 785–794, 2015.

[16] N. Shiraishi, K. Kitamura, T. Miyoshi et al., "Successful treatment of a patient with severe calcific uremic arteriolopathy (calciphylaxis) by etidronate disodium," *American Journal of Kidney Diseases*, vol. 48, no. 1, pp. 151–154, 2006.

[17] J. B. Catterall and T. E. Cawston, "Drugs in development: Bisphosphonates and metalloproteinase inhibitors," *Arthritis Research & Therapy*, vol. 5, no. 1, pp. 12–24, 2003.

[18] P. W. Santos, J. He, A. Tuffaha, and J. B. Wetmore, "Clinical characteristics and risk factors associated with mortality in calcific uremic arteriolopathy," *International Urology and Nephrology*, vol. 49, no. 12, pp. 2247–2256, 2017.

9

Simultaneous Pancreas-Kidney Transplant Complicated by Kidney Allograft Torsion and Pseudoaneurysms of the *Y*-Allograft: A Case Report and Review of the Literature

Sarah L. Tan[1,2] **Rachel Y. P. Tan**[1,2] **Gabrielle Cehic**[3,4] **Michael Wu,**[5,6] **John Kanellis**[7,8] **and Jeffrey Barbara**[1,2]

[1]*Department of Nephrology, Flinders Medical Centre, Flinders Drive, Bedford Park, South Australia 5042, Australia*
[2]*College of Medicine and Public Health, Flinders University, Sturt Road, Bedford Park, South Australia 5042, Australia*
[3]*Department of Nuclear Medicine, Flinders Medical Centre, Flinders Drive, Bedford Park, South Australia 5042, Australia*
[4]*Centre for Translational Cancer Research, University of South Australia (Cancer Research Institute), 101 Currie Street, Adelaide, South Australia 5001, Australia*
[5]*Department of Surgery and School of Clinical Sciences, Monash Health, 246 Clayton Road, Clayton, Victoria 3168, Australia*
[6]*Monash University, Wellington Road, Clayton, Victoria 3800, Australia*
[7]*Department of Nephrology, Monash Health, 246 Clayton Road, Clayton, Victoria 3168, Australia*
[8]*Centre for Inflammatory Diseases and Department of Medicine, Monash University, Wellington Road, Clayton, Victoria 3800, Australia*

Correspondence should be addressed to Rachel Y. P. Tan; rachel.tan2@sa.gov.au

Academic Editor: David Mudge

Background. We report and review the literature of two rare complications of simultaneous pancreas-kidney transplantation (SPKT) occurring in one patient. *Case Report.* A 39-year-old man with dialysis-dependent kidney failure secondary to type 1 diabetes mellitus underwent successful SPKT in October 2018. Three months later, he presented with an acute kidney injury (AKI) and returned to dialysis. Kidney scintigraphy showed a central photopenic region, and angiograms showed absent flow in the kidney transplant artery without treatable thrombus and the incidental finding of two pseudoaneurysms of the pancreatic *Y*-graft. He remained dialysis-dependent for three weeks before spontaneous partial recovery of allograft function; repeat kidney scintigraphy showed significant improvement in perfusion. However, in April 2019 he was readmitted with a sudden deterioration in kidney allograft function again necessitating haemodialysis. Repeat imaging confirmed that the kidney allograft had shifted from the left iliac fossa to the midline. He underwent surgical exploration, during which torsion of the kidney allograft was confirmed and a nephropexy was performed. The kidney allograft was originally implanted in the left retroperitoneum via a midline transperitoneal approach, which likely predisposed it to torsion. The pseudoaneurysms of the pancreatic *Y*-graft were managed conservatively, and surveillance imaging demonstrated that they remained stable in size. The patient regained reasonable kidney allograft function (estimated glomerular filtration rate, eGFR, of 45 mL/min) and maintained normal pancreatic allograft function. *Conclusion.* Kidney allograft torsion should be considered post-SPKT in patients with AKI and absent arterial flow. Although most case reports describe surgical management of pseudoaneurysms post-SPKT, our case demonstrates successful conservative management.

1. Introduction

SPKT is an established treatment option for patients with type 1 diabetes who are dialysis-dependent. There were 38 SPKT recipients in Australia in 2019 [1]. Although SPKT offers numerous benefits, including improved patient survival; recipients tend to experience surgical complications at a relatively higher rate in comparison to kidney-only recipients, without impact on longer-term allograft function [2–4].

We describe and review the literature of two rare complications of SPKT occurring in the same patient: torsion of the kidney allograft and pseudoaneurysms of the pancreatic *Y*-graft.

2. Case Presentation

A 39-year-old man with kidney failure secondary to type 1 diabetes mellitus received a simultaneous pancreas-kidney transplant in October 2018 after four years on haemodialysis. Via a transperitoneal approach, the donor's left kidney was placed in the left iliac fossa. The single transplant renal artery was anastomosed end-to-side to the left external iliac artery; the single transplant renal vein was anastomosed to the left external iliac vein, and the transplant ureter to the recipient's bladder. The donor pancreas was vascularised via a *Y*-graft from the donor splenic and superior mesenteric arteries to the recipient's right common iliac artery; the donor portal vein anastomosed to the recipient's inferior vena cava. The donor duodenum was anastomosed to the recipient's jejunum for exocrine drainage.

Postoperatively, he returned to theatre on day 0 post-transplant. A repeat laparotomy demonstrated bleeding around the venous anastomosis of the kidney allograft and a small branch off the inferior vena cava (IVC), with haemostasis being achieved.

The patient made an excellent recovery and was discharged two weeks post-transplant on triple immunosuppressive therapy: tacrolimus, mycophenolate, and prednisolone. Prior to discharge, he was euglycaemic with a creatinine of 94 μmol/L and lipase of 33 U/L. A contrast computed tomography (CT) scan performed on day 22 post-SPKT showed patent transplant vessels of both the pancreatic and kidney allografts with no abnormalities of the vasculature. No abnormal positioning of either allograft was noted.

He presented three months later (day 95 post-transplant) with AKI - creatinine 403 μmol/L and lactate dehydrogenase of 2301 U/L. He was asymptomatic. Three days prior to admission, his creatinine had been 104 μmol/L. He remained euglycaemic with a normal lipase. Kidney scintigraphy showed a central photopenic region (Figure 1), and subsequent angiography confirmed minimal flow in the transplant renal artery with a nonperfused kidney allograft and no thrombus amenable to intervention. Torsion of the vessels was not observed at the angiogram. A further contrast CT scan demonstrated no differential enhancement of the transplant kidney between the arterial and portal venous phases, and the diagnosis was presumed kidney allograft loss secondary to infarction. The placement of the kidney allograft was not commented on.

The CT also revealed the development of two pseudoaneurysms of the superior iliac artery of the *Y*-graft (Figure 2) measuring 12 × 4 mm and 3 mm, respectively.

Extensive investigation looking for infection and vasculitis (including blood cultures, antineutrophil cytoplasmic antibodies, antinuclear antibody, extractable nuclear antigen antibodies, and an antiphospholipid antibody screen) as potential causes of the pseudoaneurysms returned negative results and a decision was made to opt for conservative management. The creatinine peaked at 766 μmol/L and he was re-established on haemodialysis and discharged to home.

The patient underwent 11 sessions of haemodialysis over 3 weeks. A repeat kidney scintigraphy was performed after he reported increasing urine output and this revealed improvement in kidney perfusion with no evidence of vascular insult (Figure 3).

He was trialled off dialysis and achieved a baseline creatinine of 250 μmol/L. Pancreatic allograft function remained stable throughout this time. Mobility of the kidney allograft was suspected to be the underlying cause and a semiurgent nephropexy was planned. However, one day prior to his planned surgery, he represented on day 158 post-transplant, again with AKI (creatinine 532 μmol/L from 249 μmol/L two days prior). A third nuclear scan was performed, this time demonstrating reduced perfusion of the kidney allograft with displacement from the left iliac fossa to the central abdomen (Figure 4).

He received a single session of haemodialysis before undergoing urgent surgical correction with nephropexy. This involved surgical fixation of the kidney allograft by creating an extraperitoneal pocket to place the kidney behind the retroperitoneum. A biopsy showed acute tubular necrosis with no evidence of rejection.

The patient has since maintained reasonable allograft function with a baseline creatinine 170 μmol/L (eGFR of 45 mL/min). His pancreatic function remains stable, with no insulin requirement and normal lipase levels. An ultrasound of the pancreatic allograft at 19 months post-transplant revealed that the pseudoaneurysm was not larger at 6.5 × 5.9 mm in size; the smaller pseudoaneurysm could not be visualised. A CT with contrast at 25 months post-transplant demonstrated a pancreatic transplant of normal appearance. Regular imaging surveillance of the pseudoaneurysms will continue at 6–12 monthly intervals, or earlier in the event of symptoms.

3. Discussion

This is the first case report to describe two rare complications of SPKT — kidney allograft torsion and pseudoaneurysms of the *Y*-allograft — occurring in one patient.

Kidney torsion is an uncommon cause of allograft failure and requires a high degree of diagnostic suspicion due to its nonspecific symptomatology and variable timing of presentation. At the time of writing, there were26 published cases of kidney transplant torsion, 18 of which involved SPKT with intraperitoneal placement of the kidney. These are summarised in Table 1.

Among the SPKT recipients, for whom the kidney allograft is typically placed intraperitoneally, the timing of the occurrence of kidney allograft torsion was highly variable, ranging from the early postoperative period to ten years post-transplant [7, 11]. Interestingly, of the 8 kidney transplants performed without pancreatic transplantation, 3 of these allografts were placed extraperitoneally and experienced torsion in the early postoperative period [14–16].

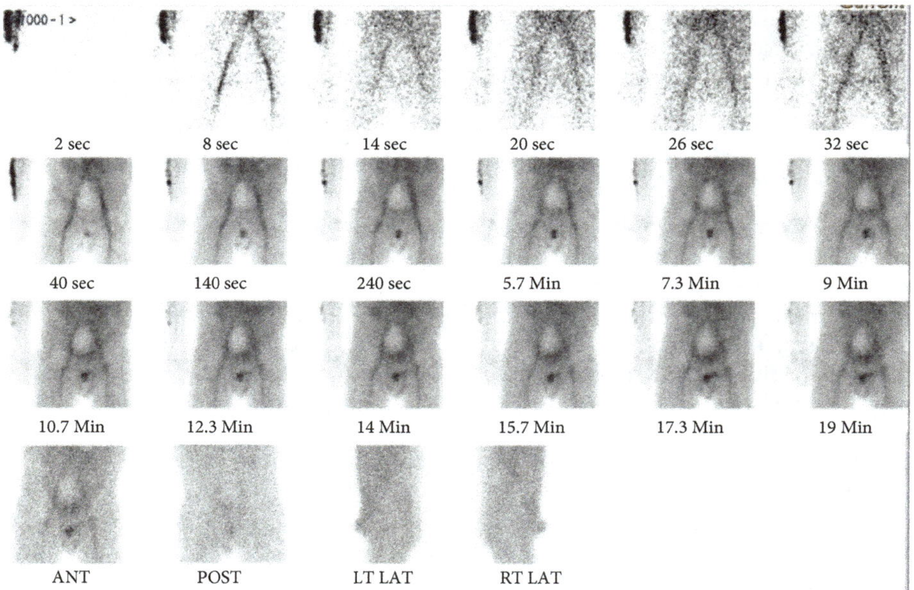

FIGURE 1: Kidney scintigraphy on day 95 post-transplantation demonstrating a central photopenic region, suggesting absent perfusion of the kidney allograft.

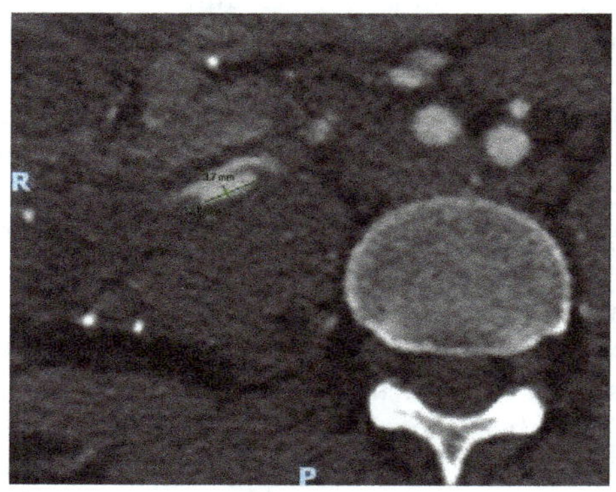

FIGURE 2: Contrast computed tomography scan of the abdomen showing one of the two pseudoaneurysms of the superior artery of the *Y*-graft.

Some clinicians have proposed that intraperitoneal placement increases the risk of mobility with subsequent torsion and recommend that prophylactic nephropexy should be performed for patients who require an intraperitoneal kidney transplant [12, 21].

Kidney allograft torsion results in a high rate of allograft loss, with only 58% of allografts salvaged (15 of 26) [7, 8, 11–21]. Successful management depends on rapid diagnosis and surgical correction to limit ischaemic time and, as in our case, can result in a favourable allograft outcome.

Pseudoaneurysm development is a rare complication of SPKT and can present as a medical emergency. Patients may present with rupture leading to significant haemodynamic instability necessitating urgent intervention [22–24]. Asymptomatic presentations such as in our patient are infrequently described [25–28]. Proposed aetiologies for pseudoaneurysm development include infection, vascular damage during transplantation, pancreatitis, and as a complication of biopsy [28–31]. Pseudoaneurysms developing in the setting of previous failed pancreas allografts have also been described [31]. The aetiology of our patient's pseudoaneurysms remains uncertain. We hypothesise that they may have developed as a consequence of vascular injury given the need for a second laparotomy to establish haemostasis.

The current literature guiding management of this uncommon complication comprises case reports and small case series. Most centres reporting their outcomes of pseudoaneurysms describe management via surgical intervention and, in more recent times, an endovascular approach [26, 31–33]. Of the three case reports describing patients with asymptomatic pseudoaneurysms, one patient went on to develop haemorrhage in the setting of anticoagulation and required endovascular intervention, and one underwent surgical exploration due to the large size of the pseudoaneurysm (8 cm) with the final patient declining intervention [26–28]. Our patient, for whom no infective cause for the pseudoaneurysms could be identified, remains

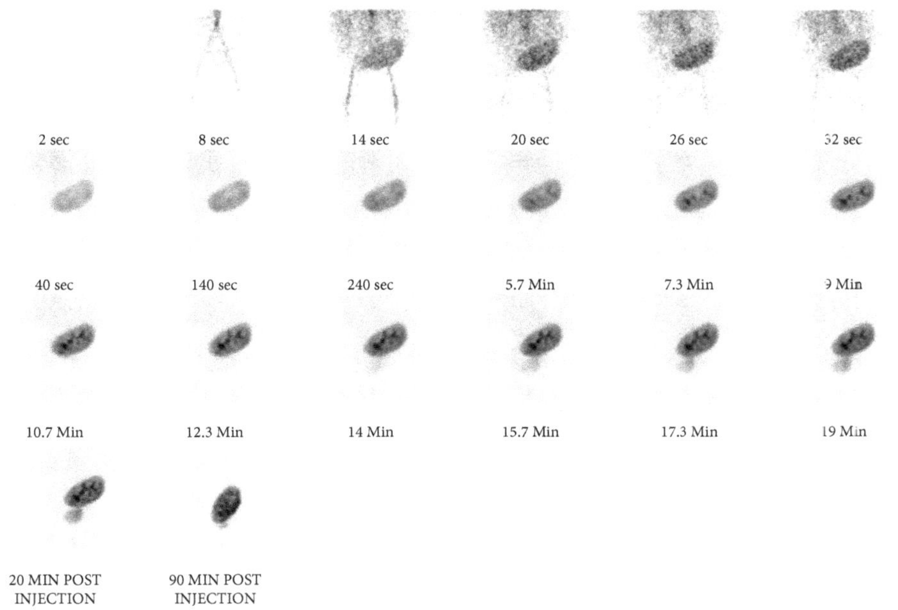

FIGURE 3: Kidney scintigraphy performed on day 115 post-transplantation demonstrating a return of perfusion to the kidney allograft.

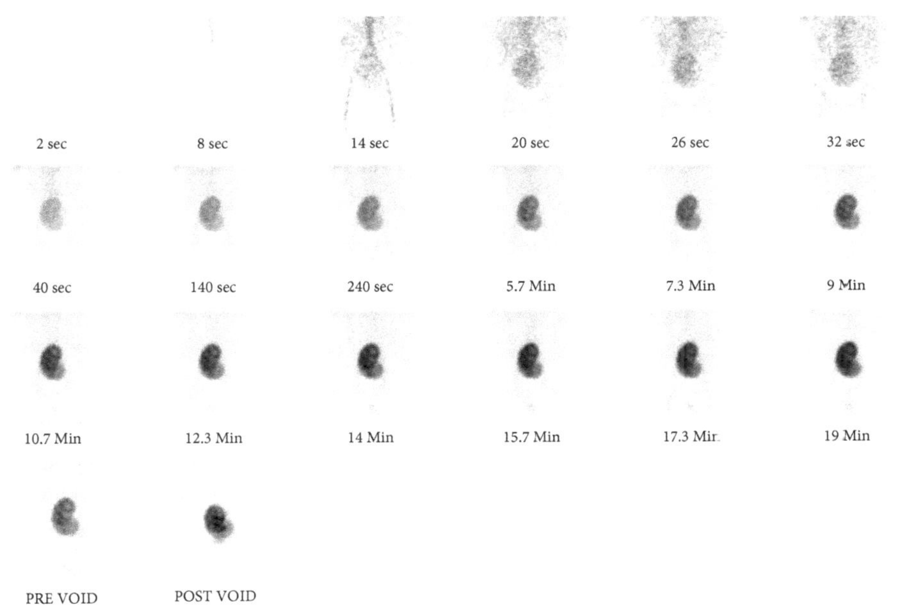

FIGURE 4: Kidney scintigraphy performed on day 158 post-transplant showing displacement of the transplant kidney to the midline, still with some perfusion present.

asymptomatic following a conservative approach at 40 months post-transplant, and imaging (ultrasound and CT with contrast) indicates that the pseudoaneurysms have remained stable in size, though ongoing surveillance will continue. For our case, conservative management with regular imaging surveillance was felt to be a reasonable option due to the relatively small size of the pseudoaneurysms, lack of clinical symptoms, and absence of an identified aetiology that clearly warranted intervention, such as infection.

In conclusion, kidney allograft torsion, though rare, is an important differential in SPKT recipients with AKI. Swift diagnosis increases the likelihood of allograft salvage, as operative correction is essential. Some transplant specialists recommend prevention via nephropexy [12]. Our case is notable in that there were two significant

Table 1: Summary table of published cases of kidney allograft torsion.

Case report	Placement of kidney allograft	Transplant type	Timing of torsion	Outcome
Marvin et al. 1995 [5]	Intraperitoneal	Kidney (intraperitoneal adult kidney donor to paediatric recipient)	6 weeks	Transplant nephrectomy
Roza et al. 1998 [6]	Intraperitoneal	2 SPKT[$]	11 and 16 months	Transplant nephrectomy
Wong-You-Cheong et al. 1998 [7]	Intraperitoneal	3 SPKT + 2 dual (en bloc) kidney transplants (paediatric donors)	Ranging from 6 to 180 days	2 SPKT + 1 dual kidney transplant had nephropexy; 2 of the 3 were retransplanted The remaining SPKT + dual kidney transplant patients required nephrectomy
West et al. 1998 [8]	Intraperitoneal	4 SPKT	3 weeks, 5 months, 22 months and 2 years	3 allografts salvaged and nephropexy performed, 1 underwent transplant nephrectomy
Badet et al. 2003 [9]	Intraperitoneal	SPKT	7 months	Allograft salvaged and nephropexy performed
Rodrigues et al. 2008 [10]	Intraperitoneal	SPKT	120 days	Transplant nephrectomy
Nangia and Saad 2009 [11]	Intraperitoneal	SPKT	10 years	Allograft salvaged and nephropexy performed
Lucewicz et al. 2011 [12]	Intraperitoneal	Living donor kidney transplant	10 weeks	Transplant nephrectomy
Kaynar et al. 2013 [13]	Intraperitoneal	Living donor kidney transplant + simultaneous bilateral nephrectomies (for polycystic kidney disease)	Two years	Allograft salvaged and nephropexy performed
Ozmen et al. 2013 [14]	Extraperitoneal	Living donor kidney transplant	4 days	Allograft salvaged and nephropexy performed
Winter et al. 2013 [15]	Extraperitoneal	Deceased donor kidney transplant	4 hours	Allograft salvaged, nephropexy not performed
Sosin et al. 2014 [16]	Extraperitoneal	Deceased donor kidney transplant	Day 0	Allograft salvaged and nephropexy performed
Sofue et al. 2015 [17]	Intraperitoneal	2 SPKT	1 month and 3months	Allografts salvaged and nephropexies performed
Dewan et al. 2016 [18]	Intraperitoneal	SPKT	2 years	Allograft salvaged and nephropexy performed
Serrano et al. 2017 [19]	Intraperitoneal	Simultaneous living donor kidney transplant + deceased donor pancreas transplant	3 years	Allograft salvaged and nephropexy performed
Narasimhan et al. 2017 [20]	Intraperitoneal	SPKT	5 weeks	Allograft salvaged and nephropexy performed
Torabi et al. 2018 [21]	Intraperitoneal	SPKT	7 months	Allograft salvaged and nephropexy performed
Tan et al.	Intraperitoneal	SPKT	3 months	Allograft salvaged and nephropexy performed

[$]SPKT, simultaneous pancreas-kidney transplantation.

kidney torsion events both requiring haemodialysis. The first episode resolved spontaneously, and the second required surgical correction.

The occurrence of pseudoaneurysms following SPKT is also unusual, and its management in the literature is variable. Our case is different in a number of aspects, but particularly in our decision to opt for conservative management in light of his asymptomatic presentation.

Consent

Written informed consent was obtained from the patient by the authors.

Disclosure

This case report was presented in the Transplantation Society of Australia and New Zealand Society of Nephrology (TSANZ) 2021 Annual Scientific Meeting as a poster and the abstract was included in supplementary journal in *Transplantation Direct.*

References

[1] ANZOD, *Monthly report on deceased organ donation in Australia*, Australia and New Zealand Organ Donation Registry, Adelaide, Australia, 2019.

[2] N. Banga, V. G. Hadjianastassiou, N. Mamode et al., "Outcome of surgical complications following simultaneous pancreas-kidney transplantation," *Nephrology Dialysis Transplantation*, vol. 27, no. 4, pp. 1658–1663, 2012.

[3] K. Esmeijer, E. K. Hoogeveen, P. J. M. van den Boog et al., "Superior long-term survival for simultaneous pancreas-kidney transplantation as renal replacement therapy: 30-yearfollow-up of a nationwide cohort," *Diabetes Care*, vol. 43, no. 2, pp. 321–328, 2020.

[4] A. O. Ojo, H. U. Meier-Kriesche, J. A. Hanson et al., "The impact of simultaneous pancreas-kidney transplantation on long-term patient survival," *Transplantation*, vol. 71, no. 1, pp. 82–89, 2001.

[5] R. G. Marvin, G. A. Halff, and I. Elshihabi, "Renal allograft torsion associated with prune-belly syndrome," *Pediatric Nephrology*, vol. 9, no. 1, pp. 81-82, 1995.

[6] A. M. Roza, C. P. Johnson, and M. Adams, "Acute torsion of the reanl transplant after combined kidney-pancreas transplant," *Transplantation*, vol. 67, no. 3, pp. 486–488, 1999.

[7] J. J. Wong-You-Cheong, K. Grumbach, T. L. Krebs et al., "Torsion of intraperitoneal renal transplants: imaging appearances," *American Journal of Roentgenology*, vol. 171, no. 5, pp. 1355–1359, 1998.

[8] M. S. West, B. R. Stevens, P. Metrakos et al., "Renal pedicle torsion after simultaneous kidney-pancreas transplantation," *Journal of the American College of Surgeons*, vol. 187, no. 1, pp. 80–87, 1998.

[9] L. Badet, P. Petruzzo, N. Lefrancois, M. Colombel, H. Fassi-Fehri, and X. Martin, "Torsion of the renal pedicle after kidney luxation after simultaneous double kidney and pancreas transplantation," *Progrès en Urologie*, vol. 13, no. 4, pp. 675–678, 2003.

[10] P. Rodrigues, F. Hering, and A. Gil, "A well-documented case of chronic renal failure due to misplacement of the transplanted kidney," *Clinics*, vol. 63, no. 1, pp. 147-148, 2008.

[11] S. Nangia and E. R. Saad, "Torsion of renal transplant 10 years after simultaneous kidney-pancreas transplantation: imaging as a diagnostic tool," *Transplantation*, vol. 87, p. 1590, 2009.

[12] A. Lucewicz, A. Isaacs, R. D. M. Allen, V. W. T. Lam, S. Angelides, and H. C. C. Pleass, "Torsion of intraperitoneal kidney transplant," *ANZ Journal of Surgery*, vol. 82, no. 5, pp. 299–302, 2012.

[13] K. Kaynar, B. Sonmez, O. Kutlu et al., "A case of recurrent episodes of acute renal allograft failure caused by renal pedicle tortion," *Renal Failure*, vol. 35, no. 4, pp. 556–559, 2013.

[14] M. M. Ozmen, I. Bilgic, I. Ziraman, and M. Koc, "Torsion of extraperitoneally transplanted kidney: an unusual complication," *Exp Clin Transplant*, vol. 11, no. 2, pp. 186–190, 2013.

[15] T. C. Winter, A. L. Clarke, and J. Campsen, "Acute torsion of a retroperitoneal renal transplant mimicking renal vein thrombosis," *Ultrasound Quarterly*, vol. 29, no. 3, pp. 203-204, 2013.

[16] M. Sosin, W. Lumeh, and M. Cooper, "Torsion of the retroperitoneal kidney: uncommon or underreported?" *Case Reports in Transplantation*, vol. 2014, pp. 1–4, 2014.

[17] K. Sofue, D. S. Vikraman, T. A. Jaffe, G. N. Chaubal, and M. R. Bashir, "Graft kidney torsion after simultaneous kidney-pancreas transplant: report of 2 cases and literature review," *Journal of Computer Assisted Tomography*, vol. 39, no. 4, pp. 506–509, 2015.

[18] R. Dewan, A. K. Dasyam, H. Tan, and A. Furlan, "Renal allograft torsion: US and CT imaging findings of a rare posttransplant complication," *Case Reports in Radiology*, vol. 2016, pp. 1–3, 2016.

[19] O. K. Serrano, A. S. Olowofela, R. Kandaswamy, and S. Riad, "Long-term graft survival after kidney allograft torsion: rapid diagnosis and surgical management key to reversibility of injury," *Transplantation Proceedings*, vol. 49, no. 7, pp. 1565–1569, 2017.

[20] E. Narasimhan, A. Kennedy, and J. Campsen, "Transplant with a twist: a pitfall in sonographic diagnosis of renal transplant torsion," *Journal of Clinical Ultrasound*, vol. 45, no. 8, pp. 528–530, 2017.

[21] J. Torabi, J. P. Rocca, K. Choinski, K. A. Lorenzen, M. Ajaimy, and J. A. Graham, "Renal allograft torsion following simultaneous pancreas kidney transplant should Be suspected with sustained kidney injury with normal pancreas function," *Progress in Transplantation*, vol. 28, no. 4, pp. 396-397, 2018.

[22] R. D. Valle, E. Capocasale, M. P. Mazzoni et al., "Embolization of a ruptured pseudoaneurysm with massive hemorrhage following pancreas transplantation: a case report," *Transplantation Proceedings*, vol. 37, no. 5, pp. 2275–2277, 2005.

[23] P. Yiannoullou, D. van Dellen, E. Khambalia et al., "Successful management of a ruptured mycotic pseudoaneurysm following pancreas transplantation using bovine pericardial patch: a case report," *Transplantation Proceedings*, vol. 46, no. 6, pp. 2023–2025, 2014.

[24] M. Z. Akhtar, A. Jones, E. Sideso, S. Sinha, A. Vaidya, and C. Darby, "Management of a ruptured mycotic pseudoaneurysm following pancreas-kidney transplantation," *Annals of Transplantation*, vol. 16, no. 4, pp. 122–125, 2011.

[25] G. J. Jaffers, W. T. Bohannon, and C. Buckley, "Endovascular repair of a pancreatic allograft mycotic aneurysm: two-yearfollow-up," *Journal of Endovascular Therapy*, vol. 18, no. 4, pp. 607–610, 2011.

[26] N. Lubezky, Y. Goykhman, R. Nakache et al., "Early and late presentations of graft arterial pseudoaneurysm following pancreatic transplantation," *World Journal of Surgery*, vol. 37, no. 6, pp. 1430–1437, 2013.

[27] V. A. L. Huurman and J. H. P. Lardenoye, "Pancreas graft salvage after successful endovascular treatment of Y graft pseudoaneurysm," *Journal of Surgical Case Reports*, vol. 2019, no. 5, p. rjz124, 2019.

[28] M. P. Verni, J. P. Leone, and A. DeRoover, "Pseudoaneurysm of the Y-graft/iliac artery anastomosis following pancreas transplantation: a case report and review of the literature," *Clinical Transplantation*, vol. 15, no. 1, pp. 72–76, 2001.

[29] S. Fujita, T. Fujikawa, K. L. Mekeel et al., "Successful endovascular treatment of a leaking pseudoaneurysm without graft loss after simultaneous pancreas and kidney transplantation," *Transplantation*, vol. 82, no. 5, pp. 717-718, 2006.

[30] B. T. Green, J. Tuttle-Newhall, P. Suhocki, S. R. Smith, and J. 'Barry O'Connor, "Massive gastrointestinal hemorrhage due to rupture of a donor pancreatic artery pseudoaneurysm in a pancreas transplant patient," *Clinical Transplantation*, vol. 18, no. 1, pp. 108–111, 2004.

[31] K. Yadav, S. Young, E. B. Finger et al., "Significant arterial complications after pancreas transplantation-Asingle-center experience and review of literature," *Clinical Transplantation*, vol. 31, no. 10, 2017.

[32] S. Mafeld, J. A. Logue, S. Masson et al., "Treatment of visceral transplant pseudoaneurysms using physician-modified fenestrated stent grafts: initial experience," *CardioVascular and Interventional Radiology*, vol. 42, no. 6, pp. 920–926, 2019.

[33] J. A. Fridell, M. S. Johnson, W. C. Goggins et al., "Vascular catastrophes following pancreas transplantation: an evolution in strategy at a single center," *Clinical Transplantation*, vol. 26, no. 1, pp. 164–172, 2012.

10

Clinical Resolution of Osmotic Demyelination Syndrome following Overcorrection of Severe Hyponatremia

Ruhin Yuridullah, Vinod Kumar, Sushant Nanavati, Monisha Singhal, and Chandra Chandran

Saint Joseph's University Medical Center, USA

Correspondence should be addressed to Ruhin Yuridullah; ryuridul@gmail.com

Academic Editor: Yoshihide Fujigaki

Osmotic Demyelination Syndrome (ODS) occurs after rapid overcorrection of severe chronic hyponatremia usually in those with a predisposition such as chronic alcoholism, malnutrition, or liver disease. Rarely, do patients make a full recovery. We report a case of ODS secondary to overcorrection of severe hyponatremia with pathognomonic clinical and radiologic signs making a complete neurological recovery. A detailed course of events, review of literature, and optimal and aggressive management strategies are discussed. There is some controversy in the literature regarding the prognosis of these patients. Our aim here is to show that, with aggressive therapy and long-term care, recovery is possible in these patients.

1. Introduction

Osmotic Demyelination Syndrome (ODS) also known as central pontine myelinolysis (CPM) was first described by Adams et al. in 1958 in alcoholics and malnourished who then developed spastic quadriplegia, pseudobulbar palsy, and varying degrees of encephalopathy or coma from acute, noninflammatory demyelination of the pons [1]. The ODS primarily occurs with overly rapid correction of severe hyponatremia (serum sodium <120 mEq/L) that has been present for more than two to three days [2–7]. The majority of ODS cases occur when initial sodium concentrations are ≤105 mEq/L [4, 5, 7, 8]. Sterns et al. showed that correction by >12 mEq/L in 24 hours or >18 mEq/L in 48 hours was associated with posttherapeutic neurologic complications when initial sodium concentration was ≤105 mEq/L [5].

Several factors appear to increase susceptibility to ODS including alcoholism, malnutrition, liver disease, and hypokalemia and the duration of hyponatremia [4, 5, 8–12]. Studies in animals have shown that brain damage does not occur when hyponatremia of <1 day duration is rapidly corrected. However, the same treatment results in fatal demyelination if hyponatremia has persisted for >2 days [9, 13–15].

The clinical manifestations of ODS are typically delayed for 2-6 days after rapid overcorrection of severe hyponatremia [5, 7, 8, 16]. The symptoms, often irreversible or partially reversible include dysarthria, dysphagia, paraparesis or quadriparesis, movement disorders, confusion, disorientation, obtundation, and coma [3, 5–7, 17]. Severely affected patients may become "locked in"; they are awake but unable to move or communicate.

Treatment often involves relowering of the sodium concentration and aggressive supportive management usually in the intensive care setting [16, 18, 19]. Death is common usually secondary to associated complications (ventilator dependency, pneumonia, venous thrombosis, pulmonary embolism, and muscle wasting) with recovery, often partial, following several months [20, 21].

2. Case Presentation

A 54-year-old male with chronic alcoholism presented with altered mental status. He had no other past medical history

TABLE 1: Serum sodium, potassium, chloride, and bicarbonate concentrations over time.

Time	Sodium (mEq/L)	Potassium (mEq/L)	Chloride (mEq/L)	Bicarbonate (mEq/L)
0 hour	102	2.4	54	38
8 hours	106	2.9	63	33
16 hours	112	2.4	71	33
24 hours	118	3.0	82	28
48 hours	119	3.8	86	24
12 days	141	4.1	107	20

apart from multiple presentations to emergency services for alcohol intoxication/withdrawal symptoms. He was not on any medications. On presentation, his vital signs were within normal limits. His Glasgow Coma Scale (GCS) was 15. He was alert, awake, but disoriented to time. Physical examination was unrevealing. CT scan of the brain was negative for any acute pathology. Laboratory evaluation revealed serum alcohol level of <10 mg/dL and urine drug toxicology was negative.

His complete metabolic panel revealed a serum sodium concentration of 102 mEq/L, potassium 2.4 mEq/L, chloride 54 mEq/L, bicarbonate 38 mEq/L, blood urea nitrogen 8 mg/dL, creatinine 0.62 mg/dL, magnesium 2.2 mg/dL, phosphorous 2.3 mg/dL, albumin 3.6 g/dL, alkaline phosphatase 116 U/L, aspartate aminotransferase 117 U/L, alanine aminotransferase 122 U/L, and bilirubin 0.9 mg/dL. His plasma osmolality was 212 mOsm/kg.

In the emergency department, he received two 1-liter boluses of 0.9% saline intravenously. His serum potassium was replete with potassium chloride 40 mEq intravenously and 80 mEq orally. He was then started on intravenous 0.9% saline infusion at a rate of 100 mL/hr. Serum sodium concentrations and other electrolytes were monitored periodically (Table 1). His serum sodium concentration was 106 mEq/L by 8 hours but increased to 112 mEq/L by 16 hours, at which point 0.9% saline infusion rate was decreased to 60 mL/hr. Patient had remained at baseline, and regular diet was started. By 24 hours, his serum sodium concentration had reached 118 mEq/L. Attempts to relower the sodium concentration were made by starting 5% dextrose in water intravenously at 200 mL/hour. Sodium concentration fluctuated in the range of 114-119 mEq/L over the next 48 hours. Serum sodium concentrations gradually increased by 3-4 mEq/L per day to 123-128 mEq/L from day 4-7 before normal values were noted by day 12.

During the initial 6 days of the presentation, patient remained awake, alert, oriented to person and place. However, he then became somnolent and uncooperative with physical examination, experienced urinary incontinence, and ultimately developed changes in speech, increased tone of the upper extremities, and paraplegia by day 13 of the presentation. During this time, he also failed swallow evaluation requiring nasogastric tube (NGT) placement. CT of the brain without contrast was repeated which did not show any acute pathology. MRI of the brain could not be performed initially due to technical reasons. Over the ensuing days, he lost the ability to vocalize any words, could only answer by nodding,

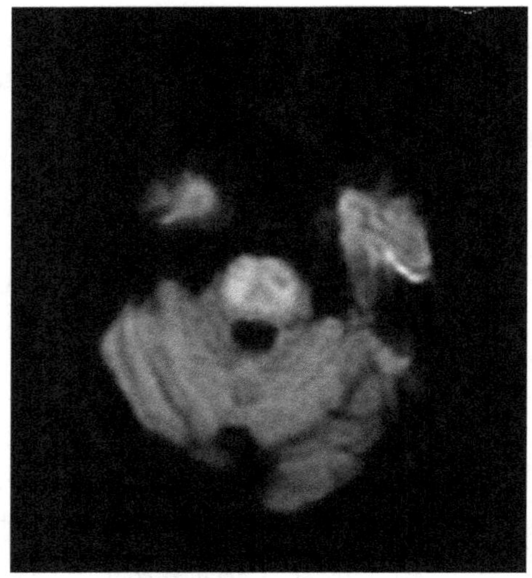

FIGURE 1: Magnetic Resonance Imaging of the brain without contrast showed high T2 signal and low T1 signal with restricted diffusion along with sparing of the bilateral peripheral pons, classic for central intrapontine, and extrapontine myelinolysis.

and was unable to elevate his upper extremities initially before losing the ability in the lower extremities. MRI of the brain performed on the third week of presentation revealed changes pathognomonic for central pontine myelinolysis sparing the periphery of the pons confirming clinical suspicion [Figures 1-2].

Over the ensuing weeks to months, aggressive physical therapy, speech therapy, and nutritional support were continued on general neurological ward. One month from symptoms onset, he gradually started to show signs of improvement and was initially only able to form single words, then phrases, and then sentences. By one and a half months, except for dysphagia for which he relied on NGT feedings, he displayed marked improvement in tetraparesis. Modified barium swallow revealed silent aspiration with liquids with no reflexive response to aspiration events, requiring placement of Percutaneous Endoscopic Gastric (PEG) tube 2 months from presentation. He failed repeated swallow evaluations and the PEG tube remained in place for a period of 80 days until he was finally able to tolerate oral pureed diet.

3. Discussion

ODS is a rare neurological condition described by Adams et al. in 1950s. Most commonly ODS is seen following rapid

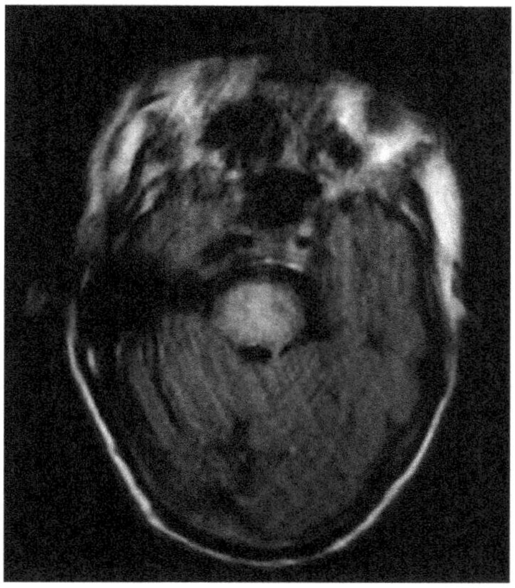

FIGURE 2: Magnetic Resonance Imaging of the brain without contrast showed high T2 signal and low T1 signal with restricted diffusion along with sparing of the bilateral peripheral pons, classic for central intrapontine, and extrapontine myelinolysis.

overcorrection of serum sodium in patients with severe chronic hyponatremia (serum sodium <120 mEq/L). The majority of ODS cases occur with initial serum sodium concentrations of <105 mEq/L. Alcoholism, malnutrition, liver disease, hypoxia, and hypokalemia predispose these patients in developing ODS. In our patient, chronic alcoholism and malnutrition were likely contributing factors.

Hyponatremia is defined by the relative excess of water to the serum sodium concentration. Hypotonic hyponatremia affects the brain by causing entry of water into the brain resulting in cerebral edema [3]. However, cellular adaptation by the brain restores the brain volume by initially causing loss of electrolytes within a few hours ("rapid adaptation") and then ultimately normalizing brain volume through the loss of organic osmolytes over several days ("slow adaptation") [3]. In the case of chronic hyponatremia, rapid correction of the serum sodium leads to increased extracellular tonicity, fluid shift to the extracellular compartment, and dehydration of the brain cells due to little adjustment time [3, 17]. Since oligodendrocyte is more susceptible to this type of damage, it leads to degeneration and destruction of the myelin [14].

The clinical manifestations of ODS are typically delayed for 2-6 days following the insult. As with our patient, initial symptoms may present with depressed level of awareness, dysarthria or mutism, and additional symptoms onset over the ensuing 1-2 weeks including quadriparesis, impaired sensation, and difficulty with coordination. At its most severe state, myelinolysis can lead to coma, "locked-in" syndrome, and death.

MRI is often the imaging of choice. In our patient, T2-weighted MRI revealed classic hyperintense or areas of demyelination of the pons consistent with ODS. Unfortunately, we initially could not perform the MRI until third week of symptoms onset due to technical reasons. However, our suspicion remained high and we continued with aggressive supportive measures in view of the symptoms. Delayed imaging is preferred to confirm the diagnosis since conventional imaging (MRI and CT) lag clinical manifestations in the first two weeks [10].

Our patient's unique presentation makes this case noteworthy with respect to detailed timing of the events. Following the initial pathognomonic symptoms described, he gradually displayed improvement and ultimately, making a remarkable, full recovery of tetraparesis by one and a half months. Despite marked improvements in motor and speech, dysphagia persisted for almost four and a half months and he remained dependent on NGT feedings and later PEG tube feeds. However, repeated swallow evaluations were performed periodically despite multiple failed attempts. As Louis G et al. demonstrated in a cohort of 36 patients with ODS managed in critical care setting, 32 of the patients required mechanical ventilation, 69 percent survived, and 56 percent of the survivors were left with only minimal neurologic sequelae. Furthermore, the initial severity of the illness was not a predictor of long-term prognosis [21]. Singh et al. performed a thorough search of the literature using multiple databases to identify all case series of ODS patients published from 1959 to January 2013. 2602 articles were identified comprising of 541 patients with ODS of whom 51.9% had favorable recovery and death in 24.8% [2].

Therefore, regardless of the initial severity of symptoms, we urge for aggressive early management including daily physical therapy, speech therapy, and optimal nutritional support including early PEG tube placement as opposed to seeking early comfort measures. The incremental improvements in mentation and functional capacity take months to be noticed. We strongly suggest that similar patients' needs to be aggressively cared for since complete recovery are possible.

References

[1] R. D. Adams, M. Victor, and E. L. Mancall, "Central pontine myelinolysis: a hitherto undescribed disease occurring in alcoholic and malnourished patients," *Archives of Neurology & Psychiatry*, vol. 81, no. 2, pp. 154–172, 1959.

[2] T. D. Singh, J. E. Fugate, and A. A. Rabinstein, "Central pontine and extrapontine myelinolysis: a systematic review," *European Journal of Neurology*, vol. 21, no. 12, pp. 1443–1450, 2014.

[3] H. J. Adrogué and N. E. Madias, "Hyponatremia," *The New England Journal of Medicine*, vol. 342, no. 21, pp. 1581–1589, 2000.

[4] R. H. Sterns, "Severe symptomatic hyponatremia: Treatment and outcome. A study of 64 cases," *Annals of Internal Medicine*, vol. 107, no. 5, pp. 656–664, 1987.

[5] R. H. Sterns, J. D. Cappuccio, S. M. Silver, and E. P. Cohen, "Neurologic sequelae after treatment of severe hyponatremia: a multicenter perspective," *Journal of the American Society of Nephrology*, vol. 4, p. 1522, 1994.

[6] R. H. Sterns, J. E. Riggs, and S. S. Schochet Jr., "Osmotic demyelination syndrome following correction of hyponatremia," *The New England Journal of Medicine*, vol. 314, no. 24, pp. 1535–1542, 1986.

[7] J. G. Verbalis, S. R. Goldsmith, A. Greenberg et al., "Diagnosis, evaluation, and treatment of hyponatremia: expert panel recommendations," *The American Journal of Medicine*, p. 126, 2013.

[8] J. C. George, W. Zafar, I. D. Bucaloiu, and A. R. Chang, "Risk factors and outcomes of rapid correction of severe hyponatremia," *Clinical Journal of American Society of Nephrology*, vol. 13, p. 984, 2018.

[9] R. S. Tanneau, A. Henry, F. Rouhart et al., "High incidence of neurologic complications following rapid correction of severe hyponatremia in polydipsic patients," *Journal of Clinical Psychiatry*, vol. 55, no. 8, pp. 349–354, 1994.

[10] R. H. Sterns, S. U. Nigwekar, and J. K. Hix, "The treatment of hyponatremia," *Seminars in Nephrology*, vol. 29, no. 3, pp. 175–318, 2009.

[11] R. J. Martin, "Central pontine and extrapontine myelinolysis: the osmotic demyelination syndromes," *Neurology in Practice*, vol. 75, 3, pp. iii22–iii28, 2004.

[12] J. W. Lohr, "Osmotic demyelination syndrome following correction of hyponatremia: association with hypokalemia," *American Journal of Medicine*, vol. 96, no. 5, pp. 408–413, 1994.

[13] B. K. Kleinschmidt-Demasters, A. M. Rojiani, and C. M. Filley, "Central and extrapontine myelinolysis : then and now," *Journal of Neuropathology & Experimental Neurology*, vol. 65, no. 1, pp. 1–11, 2006.

[14] R. H. Sterns, D. J. Thomas, and R. M. Herndon, "Brain dehydration and neurologic deterioration after rapid correction of hyponatremia," *Kidney International*, vol. 35, no. 1, pp. 69–75, 1989.

[15] A. Soupart, R. Penninckx, A. Stenuit, O. Perier, and G. Decaux, "Reinduction of hyponatremia improves survival in rats with myelinolysis-related neurologic symptoms," *Journal of Neuropathology & Experimental Neurology*, vol. 55, no. 5, pp. 594–601, 1996.

[16] R. H. Sterns, J. K. Hix, and S. Silver, "Treatment of hyponatremia," *Current Opinion in Nephrology and Hypertension*, vol. 19, p. 493, 2010.

[17] M. L. Moritz and J. C. Ayus, "The pathophysiology and treatment of hyponatraemic encephalopathy: an update," *Nephrology Dialysis Transplantation* , vol. 18, no. 12, pp. 2486–2491, 2003.

[18] A. Soupart, M. Ngassa, and G. Decaux, "Therapeutic relowering of the serum sodium in a patient after excessive correction of hyponatremia," *Clinical Nephrology*, vol. 51, no. 6, pp. 383–386, 1999.

[19] S. Oya, K. Tsutsumi, K. Ueki, and T. Kirino, "Reinduction of hyponatremia to treat central pontine myelinolysis," *Neurology*, vol. 57, no. 10, pp. 1931-1932, 2001.

[20] H. Menger and J. Jörg, "Outcome of central pontine and extrapontine myelinolysis," *Journal of Nephrology*, vol. 246, p. 700, 1999.

[21] G. Louis, B. Megarbane, S. Lavoué et al., "Long-term outcome of patients hospitalized in intensive care units with central or extrapontine myelinolysis," *Critical Care Medicine*, vol. 40, p. 970, 2012.

11

Roseomonas mucosa-Induced Peritonitis in a Patient Undergoing Continuous Cycler Peritoneal Dialysis: Case Report and Literature Analysis

Sasmit Roy,[1] Sumit Patel,[2] Hardhik Kummamuru,[3] Amarinder Singh Garcha,[4] Rohan Gupta,[5] and Sreedhar Adapa[4]

[1]*Department of Medicine, Centra Health, Lynchburg, VA 24501, USA*
[2]*Department of Internal Medicine, Adventist Health Community Care, Hanford, CA 93230, USA*
[3]*University of Texas, Arlington, TX 76019, USA*
[4]*Kaweah Delta Health Care District, Visalia, CA 93291, USA*
[5]*Community Regional Medical Center, Fresno, CA 93721, USA*

Correspondence should be addressed to Sasmit Roy; docsasmit@gmail.com

Academic Editor: Yoshihide Fujigaki

Roseomonas species, a rare Gram-negative microorganism, has seldom been reported to cause peritonitis in end-stage renal disease patients on peritoneal dialysis. Only seven cases of peritonitis by this rare microorganism have been reported worldwide. Treatment options can be challenging if not detected early and can lead to significant morbidity and mortality along with the switching of the dialysis modality to hemodialysis which is highly undesirable. Our patient is a 65-year-old Caucasian female who needed to be changed to emergency hemodialysis due to inability to perform peritoneal dialysis from suspected peritonitis and was subsequently discovered to have peritonitis from *Roseomonas mucosa*. She recovered with a prolonged antibiotics course and returned to peritoneal dialysis in 3 months following her treatment completion. Prompt diagnosis and prolonged antibiotics are a cornerstone in the management of this rare microorganism to prevent mortality and morbidity from peritonitis.

1. Introduction

Peritonitis, caused by infectious microorganisms, is a hazardous outcome in end-stage renal disease (ESRD) patients undergoing peritoneal dialysis. It can lead to a high rate of morbidity and mortality if not treated properly and timely [1]. *Roseomonas* species, a rare Gram-negative, pink pigmented, oxidized coccobacillus, is normally identified as environmental commensal in water and soil and was first reported as infectious etiology in clinical medicine by Rihs et al. in 1993 [2]. First reported case of *Roseomonas* peritonitis was documented by JA Sandoe et al. in 1997 [3]. Only a handful of cases of *Roseomonas*-induced peritonitis in peritoneal dialysis patients have been reported worldwide, seven to be exact [3–9]. The most affected mode of infection can be bloodstream, musculoskeletal, skin, and soft tissue with peritonitis being extremely rare [10]. The treatment can be challenging if proper antibiotics are not initiated timely and thus may delay the course of clinical recovery and can even lead to serious ill-fated consequences.

2. Case Report

A 65-year-old Caucasian female patient who was on peritoneal dialysis (PD) for end-stage renal disease (ESRD) presented to the emergency room (ER) with shortness of breath for 3 days. The PD catheter stopped draining for the last 5 days, and the patient was waiting to see the surgeon adjust the position of it. The medical history was significant for hypertension, hyperlipidemia, and ESRD. She had no recent history of going anywhere for swimming or taking bath in a hot tub. Home medication included amlodipine 10 mg daily, clonidine 0.1 mg three times a day, furosemide 40 mg daily, metoprolol succinate 50 mg daily, renal vitamin 1 tablet daily, pravastatin 10 mg at nighttime, and potassium chloride 20 milliequivalents daily. She was doing continuous cycler peritoneal dialysis at home with a total of 4 exchanges of 2.5% dextrose solution bags, each exchange for 2 hours and with 2 Liters fill during the exchanges. Her total PD duration was 9 hours at night with no daytime dwell. She was doing PD for the last 2 years with no issues of infection before. Her PD was not accompanied by any major issues of constipation or diarrhea in recent past. There was no major social shift in home dynamics, with her primary care giver, i.e., her husband staying with her since she started PD and helping her with the treatment throughout. She did not have any pets at home neither did she have any recent visit from any sick relatives or any pets from neighbors or friends.

Vital signs revealed a temperature of 97.7 Fahrenheit (F), pulse rate of 82 beats per minute (bpm), blood pressure of 170/106 mm Hg, and respiratory rate of 24 breaths per minute with oxygen saturation of 90% on room air. Physical examination showed that the patient was in visible respiratory distress. Lung examination was significant for decreased air entry in bilateral lung fields and basal crackles, and the patient had bilateral pitting pedal edema. The rest of the physical examination was insignificant. Initial admission labs are as given in Table 1.

Attempts to access the PD catheter in ER were unsuccessful with no drainage of dialysate. Because of hyperkalemia and significant volume overload, she underwent emergent hemodialysis after getting a temporary left internal jugular dialysis catheter placed urgently. General surgery was consulted for the malfunctioning PD catheter, and the patient underwent diagnostic laparoscopy. The PD catheter was noted to be clogged with fibrin glue and mispositioned to the right lower quadrant. The catheter was unclogged followed by repositioning to the most dependent part of the peritoneal cavity in the pelvis. The peritoneal fluid was noted to be cloudy, and the fluid was sent for cell count, Gram stain, and culture. The patient was also started on empiric intraperitoneal (IP) vancomycin and aztreonam for suspected peritonitis. PD fluid cell count revealed white blood cell (WBC) count of 209/microliter (μL) with 72% neutrophils and red blood cells (RBC) count of 2337/μL, and Gram stain revealed >100 WBC/low power field (lpf) with no organism. Aerobic bottle grew Gram-negative bacilli at 48 hours, and the organism was identified as *Roseomonas mucosa* at 96 hours by matrix-assisted laser desorption/ionization-time of flight (MALDI-TOF) mass spectrometry (MS). The organism was resistant to cephalosporin and sensitive to gentamicin. After clinical stability in 3 days, the patient was discharged from the hospital with intraperitoneal gentamicin for a total of 3 weeks. The patients continued to have drainage issues and persistently elevated PD fluid WBC counts despite being on antibiotics. The PD catheter was removed, and the modality was changed to hemodialysis. 3 months after the episode, she reverted to peritoneal dialysis again. She continues to be on PD now with no recurrence of peritonitis from *Roseomonas* or any other species as per subsequent serial negative PD fluid cultures.

3. Discussion

Peritonitis, described as an inflammation of the peritoneum, is a serious complication for ESRD patients undergoing PD and is usually caused by bacteria or fungi. Peritonitis maybe secondary to nondialytic-related systemic or intraabdominal processes or related to peritoneal dialysis itself. Tzamaloukas AH et al. in one review article demonstrated that less than 6% of cases are related to secondary causes, while the rest 94% cases are due to peritoneal dialysis itself in patients undergoing continuous ambulatory peritoneal dialysis (CAPD) [11]. Common clinical features are abdominal pain with cloudy effluent, fever, nausea/vomiting, and hypotension. Common diagnostic methods employed are to obtain cell type and count and peritoneal fluid culture. The major laboratory parameter that is highly suggestive of bacterial infection is peritoneal fluid leukocyte count above 100 cells/mm^3. Less than 8 leucocytes/mm^3 go against a diagnosis of peritonitis [12]. Peritoneal fluid culture is positive in 80–95% of cases of peritonitis if proper technique is performed [13].

Most of the peritonitis is caused by bacteria. 45–65% of bacteria being a Gram-positive organism, while 15–35% representing Gram-negative ones [14, 15]. Coagulase-negative *Staphylococcus* is the commonest cause of peritonitis. In one of the most recent extensive studies by Whitty et al., *Staphylococcus* accounted for 60% of infectious etiology by Gram-positive organisms and 39% overall causative organisms [16]. *Streptococcus* species caused 20% of infection, while other common Gram-positive organisms were *Staphylococcus aureus*, *Enterococcus*, and *Corynebacterium* spp. Common Gram-negative organisms are *Escherichia coli*, *Pseudomonas*, and *Klebsiella* species [16]. Among other species, fungal infection with *Candida albicans* and *Candida parapsilosis* is becoming more and more prevalent [17].

As per the 2016 International Society of Peritoneal Dialysis (ISPD) guidelines [18], initial empiric treatment includes a combination of vancomycin or first generational cephalosporins such as cefazolin and third or fourth generational cephalosporins such as ceftazidime or cefepime or an aminoglycoside such as gentamicin or aztreonam to cover both Gram type species. Though commonly not needing removal of the dialysis catheter if infected by Gram-negative organisms, sometimes, rare infections occur resulting in a change in modality of dialysis to hemodialysis or the removal of the catheter [19]. Worse complications of PD could result in hospitalization, morbidity, or death [19].

In a study concluded recently, the incidence rate for peritonitis episodes was found through observation in a large-scale patient population worldwide [20]. This was conducted in 209 facilities across seven countries (New Zealand, Australia, Canada, Japan, Thailand, the United States, and the United Kingdom). Here, it was reported that out of 7,051 patients on peritoneal dialysis, a count of 2,272 episodes of peritonitis was recorded in total. This calculates to be a rate of about 0.28 per patient per year. In the United

Table 1: Admission labs.

Lab values	Reference range	On presentation
Sodium (millimole/liter)	135–145	131
Potassium (millimole/liter)	3.5–5.1	7.1
Chloride (millimole/liter)	98–106	100
CO_2 (millimole/liter)	23–29	22
Blood urea nitrogen (BUN) (milligram/deciliters)	8–24	119
Creatinine (milligrams/deciliters)	0.7–1.3	9.43
Calcium (milligram/deciliters)	8.8–10.2	9.3
Glucose (milligram/deciliters)	70–105	99
White blood cells (thousand/millimiters^3)	4–10	6.9
Hemoglobin (gram/deciliters)	14–16	10.6
Platelets (thousand/millimiters^3)	150–450	183

Table 2: Summary of all cases reported to have *Roseomonas* spp. peritonitis with outcome.

Author	Year	Patient age/ gender	Study country	*Roseomonas* species	Dialysis modality	Dialysis culture	Treatment received	Outcome	Modality changed
Sandoe et al. [3]	1997	62/F	UK	*R. gilardii*	CAPD	Positive	IP vancomycin and then IP netilmicin	Resolved	No
Bibashi et al. [4]	2000	65/F	Greece	*R. fauriae*	CAPD	Positive	IP vancomycin plus IP netilmicin and then ciprofloxacin	Resolved	No
Tsai et al. [5]	2012	48/M	Taiwan		CCPD	Positive	IP ceftazidime plus IP cefazolin and then PO ciprofloxacin	Resolved	No
Boyd et al. [6]	2012	19/M	USA	*R. mucosa*	CCPD	Positive	IP ceftazidime and then IP ciprofloxacin	Resolved	No
Matsukuma et al. [7]	2014	61/M	Japan	*R. mucosa*	CAPD	Positive	IP ceftazidime and then IP ciprofloxacin	Resolved	Yes, to HD
Malini et al. [8]	2016	61	Malaysia	*R. gilardii*	CAPD	Positive	IP ceftazidime plus IP cloxacillin and then IP meropenem	Resolved	Yes, to HD
Burstahler et al. [9]	2021	73/M	Russia	*R. gilardii*	CCPD	Positive	IP ceftazidime plus IP vancomycin and then IP ciprofloxacin	Resolved	No

F, female; M, male; R, *Roseomonas*; UK, the United Kingdom; USA, the United States of America; IV, intravenous; IP, intraperitoneal; PO, per oral; CAPD, continuous ambulatory peritoneal dialysis; CCPD, continuous cycler peritoneal dialysis; HD, hemodialysis.

States, it is reported as 0.26 episodes per patient per year, with a given range of 0.24–0.27 episodes.

Roseomonas is a pink segmented, coccoid rod. It is a Gram-negative bacterium that has four named subspecies, known as *R. gilardii, R. cervicalis, R. mucosa*, and *R. fauriae* [3]. This was first reported by Rihs et al. [2] in 1993 as a species different from the initial thought genus of *Methylobacterium. Roseomonas* is found naturally and is accessible through water and soil. Reported infection through *Roseomonas* has been documented in bloodstream, as well as in cerebrospinal fluid, skin and soft tissues [10]. The route of *Roseomonas* infection is uncertain. It is theorized that the infection could occur through water, such as water from contaminated faucets. There are very few cases of peritonitis in PD patients that have been reported with *Roseomonas* as a causative organism. As per PubMed Central literature search, worldwide there have been only seven recorded cases with the different subspecies of *Roseomonas* infection in PD patients [3–9]. They are summarized in Table 2. The first reported case in PD patients came out of the UK by Sandoe et al. in 1997. Out of the seven patients recorded for *Roseomonas* in PD, three patients were affected by *R. gilardii*, one with *R. fauriae*, one with *Roseomonas* genus, and two with *R. mucosa*. Out of the 7 cases, 4 cases were on CAPD, while 3 were on CCPD.

Treatment methods for *Roseomonas* peritonitis are broad-spectrum antibiotics, given through intraperitoneal administration. In a systemic review of all published *Roseomonas* cases recently conducted by Ioannou et al. [10], beta-lactams resistance was discovered to be significantly elevated with respective penicillin, piperacillin/tazobactam, and cephalosporin resistance being at 96.6%, 90.7%, and 77.8%. Carbapenems and quinolones are most effective in treating this rare organism [10]. Overall mortality to *Roseomonas* species was reported by them to be at 1%. Because it is still a rare organism and due to paucity of clinical evidence, it is suggested that treatment duration be stretched to 3 weeks of antibiotics [8]. Hopefully, this will prevent the change in modality to hemodialysis which is always undesirable to patients.

4. Conclusions

Due to the rarity of this microorganism causing infectious peritonitis and the high rate of resistance to cephalosporin which is considered a first-time empiric therapy in peritonitis management, *Roseomonas* species needs to be inculcated in medical literature more. This will help nephrologists broaden their differential of peritonitis, especially in cases of nonresolving clinical peritonitis.

Consent

The patient consented for publication of this study and the written consent form is available to authors for submission if requested.

References

[1] S. Adapa, S. Naramala, D. Boken, A. Moreno, and V. M. Konala, "Peritonitis from anaerobic gram-positive cocci likely due to translocation of bacteria from gut in a patient undergoing peritoneal dialysis," *Cureus*, vol. 11, no. 11, Article ID e6060, 2019.

[2] J. D. Rihs, D. J. Brenner, R. E. Weaver, A. G. Steigerwalt, D. G. Hollis, and V. L. Yu, "Roseomonas, a new genus associated with bacteremia and other human infections," *Journal of Clinical Microbiology*, vol. 31, no. 12, pp. 3275–3283, 1993.

[3] J. A. Sandoe, H. Malnick, and K. W. Loudon, "A case of peritonitis caused by Roseomonas gilardii in a patient undergoing continuous ambulatory peritoneal dialysis," *Journal of Clinical Microbiology*, vol. 35, no. 8, pp. 2150–2152, 1997.

[4] E. Bibashi, D. Sofianou, K. Kontopoulou, E. Mitsopoulos, and E. Kokolina, "Peritonitis due to *Roseomonas fauriae* in a patient undergoing continuous ambulatory peritoneal dialysis," *Journal of Clinical Microbiology*, vol. 38, no. 1, pp. 456-457, 2000.

[5] S.-F. Tsai, C.-H. Chen, K.-H. Shu, and M.-J. Wu, "Peritonitis caused by Roseomonas in a patient undergoing automated peritoneal dialysis: case report and literature review," *Internal Medicine*, vol. 51, no. 13, pp. 1721–1724, 2012.

[6] M. A. Boyd, M. B. Laurens, P. D. Fiorella, and S. R. Mendley, "Peritonitis and technique failure caused by Roseomonas mucosa in an adolescent infected with HIV on continuous cycling peritoneal dialysis," *Journal of Clinical Microbiology*, vol. 50, no. 11, pp. 3801–3804, 2012.

[7] Y. Matsukuma, K. Sugawara, S. Shimano et al., "A case of bacterial peritonitis caused by Roseomonas mucosa in a patient undergoing continuous ambulatory peritoneal dialysis," *CEN Case Reports*, vol. 3, no. 2, pp. 127–131, 2014.

[8] S. Malini, B. L. Goh, and T. S. Lim, "A rare case of Roseomonas gilardii peritonitis in a patient on continuous ambulatory peritoneal dialysis," *Peritoneal Dialysis International: Journal of the International Society for Peritoneal Dialysis*, vol. 36, no. 5, p. 578, 2016.

[9] M. S. Burgstahler, S. D. Bieber, and D. C. Pfeiffer, "A case of *Roseomonas gilardii* peritonitis associated with a flooded peritoneal dialysis treatment space," *Annals of Clinical and Laboratory Science*, vol. 51, no. 2, pp. 255–257, 2021.

[10] P. Ioannou, V. Mavrikaki, and D. P. Kofteridis, "*Roseomonas* species infections in humans: a systematic review," *Journal of Chemotherapy*, vol. 32, no. 5, pp. 226–236, 2020.

[11] A. H. Tzamaloukas, L. E. Obermiller, L. J. Gibel et al., "Peritonitis associated with intra-abdominal pathology in continuous ambulatory peritoneal dialysis patients," *Peritoneal Dialysis International*, vol. 13, no. Suppl 2, pp. S335–S337, 1993.

[12] A. Tranaeus, O. Heimbürger, and B. Lindholm, "Peritonitis in continuous ambulatory peritoneal dialysis (CAPD): diagnostic findings, therapeutic outcome and complications," *Peritoneal Dialysis International: Journal of the International Society for Peritoneal Dialysis*, vol. 9, no. 3, pp. 179–190, 1989.

[13] P. K.-T. Li, C. C. Szeto, B. Piraino et al., "Peritoneal dialysis-related infections recommendations: 2010 update," *Peritoneal Dialysis International: Journal of the International Society for Peritoneal Dialysis*, vol. 30, no. 4, pp. 393–423, 2010.

[14] S. Mujais, "Microbiology and outcomes of peritonitis in North America," *Kidney International*, vol. 70, no. 103, pp. S55–S62, 2006.

[15] T. N. Oo, T. L. Roberts, and A. J. Collins, "A comparison of peritonitis rates from the United States Renal Data System database: CAPD versus continuous cycling peritoneal dialysis patients," *American Journal of Kidney Diseases*, vol. 45, no. 2, pp. 372–380, 2005.

[16] R. Whitty, J. M. Bargman, A. Kiss, L. Dresser, and P. Lui, "Residual kidney function and peritoneal dialysis-associated peritonitis treatment outcomes," *Clinical Journal of the American Society of Nephrology*, vol. 12, no. 12, pp. 2016–2022, 2017.

[17] S. Roy, P. Vantipalli, A. Garcha, M. Pokal, and S. Adapa, "The emerging uncommon non-albicans Candida: Candida parapsilosis peritonitis in a peritoneal dialysis patient," *Cureus*, vol. 13, no. 8, Article ID e17083, 2021.

[18] P. K.-T. Li, C. C. Szeto, B. Piraino et al., "ISPD peritonitis recommendations: 2016 update on prevention and treatment," *Peritoneal Dialysis International: Journal of the International Society for Peritoneal Dialysis*, vol. 36, no. 5, pp. 481–508, 2016.

[19] S. Adapa, S. Naramala, B. R. Madhira, V. Gayam, P. Sahasranam, and V. M. Konala, "Peritonitis secondary to uncommon gram-negative coccobacillus transmitted from a cat in a patient on peritoneal dialysis," *Journal of Investigative Medicine High Impact Case Reports*, vol. 7, Article ID 232470961989516, 2019.

[20] J. Perl, D. S. Fuller, B. A. Bieber et al., "Peritoneal dialysis-related infection rates and outcomes: results from the peritoneal dialysis outcomes and practice patterns study (PDOPPS)," *American Journal of Kidney Diseases*, vol. 76, no. 1, pp. 42–53, 2020.

12

A Rare Case of Extensive Eggshell Intestinal Wall Peritoneal Calcification in a Long-Term Continuous Peritoneal Dialysis Patient

Erasmia Sampani, Chrysostomos Dimitriadis, Efstratios Kasimatis, Evangelos Memmos, and Aikaterini Papagianni

Department of Nephrology, School of Medicine, Aristotle University of Thessaloniki, General Hospital "Hippokratio", Thessaloniki, Greece

Correspondence should be addressed to Erasmia Sampani; sampaniedoc@gmail.com

Academic Editor: Bernard G. Jaar

Encapsulating peritoneal sclerosis (EPS) is a rare but rather serious complication of long-term peritoneal dialysis. The etiology of EPS is multifactorial, with long-term peritoneal dialysis, multiple peritonitis episodes, and uncontrolled hyperparathyroidism considered to be major risk factors for this often life-threatening condition. We report a case of a 55-year-old female patient with Down syndrome and end-stage renal disease (ESRD) on long-term peritoneal dialysis (PD) with extensive intestinal peritoneal calcifications and a rather uncomplicated long follow-up.

1. Case Presentation

We present the case of a 55-year-old female with a history of Down's syndrome, vesicoureteric reflux, and recurrent urinary tract infections since age four that led to ESRD at age 30. Her initial dialysis method was continuous ambulatory peritoneal dialysis (CAPD). The initial CAPD regimen consisted of four, two-liter dwell exchanges per day, using only 1.36% dextrose, with a biocompatible solution, buffered by a mixture of lactate and bicarbonate. The patient was a low average transporter and easily achieved adequate ultrafiltration (>1.0 Lit/day). Her CAPD course was complicated by two mild episodes of peritonitis in the first 2 years. The isolated pathogens were coagulase-negative *Staphylococcus* and Streptococcus viridans, and both were successfully and easily treated with intraperitoneal administration of vancomycin and cefuroxime, respectively. The patient's clinical course was otherwise uncomplicated.

Fourteen years following the initiation of PD, she presented with mild abdominal pain and bloody effluent. There were no signs of overt malnutrition or weight loss. She appeared quite well nourished, her blood pressure was 140/70, there was no clinically evident oedema, and hemoglobin values were maintained within normal limits. PD fluid was clear, cell count < 15/mm^3, and there was no tenderness on examination. Her mother reported regular bowel movements and no fever or nausea. Abdominal computed tomography (CT) (Figure1(a)) showed a—rather expected after long-term PD—focal thickening of the peritoneal membrane suggestive of peritoneal sclerosis but no localization or distension of the bowel loops with no cocooning or signs of bowel obstruction. Inflammation markers (CRP, fibrinogen) were consistently within normal limits. We strongly recommended switching dialysis treatment to hemodialysis, but her mother considered hemodialysis practically impossible in a patient with Down's syndrome and very poor cooperation. She decided to take the risk of continuing PD for as long as possible.

The patient also had a history of secondary hyperparathyroidism. She was treated with alfacalcidol and had a fast and favorable response, with iPTH levels promptly subsiding within a year and being kept within the

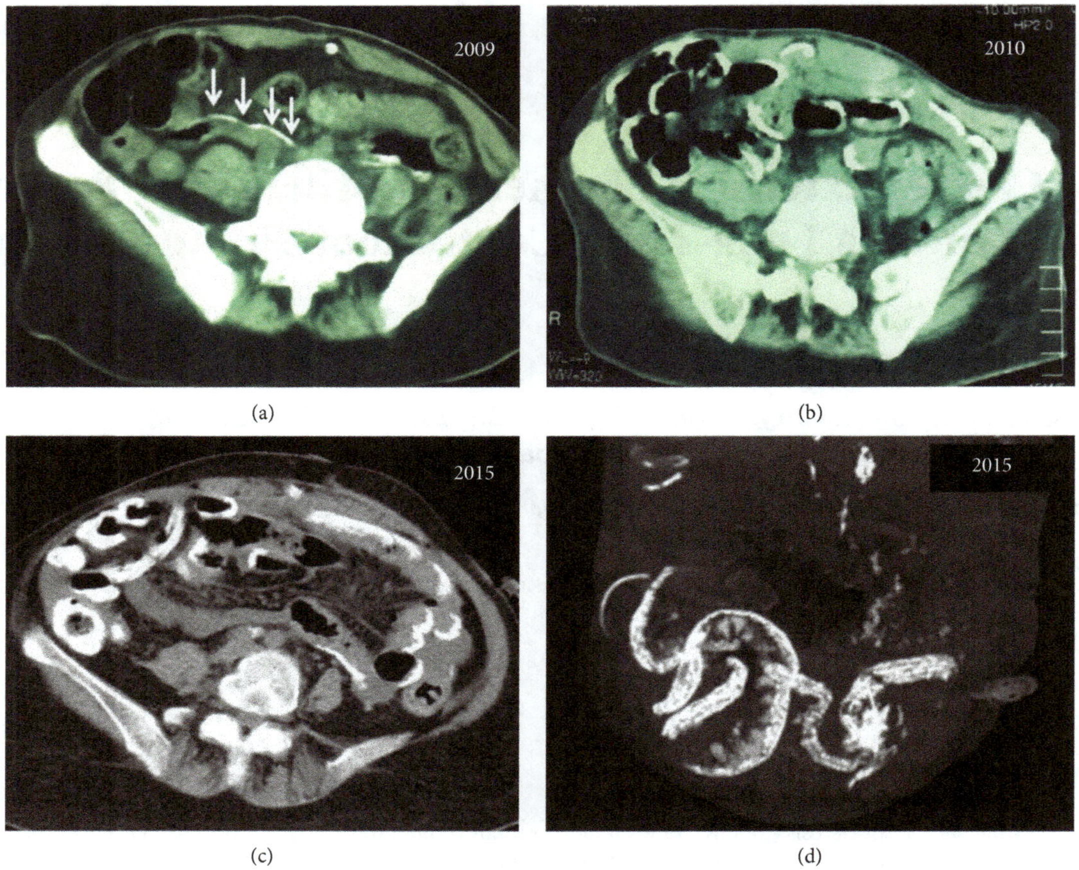

(a) (b) (c) (d)

FIGURE 1: Abdominal CT scans of the patient in 2009 (a), showing mild linear peritoneal calcifications (arrows), which became full-blown calcifications of the visceral small bowel peritoneum a year later in 2010 (b) that remained or minimally increased over the next five years (2015 (c)). (d) Processed sagittal plane image of the 2015 abdominal scan showing the extent of bowel wall calcifications.

recommended range (150–350) ever since. Both calcium and phosphate levels, as well as their product, also remained within the recommended range. One year later, she was switched to CCPD after the loss of residual renal function and loss of ultrafiltration due to a progressive change to fast peritoneal transport status.

The patient's clinical course began to deteriorate with symptoms of nausea, loss of appetite, vomiting, and frequent episodes of diffuse abdominal pain. Plain abdominal radiographs revealed extensive linear calcifications along the small intestinal wall, outlining, like a calcified eggshell (Figure 2(a)). An abdominal CT scan (Figure 1(b)) confirmed the diagnosis of calcifying peritonitis, revealing extensive eggshell calcification along the bowel wall, but again no signs of cocooning, localization of the bowel loops, or obstructive ileus were observed. Although there were no formal imaging proofs of encapsulation (EPS), she had the clinical setting and symptoms compatible with sclerosing peritonitis.

The patient and family once again refused the recommended change of dialysis method. Therefore, treatment commenced with tamoxifen 20 mg daily and methylprednisolone 8 mg OD. The patient's symptoms subsided and her clinical condition ameliorated over the next two months. Steroids were tapered to 4 mg every other day over three months, but she was kept on low-dose tamoxifen (10 mg OD) ever since with regular gynecological examination for endometrial hyperplasia every year. Follow-up abdominal CT 5 years later (Figure 1(c)) confirmed the extensive linear calcification of the small intestinal loops, affecting mostly the intestinal splanchnic peritoneum but without any signs of cocooning or intestinal obstruction. Despite the extensive small bowel calcifications, no episodes of bowel obstruction have been recorded till now and the patients' clinical condition remains impressively stable on tamoxifen and methylprednisolone until today.

2. Discussion

Peritoneal sclerosis is a rare but well-recognized complication of long-term peritoneal dialysis. Sclerosing peritonitis (SP) usually presents with symptoms of insidious peritoneal (abdominal pain, bloody effluent, and late ultrafiltration failure) and systemic inflammation (loss of appetite, cachexia, malnourishment, low albumin, and rise in CRP). When this leads to the formation of a fibrous cocoon where there is bowel localization and signs and symptoms of intestinal obstruction, the disease is considered encapsulating peritoneal sclerosis (EPS) and eventually leads to the development of full-blown obstructive ileus [1–4].

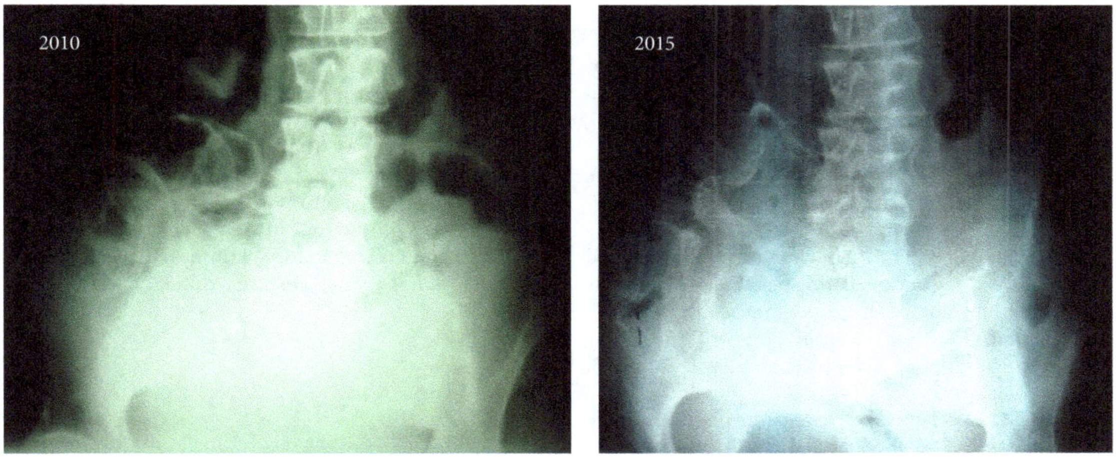

(a) (b)

FIGURE 2: Plain abdominal films of the patient, without any contrast media, showing extensive calcifications of the bowel wall in 2010 (a) and five years later, in 2015 (b).

Pathogenesis of EPS is considered to be multifactorial, and diagnosis is often based on radiological findings of sclerosis, calcification, peritoneal thickening, or encapsulation of the intestines [5].

The incidence of sclerosing peritonitis in peritoneal dialysis patients has been reported to vary in different cohorts between 0.7 and 3.3% but, rather uniformly, in all of the studies, it was clearly associated with the duration of PD [6]. Rigby and Hawley reported a prevalence of confirmed EPS that was reaching 19.4% for patients exceeding 8 years of peritoneal dialysis [4]. Nomoto et al. and Kawanishi et al. also described the major impact of time on PD on the incidence of EPS rising up to more than 17% for those treated for more than 15 years [3, 7].

It has also been suggested that systemic or local inflammation associated with factors such as uremia, malignancies, or peritonitis may be the triggering factor for metastatic peritoneal calcifications. PD-associated peritoneal calcification or calcifying peritonitis (CP) is a rare condition that has been described as an idiopathic syndrome or as part of the clinical manifestations of encapsulating peritoneal sclerosis [8]. It refers to patients with symptoms usually including abdominal pain and bloody or cloudy, sterile effluent that was not associated with formal intestinal obstruction/ileus and had a more benign course than that of "classic" EPS. Only 15 cases have been reported in the literature [8–18]. Several factors have been associated with this rare situation, including frequent peritonitis episodes, calcium-phosphate disturbances, extensive use of vitamin D and calcium products, and secondary hyperparathyroidism. However, due to the small incidence of cases, the causes of this rare condition have not yet been identified and the mechanism underlying the pathogenesis is probably multifactorial.

Clinical manifestations, as well as radiological findings, may differ from the ones seen in EPS. In CP, complete bowel obstruction has not been reported. Radiological findings may include extensive linear calcifications of the parietal and visceral peritoneum, often revealed in a plain abdominal X-ray. However, the patency of the bowel remained intact and no signs of ileus were observed in any of the reported cases. Even more uncommon are the cases in which peritoneal calcification affects mainly the visceral peritoneum. The first report in the literature was from Marichal et al. in 1987 who described two patients of whom one had extensive calcification of the intestinal visceral peritoneum [9]. Both cases were associated with extremely high peritonitis rates (up to one every four months), and the one with visceral peritoneal calcification was much longer on PD (7 years) and had secondary hyperparathyroidism. Francis et al. and Ubara et al. also reported cases of patients with extensive peritoneal calcifications that included the visceral peritoneum of the bowel [10, 18]. Calcifying peritonitis in those cases was also associated with a high number of peritonitis episodes and severe secondary hyperparathyroidism [10].

Our patient had an uncommon complication of PD as she developed extensive calcification of the bowel wall minimally affecting the parietal peritoneum. She did not have a high peritonitis incidence, and although her secondary hyperparathyroidism coincided with the initial presentation of calcification, it was rather promptly and easily controlled. Taking into account the fact that the patient was already in peritoneal dialysis for more than ten years, EPS was considered a possible diagnosis and an evolving process, and so we proceeded in therapy with steroids and tamoxifen, used rather as prophylaxis for a forthcoming progression to full-blown EPS. It seemed like a reasonable approach as rescue therapy, taking as a fact that she and her family declined to change the dialysis modality.

We were pleasantly surprised by her outcome, as it is the first case of CP reported to have acceptable survival without progressing to obstructive EPS or dying, while remaining on PD for more than 9 years since the initial diagnosis, for a total of almost 24 years on PD. A biopsy was not performed, as the patient refused any surgical procedure, so, unfortunately, we cannot support our case with histological evidence of peritoneal calcification.

References

[1] S. Campbell, P. Clarke, C. Hawley et al., "Sclerosing peritonitis: identification of diagnostic, clinical, and radiological features," *American Journal of Kidney Diseases*, vol. 24, no. 5, pp. 819–825, 1994.

[2] J. W. Dobbie, "Pathogenesis of peritoneal fibrosing syndromes (sclerosing peritonitis) in peritoneal dialysis," *Peritoneal Dialysis International*, vol. 12, no. 1, pp. 14–27, 1992.

[3] Y. Nomoto, Y. Kawaguchi, H. Kubo, H. Hirano, S. Sakai, and K. Kurokawa, "Sclerosing encapsulating peritonitis in patients undergoing continuous ambulatory peritoneal dialysis: a report of the Japanese sclerosing encapsulating peritonitis study group," *American Journal of Kidney Diseases*, vol. 28, no. 3, pp. 420–427, 1996.

[4] R. J. Rigby and C. M. Hawley, "Sclerosing peritonitis: the experience in Australia," *Nephrology Dialysis Transplantation*, vol. 13, no. 1, pp. 154–159, 1998.

[5] Y. Kawaguchi, H. Kawanishi, S. Mujais, N. Topley, and D. G. Oreopoulos, "Encapsulating peritoneal sclerosis: definition, etiology, diagnosis, and treatment," *Peritoneal Dialysis International*, vol. 20, pp. S43–S55, 2000.

[6] Z. Moinuddin, A. Summers, D. van Dellen, T. Augustine, and S. E. Herrick, "Encapsulating peritoneal sclerosis-a rare but devastating peritoneal disease," *Frontiers in Physiology*, vol. 5, p. 470, 2014.

[7] H. Kawanishi, Y. Kawaguchi, H. Fukui et al., "Encapsulating peritoneal sclerosis in Japan: a prospective, controlled, multicenter study," *American Journal of Kidney Diseases*, vol. 44, no. 4, pp. 729–737, 2004.

[8] C. W. Kuo, P. T. Lee, H. C. Fang, K. J. Chou, H. M. Chung, and C. L. Chen, "Extensive peritoneal calcification as a complication of long-term peritoneal dialysis and secondary hyperparathyroidism: a case report and review of the literature," *Peritoneal Dialysis International*, vol. 26, no. 5, pp. 609–612, 2006.

[9] J. F. Marichal, B. Faller, P. Brignon, D. Wagner, and P. Straub, "Progressive calcifying peritonitis: a new complication of CAPD? report of two cases," *Nephron*, vol. 45, no. 3, pp. 229–232, 1987.

[10] D. M. A. Francis, I. Busmanis, and G. Becker, "Peritoneal calcification in a peritoneal dialysis patient: a case report," *Peritoneal Dialysis International*, vol. 10, no. 3, pp. 237–240, 1990.

[11] B. A. Warady, V. Bahl, U. Alan, and S. Hellerstein, "Symptomatic peritoneal calcification in a child: treatment with tidal peritoneal dialysis," *Peritoneal Dialysis International*, vol. 14, no. 1, pp. 26–29, 1994.

[12] Y. W. Yoshindo, K. T. Shigematsu, H. K. Hirofumi et al., "Extensive peritoneal calcification as a complication of long-term CAPD," *Peritoneal Dialysis International*, vol. 15, no. 4, pp. 369–371, 1995.

[13] S. Fletcher, J. Gibson, and A. M. Brownjohn, "Peritoneal calcification secondary to severe hyperparathyroidism," *Nephrology Dialysis Transplantation*, vol. 10, no. 2, pp. 277–279, 1995.

[14] C. K. Farmer, D. J. Goldsmith, P. Sharpstone, and J. C. Kingswood, "Maintenance of adequate dialysis in a patient with peritoneal calcification using tidal peritoneal dialysis," *Clinical Nephrology*, vol. 49, no. 1, pp. 55–58, 1998.

[15] C. Kitoh, K. Miyagi, T. Onoe, K. Katano, T. Shimada, and T. Takegoshi, "Reversible peritoneal calcification in a patient treated by CAPD," *Clinical Nephrology*, vol. 52, no. 5, pp. 329–332, 1999.

[16] E. S. Najem, M. Webel, and J. M. Ailinani, "Reversibility of peritoneal calcification in a dialysis patient maintained on hemodialysis and total parenteral nutrition," *American Journal of Roentgenology*, vol. 172, no. 1, pp. 247-248, 1999.

[17] M. R. Clatworthy, P. Williams, C. J. Watson, and N. V. Jamieson, "The calcified abdominal cocoon," *The Lancet*, vol. 371, no. 9622, p. 1452, 2008.

[18] Y. Ubara, H. Katori, T. Tagami et al., "Severe ectopic calcification of the intestinal wall in a patient on long-term continuous ambulatory peritoneal dialysis therapy," *American Journal of Kidney Diseases*, vol. 35, no. 4, pp. 761–766, 2000.

13

Atypical Antiglomerular Basement Membrane Disease in a Pediatric Patient Successfully Treated with Rituximab

Kuang-Yu Jen[1] **and Ari Auron**[2]

[1]*Department of Pathology and Laboratory Medicine, University of California, Davis School of Medicine, Sacramento, CA, USA*
[2]*Department of Pediatric Nephrology, The Permanente Medical Group, Roseville, CA, USA*

Correspondence should be addressed to Kuang-Yu Jen; kyjen@ucdavis.edu

Academic Editor: Hiro Matsukura

Classic antiglomerular basement membrane (anti-GBM) disease is an exceedingly rare but extremely aggressive form of glomerulonephritis, typically caused by autoantibodies directed against cryptic, conformational epitopes within the noncollagenous domain of the type IV collagen alpha-3 subunit. Pathologic diagnosis is established by the presence of strong, diffuse, linear staining for immunoglobulin on immunofluorescence microscopy. Recently, patients with atypical clinical and pathologic findings of anti-GBM disease have been described. These patients tend to have an indolent clinical course, without pulmonary involvement, and laboratory testing rarely reveals the presence of anti-GBM antibodies. Specific guidelines for the treatment and management of these patients are unclear. Here, we describe a case of atypical anti-GBM disease in a young child who presented with hematuria and prominent proteinuria. Throughout the course of his illness, creatinine remained normal. He was conservatively treated with steroids and rituximab, resulting in resolution of his clinical symptoms and normalization of laboratory findings.

1. Introduction

Antiglomerular basement membrane (anti-GBM) disease is an autoimmune disorder that is widely viewed as one of the most aggressive forms of glomerulonephritis. It can be accompanied by concurrent pulmonary hemorrhage, in which case the term Goodpasture syndrome is preferred. Anti-GBM disease is extremely rare in adults, with an estimated incidence of 0.5–1.64 cases per million per year, and even more so in children with under 30 cases ever reported in the literature [1–5]. A bimodal age distribution has been observed in larger series, showing peak incidences in the third decade and in the sixth to seventh decades [4, 6–8]. Those in the younger age group tend to present with Goodpasture syndrome and are more often males, whereas those in the older age group tend to experience disease limited to the kidneys.

Correlating to the rapidly progressive nature of this condition, crescents and necrotizing lesions are nearly always identified on biopsy, often showing diffuse glomerular involvement. Pathologic diagnosis necessitates the presence of diffuse, linear glomerular basement membrane staining for immunoglobulin (typically immunoglobulin G) on immunofluorescence microscopy, which is most commonly caused by the presence of autoantibodies directed against cryptic, conformational epitopes within the noncollagenous domain of the type IV collagen alpha-3 subunit (α3NC1) [9, 10].

More recently, it has become apparent that approximately 10% of patients with immunofluorescence findings of anti-GBM disease present with atypical clinical and pathological findings, often characterized by an indolent clinical course [11, 12]. Such patients show no pulmonary involvement, and laboratory testing rarely reveals anti-GBM antibodies against α3NC1. Nearly all cases thus far reported have been in adults, with very rare instances in the pediatric population [13, 14]. Here, we describe a case of atypical anti-GBM disease in a young child, who was conservatively treated with steroids and rituximab, resulting in resolution of clinical symptoms and normalization of laboratory findings.

2. Case Report/Case Presentation

A 4-year-old Caucasian boy with no significant past medical history developed nonspecific gastrointestinal and respiratory symptomatology, including vomiting, rhinorrhea, and cough that lasted for 4-5 weeks. Subsequently, he developed a fever followed by multiple episodes of painless gross hematuria that lasted for a few days. At that point, he was referred to pediatric nephrology for further workup. Initial physical examination was unremarkable with the exception of mild pallor. He was normotensive, afebrile, and did not have any rashes or joint pain. Pulmonary examination was normal. Urinalysis revealed the presence of blood with active urinary sediment on urine microscopy, as well as nephrotic range proteinuria of approximately 5.4 g/g based on a spot urine protein-to-creatinine ratio. Other laboratory findings were normal, including normal serum creatinine of 0.34 mg/dL. Computed tomography of the chest was normal. Renal ultrasonography revealed bilateral echogenic kidneys that were of normal size.

Subsequently, a renal biopsy was performed. The light microscopy sections contained more than 36 glomeruli with 7 additional glomeruli on toluidine blue-stained thick sections, of which none were globally sclerotic. Two glomeruli showed subtle segmental scars, one of which was associated with karyorrhectic nuclear debris. Deeper level sections disclosed a single glomerulus with segmental endocapillary hypercellularity, karyorrhexis, and a small cellular crescent (Figure 1(a)). A few glomeruli exhibited prominent visceral epithelial cells with protein resorption droplets, while others demonstrated tubularization of the parietal epithelium. Aside from these glomerular changes, the remaining glomeruli appeared unremarkable (Figure 1(b)). The tubulointerstitium and vessels were also unremarkable, except for a few scattered red blood cell casts. Immunofluorescence revealed strong, diffuse, global, linear glomerular basement membrane staining for IgG as well as moderate kappa and lambda light chain staining in the same pattern (Figure 1(c)). Other immunoreactants including IgM, IgA, C3, C1q, fibrinogen, and albumin were negative. Electron microscopy disclosed widespread mild subendothelial widening, without the presence of electron-dense immune deposits (Figure 1(d)). Given the rare finding of active glomerulonephritis along with the strong linear IgG glomerular basement membrane staining on immunofluorescence, the diagnosis of atypical anti-GBM disease was made.

The biopsy findings prompted further laboratory studies, including serologies for anti-GBM antibody, which was positive at 6.3 AI (normal < 1.0 AI) by multiplex flow immunoassay. All other serologies including antinuclear antibodies and antineutrophil cytoplasmic antibodies were negative. Complements C3 and C4 were within normal range.

The patient was treated with intravenous methylprednisolone (30 mg/kg) daily for 3 days followed by oral prednisone (2 mg/kg) daily for 6 weeks. Concurrently, he received 4 weekly doses of rituximab at 375 mg/m^2 per dose, which were well-tolerated. This decision to use rituximab instead of plasmapheresis was made given the patient's normal serum creatinine and minimal pathology by light microscopy. His prednisone was then tapered off over the next 5 months. Once his oral steroid taper started, the patient was prescribed mycophenolate mofetil at 600 mg/m^2 per dose, twice daily.

One week after receiving the fourth and final rituximab dose, the patient's anti-GBM antibody titers became undetectable and has stayed negative to date (Figure 2). Furthermore, one month after completing the rituximab course, the patient's proteinuria completely resolved and has remained negative to date (Figure 2). The patient's renal function throughout the course of his illness remained normal. Nine months after his initial presentation, the patient was asymptomatic, and at that point, slow tapering of mycophenolate mofetil was initiated and completely stopped 12 months after his initial presentation. He experienced no complications, such as infections or any significant side-effects, due to treatment. At the latest follow-up, 15 months after initial presentation, the patient remains asymptomatic, with normal urinalysis, urine sediment, blood pressure, and renal function, as well as negative anti-GBM titers.

3. Discussion/Conclusion

In the literature, the definition or inclusion criteria for atypical anti-GBM disease has been inconsistent. Numerous case reports use the term to describe patients who have biopsy-proven anti-GBM disease with the typical finding of crescentic/necrotizing glomerulonephritis but who are serologically negative for anti-GBM antibodies. Others use the term to describe anti-GBM disease in patients with secondary etiologies, such as infection or medication. Still others use the term to describe patients with primarily pulmonary symptoms, without significant renal involvement. In this report, we follow the inclusion criteria of Nasr et al. where atypical anti-GBM disease is defined by the presence of strong, diffuse, linear immunoglobulin staining within the glomerular basement membrane on immunofluorescence microscopy, but the light microscopy lacks the typical diffuse crescentic/necrotizing glomerulonephritis pattern of glomerular injury. Based on this definition, atypical anti-GBM disease is an extremely rare form of glomerulonephritis that affects approximately 10 percent of all patients that show the diagnostic finding of anti-GBM disease. In contrast to the rapidly progressive nature of classic anti-GBM disease, patients with this atypical variant present subacutely, with only mild renal insufficiency. The clinical course is usually indolent, although few may progress to end-stage renal disease. Thus far, nearly all patients that have been included in major case series reporting this entity have been adults. In this case report, we describe a case of atypical anti-GBM disease in a 4-year-old boy.

Cases of atypical anti-GBM disease in children are summarized in Table 1. It was first reported over 4 decades ago by Wilson and Dixon within a large cohort of almost all adult patients with classic anti-GBM disease [13]; however,

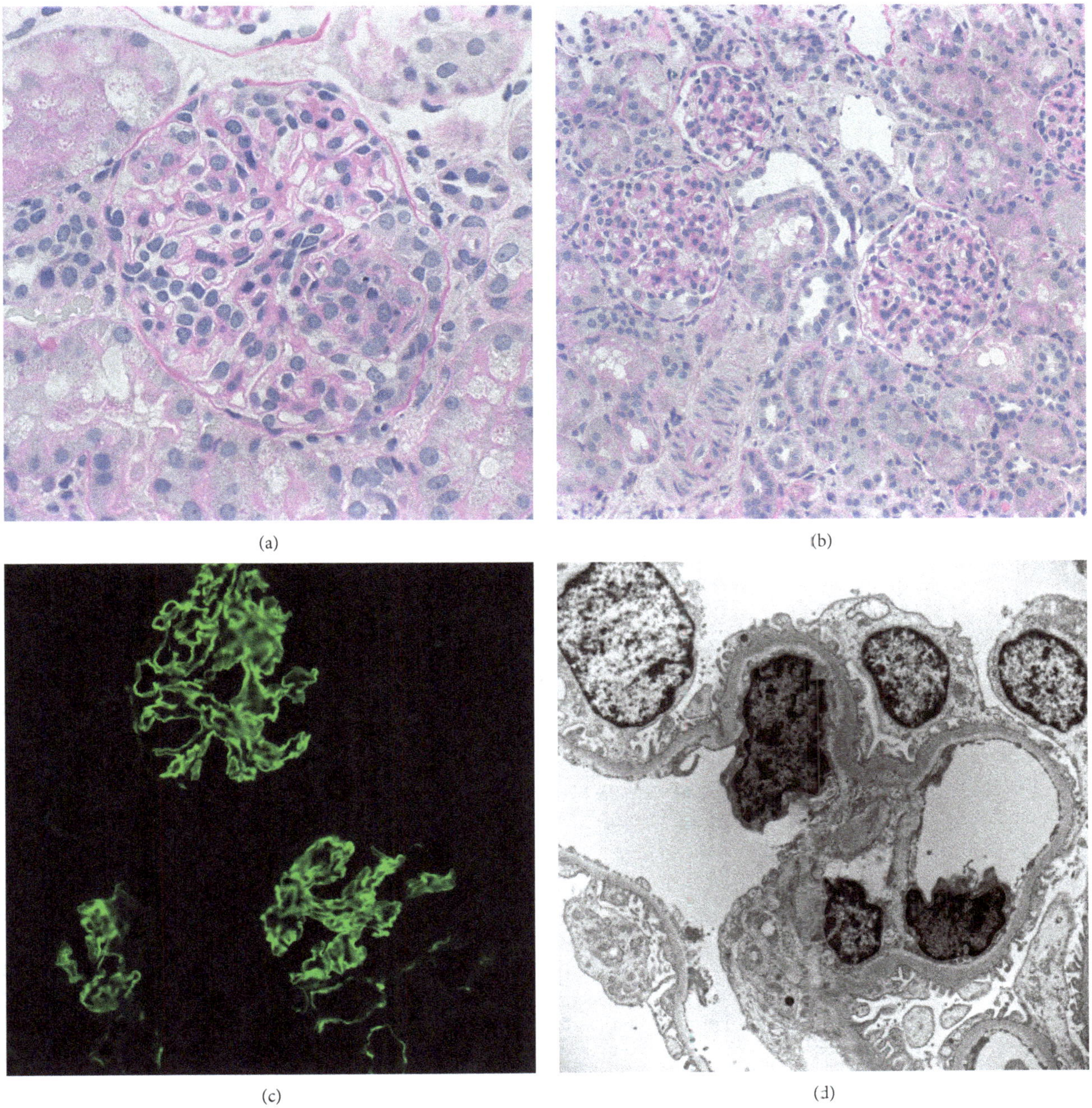

FIGURE 1: Renal biopsy findings. (a) One glomerulus showing segmental endocapillary hypercellularity, karyorrhectic nuclear debris, and a small cellular crescent (periodic acid-Schiff; original magnification: 400x). (b) Nearly, all of the remaining glomeruli demonstrate no significant abnormalities (periodic acid-Schiff; original magnification: 200x). (c) Immunofluorescence for IgG reveals diffuse, global, linear staining within the glomerular basement membrane (original magnification: 200x). (d) Widespread, subtle subendothelial widening is noted on electron microscopy, without the presence of any immune deposits (original magnification: 4800x).

specific clinical details were not provided. Other reported cases include an 8-year-old girl who was incidentally found to have anti-GBM disease based on screening urine studies that revealed nephrotic range proteinuria and hematuria. She was successfully treated with plasmapheresis, steroids, and cyclophosphamide [14]. To our knowledge, our patient is the first reported case of atypical anti-GBM disease in a child where instead of plasmapheresis, a more conservative treatment approach was taken with the use of rituximab.

Much of what is known about the clinicopathologic characteristics of atypical anti-GBM disease comes from two recently published major case series [11, 12]. The largest was reported by Nasr et al. on 20 patients, all of whom were adults [11]. Their patients often presented with heavy proteinuria as well as hematuria and mild renal insufficiency. None of them showed pulmonary involvement, and no circulating anti-α3NC1 antibodies were detected by conventional enzyme-linked immunosorbent assay (ELISA) or

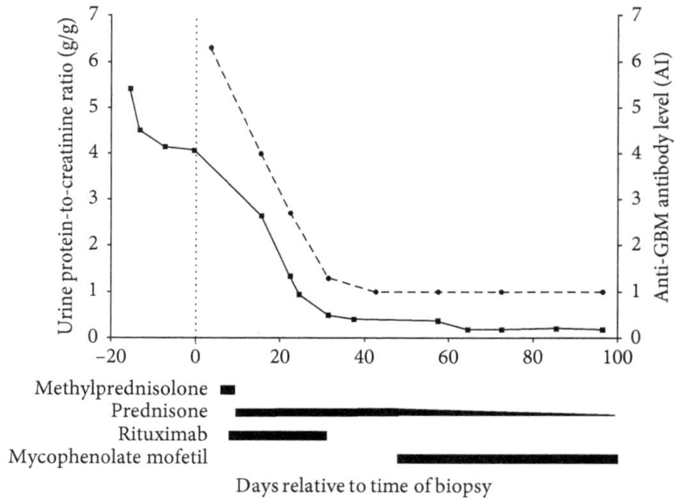

FIGURE 2: Degree of proteinuria and antiglomerular basement membrane (anti-GBM) antibody levels during the course of illness. Spot urine protein-to-creatinine ratio (solid line) and anti-GBM antibody levels (dotted line) are shown relative to the time of biopsy. *Limit of detection for anti-GBM antibody levels is 1.0 AI, which has remained <1.0 AI since day 43. **Limit of detection for urine protein-to-creatinine ratio is 0.19, which has remained between <0.19 and 0.25 since day 64. Data extend to day 334 at the latest follow-up. Length of treatment is indicated by black bars below the X-axis.

TABLE 1: Pediatric cases of atypical antiglomerular basement membrane disease in the literature.

Publication	Age/ gender	Presentation	Biopsy findings	α3NC1 antibodies	Treatment	Outcome
Jen and Auron (present case)	4/M	Nephrotic-range proteinuria, hematuria, normal renal function	One glomerulus with segmental endocapillary hypercellularity, karyorrhexis, and small cellular crescent	Positive	Rituximab, steroids, MMF	Asymptomatic with normal renal function at 15 months
Wilson and Dixon [13]	14/M	No onset of renal failure within a large cohort of typical anti-GBM disease	N/A	Positive	Steroids	Living 1 yr with normal function
	13/M			Negative	Steroids, azathioprine	Living 18 mo with normal function
	5/M			Negative	Steroids, cyclophosphamide	Living 7 yr with normal function
Nagano et al. [14]	8/F	Incidental hematuria and proteinuria on screening	Mild mesangial proliferation; no crescents	Positive	Plasmapheresis, steroids, cyclophosphamide	Decreased proteinuria and antibody titers; no long-term follow-up

multiplex flow immunoassay in any of the patients. One-year patient and renal survival rates were 93% and 85%, respectively, indicating an indolent but sometimes slowly progressive clinical course. Interestingly, they noted that half of their patients showed monotypic immunoglobulin deposition, while the other half was polytypic. They reported no significant clinical or pathologic differences between the two groups except for a lower rate of crescents and/or fibrinoid necrosis in the monotypic cases.

The other major case series, by Troxell and Houghton, described 5 adult cases of atypical anti-GBM disease [12]. All four patients with urinalysis data presented with hematuria, and 2 of 3 patients with data on proteinuria status showed >1 g/g urine protein-to-creatinine ratio, although they excluded patients with heavy proteinuria from their series. In contrast to Nasr et al., 3 of their patients showed positive anti-GBM antibody serologies, of which one reported hemoptysis. This latter patient had a more unusual clinical course given that he initially exhibited features of Goodpasture syndrome with minimal renal involvement but 3 months later presented with more typical/classic features of anti-GBM disease, suggesting that an atypical presentation may indicate a prodrome to outright expression of classic anti-GBM disease.

Our patient's clinical presentation was similar to most of the reported cases of atypical anti-GBM disease, mainly consisting of proteinuria (nephrotic range by urine protein-to-creatinine ratio) and hematuria (both macroscopic and microscopic). However, in our case, the renal function on presentation and throughout the observation period remained normal. His biopsy revealed focal/rare endocapillary proliferative glomerulonephritis with small crescent formation involving <5% of the glomeruli, a pattern that was most frequently encountered in the case series summarized above. Interestingly, electron microscopy in our case exhibited widespread mild subendothelial widening, a common but nonspecific finding that can be seen in the setting of classic anti-GBM disease. Immunofluorescence microscopy revealed the presence of polytypic anti-GBM IgG given that both kappa and lambda light chains were positive. In contrast to the patients in the series by Nasr et al., our patient had detectable anti-GBM antibodies, which rapidly decreased to undetectable levels following treatment. Given that the anti-GBM antibodies in our patient were detected via multiplex flow immunoassay, these antibodies were most likely directed against the most common epitope typically seen in classic anti-GBM disease, namely, the type IV collagen α3NC1 domain. It is unclear why our patient experienced relatively mild renal symptoms even with appreciably high initial levels of anti-GBM antibodies. Possibilities include low epitope affinity by our patient's autoantibodies or a low degree of complement activation. To the latter point, it should be noted that C3 and C1q were negative by immunofluorescence microscopy on the biopsy, and thus, a low degree of complement activation could be plausible. In the case of low epitope affinity, the ability to detect the anti-GBM antibody by multiplex flow immunoassay would also be expected to be hampered and thus would be unlikely.

In classic anti-GBM disease, initial aggressive therapy is warranted, consisting of plasma exchange, oral cyclophosphamide, and glucocorticoids for all patients with kidney involvement who do not require immediate dialysis [9, 15]. However, the proper treatment modality for atypical anti-GBM disease is uncertain given the rarity of this disease. One must weigh the possible benefits of prompt and aggressive treatment to prevent any further renal injury against the detrimental cytotoxic effects of cyclophosphamide, especially for a child in our case. Given the patient's stable and baseline serum creatinine as well as the relatively mild histologic changes seen on biopsy, we decided to conservatively manage our patient with an initial combination of rituximab and steroids followed by mycophenolate, without the use of plasmapheresis/plasma exchange or cytotoxic agents. The patient immediately responded with a dramatic decrease in proteinuria and anti-GBM antibody levels, both of which have remained undetectable at the latest follow-up approximately 1-year after initial presentation. Given the success that we observed with conservative treatment of atypical anti-GBM disease in our patient, such an approach in children should be considered if this rare entity is encountered.

Consent

The legal guardian of our subject has given her written informed consent to publish this case.

Authors' Contributions

KYJ drafted the majority of the manuscript. AA provided the clinical data and wrote portions of the manuscript. All authors contributed to the critical appraisal of the manuscript and have approved the final version of the manuscript that was submitted.

References

[1] L. Butani, "Rapidly progressive glomerulonephritis," in *Adolescents with Chronic Kidney Disease: From Diagnosis to End-Stage Disease*, M. N. Haddad, E. Winnicki, and S. Nguyen, Eds., Springer International Publishing, Cham, Switzerland, pp. 93–105, 2019.

[2] A. Bayat, K. Kamperis, and T. Herlin, "Characteristics and outcome of Goodpasture's disease in children," *Clinical Rheumatology*, vol. 31, no. 12, pp. 1745–1751, 2012.

[3] G. Dorval, M. Lion, S. Guérin et al., "Immunoadsorption in anti-GBM glomerulonephritis: case report in a child and literature review," *Pediatrics*, vol. 140, no. 5, Article ID e20161733, 2017.

[4] S. P. McAdoo and C. D. Pusey, "Anti-glomerular basement membrane disease," *Clinical Journal of the American Society of Nephrology*, vol. 12, no. 7, pp. 1162–1172, 2017.

[5] M. Canney, P. V. O'Hara, C. M. McEvoy et al., "Spatial and temporal clustering of anti-glomerular basement membrane disease," *Clinical Journal of the American Society of Nephrology*, vol. 11, no. 8, pp. 1392–1399, 2016.

[6] E. G. Fischer and D. J. Lager, "Anti-glomerular basement membrane glomerulonephritis," *American Journal of Clinical Pathology*, vol. 125, no. 3, pp. 445–450, 2006.

[7] J. B. Levy, A. N. Turner, A. J. Rees, and C. D. Pusey, "Long-term outcome of anti-glomerular basement membrane antibody disease treated with plasma exchange and immunosuppression," *Annals of Internal Medicine*, vol. 134, no. 11, pp. 1033–1042, 2001.

[8] C. O. Savage, C. D. Pusey, C. Bowman, A. J. Rees, and C. M. Lockwood, "Antiglomerular basement membrane antibody mediated disease in the British Isles 1980-4," *BMJ*, vol. 292, no. 6516, pp. 301–304, 1986.

[9] R. J. Glassock, "Atypical anti-glomerular basement membrane disease: lessons learned," *Clinical Kidney Journal*, vol. 9, no. 5, pp. 653–656, 2016.

[10] J. C. Jennette and V. Nickeleit, "Anti-glomerular basement membrane glomerulonephritis and Goodpasture syndrome," in *The Heptinstall's Pathology of the Kidney*, J. C. Jennette V. D. D'Agati, J. L. Olson, and F. G. Silva, Eds., Wolter Kluwer, Philadelphia, PA, USA, 7th edition, 2015.

[11] S. H. Nasr, A. B. Collins, M. P. Alexander et al., "The cli copathologic characteristics and outcome of atypical a glomerular basement membrane nephritis," *Kidney Inte tional*, vol. 89, no. 4, pp. 897–908, 2016.

[12] M. L. Troxell and D. C. Houghton, "Atypical anti-glome basement membrane disease," *Clinical Kidney Journal*, no. 2, pp. 211–221, 2016.

[13] C. B. Wilson and F. J. Dixon, "Anti-glomerular ba membrane antibody-induced glomerulonephritis," *International*, vol. 3, no. 2, pp. 74–89, 1973.

[14] C. Nagano, Y. Goto, K. Kasahara, and Y. Kuroyan report: anti-glomerular basement membrane antib

with normal renal function," *BMC Nephrology*, vol. 16, no. 1, p. 185, 2015.

[15] A. A. Kaplan, G. B. Appel, and C. D. Pusey, "Anti-GBM (Goodpasture) disease: treatment and prognosis," in *Plasmapheresis Plus Immunosuppressive Therapy*, T. W. Post, Ed., UpToDate, Waltham, MA, USA, 2007.

14

Acute Kidney Failure in a Young African American Male

Thuan V. Nguyen,[1] Nada M. Bader,[1] Harpreet Sidhu,[1] Caprice Cadacio,[1] Susana M. Mendoza,[1] Phuong Thu T. Pham,[2] and Phuong Chi T. Pham[1]

[1] *Olive View-UCLA Medical Center, Division of Nephrology and Hypertension, Los Angeles, CA 91342, USA*
[2] *David Geffen School of Medicine at UCLA, Kidney Transplant, Los Angeles, CA 90095, USA*

Correspondence should be addressed to Phuong Chi T. Pham; pctp@ucla.edu

Academic Editor: Kouichi Hirayama

Retroperitoneal fibrosis (RPF) is a condition characterized by chronic inflammatory and fibrotic changes in the retroperitoneum that can lead to serious complications including kidney failure, mesenteric and limb ischemia, and deep venous thrombosis among others. Affected individuals may present with nonspecific symptomology that would require a high clinical index of suspicion for prompt diagnosis. We herein discuss a case of a young African-American man with recurrent deep venous thrombosis who presents with a 4-week history of constant aching pain of abdomen and back and kidney failure. Initial noncontrast computed tomogram (CT) only revealed mild bilateral hydroureteronephrosis with inflammatory changes but without obvious mass or lymphadenopathy. At the insistence of the renal consulting team to rule out RPF, a CT-urogram was performed which revealed an infiltrative mass encasing the aorta, inferior vena cava, and common iliac vessels. Laparoscopic biopsy revealed dense fibroadipose tissue, lymphocytic aggregates, focal scattered IgG4-positive plasma cells, and fibrin deposition. Patient underwent bilateral nephrostomy placement and empirical corticosteroid therapy with resolution of kidney failure. Our case illustrates a classic presentation of RPF with relatively benign findings on noncontrast CT that could have been missed if clinicians did not keep a high index of suspicion for the condition.

1. Introduction

Idiopathic retroperitoneal fibrosis (RPF) is a relatively uncommon condition characterized by chronic inflammatory and fibrotic changes in the retroperitoneum that can lead to diffuse encasement and compression of retroperitoneal structures and a myriad of associated complications. Clinical symptomology ranges from nonspecific constitutional symptoms, vague diffuse abdominal or back pain, abdominal distension, and lower extremity edema to more serious complications including kidney failure, mesenteric and limb ischemia, and deep venous thrombosis, among others [1–3]. Prompt diagnosis of RPF may be challenging due to its nonspecific and broad clinical manifestations.

In patients who present with kidney failure from obstructive nephropathy, prompt diagnosis may be further hindered by the absence of significant hydronephrosis. It is plausible that compression of the kidneys, aorta, and renal arteries by inflammatory and fibrosing tissues leads to poor renal blood flow and low urine production, thus the appearance of relatively mild hydroureteronephrosis. Additionally, the level of RPF involvement may be more distal, which leads to hydroureters rather than overt hydronephrosis in early disease. Alternatively, kidney failure in patients with RPF may partly arise from renal ischemia due to the encasement of renal vasculature, in which case, hydronephrosis would not be observed. Finally, in the case of RPF associated with IgG4 related disease, kidney injury may be due to direct IgG4 related sclerosing interstitial nephritis independent of RPF-associated structural compromise [4].

We herein discuss a case of a young African American male who presents with relatively acute kidney failure of unknown etiology whose initial kidney ultrasound and noncontrast computed tomogram (CT) of abdomen and pelvis only revealed mild bilateral hydroureteronephrosis.

2. Case Report

Clinical History. A 27-year-old African American male with a history of unprovoked recurrent right lower extremity deep vein thrombosis and bilateral testicular hydrocele presented with a 4-week history of bilateral flank and generalized nonradiating lower abdominal pain. The pain was described as constant ache, associated with early satiety, but without nausea/vomiting, diarrhea, melena, or hematochezia. He denied weight loss or any urinary symptoms. Social history was negative for tobacco smoking and alcohol or recreational drug use. Medications included diphenhydramine as needed for sleep and apixaban.

Physical Exam. Vital vital signs revealed temperature 37.1°C, blood pressure 121/69 mmHg, pulse 96 beats/minute, and respiratory rate 16/minute. Lungs and heart exams were unremarkable. Lower half abdomen was mildly tender with palpation, but without mass, rebound, or guarding. There was mild right costovertebral angle tenderness and trace bilateral pedal edema. Genitalia were within normal limits without edema.

Initial Laboratory Data. Routine chemistry revealed serum sodium 133 mEq/L, potassium 5.0 mEq/L, chloride 98 mEq/L, bicarbonate 25 mEq/L, blood urea nitrogen 57 mg/dL, creatinine 12.6 mg/dL (baseline of 1.0 mg/dL one month prior), estimated glomerular filtration rate 6 mL/min/1.73 m^2, and calcium 8.6 mg/dL. Urinalysis revealed specific gravity 1.014, pH 8.0, no red or white blood cells, 100 mg/dL protein, and no glucose or blood. Urine protein to creatinine and albumin to creatinine ratios were 0.5 and 0.293 g/g creatinine respectively. Renal ultrasound and abdomen/pelvis CT without contrast revealed mild bilateral hydroureteronephrosis with nonspecific inflammatory changes (Figure 1).

The bland urinalysis and lack of significant proteinuria/albuminuria suggest tubulointerstitial injury (late phase of acute tubular necrosis, chronic tubulointerstitial nephritis) or obstructive uropathy. Differential diagnoses of obstructive uropathy relevant to current African American patient with unknown sickle cell history include recently passed papillary necrotic tissues or bladder stone, complicated medullary carcinoma (associated with sickle cell trait), diphenhydramine-induced neurogenic bladder, or retroperitoneal fibrosis (RPF). Rapidly progressive glomerulonephritis is thought to be less likely given the bland urinalysis.

Additional Investigations. Given the mismatched relatively benign findings of both urinalyses and imaging studies and degree of kidney failure and associated symptomology suspicious for RPF, an abdomen and pelvis CT with intravenous contrast was obtained.

Abdomen and pelvis computed tomogram with intravenous contrast revealed mild bilateral hydroureteronephrosis with point of obstruction at the level of distal abdominal aorta and inferior vena cava. There was an ill-defined, infiltrative soft tissue mass encasing both aorta, and inferior vena cava (approximately 7.2 cm). The mass appeared to infiltrate along the bilateral proximal common iliac vessels (Figure 2).

Serologies to evaluate for autoimmune diseases and infectious etiologies including C-reactive-protein, human-immunodeficiency-virus, QuantiFERON gold, and anti-nuclear-antibody were negative. Serum lactate dehydrogenase obtained for possible lymphoproliferative disorder was mildly elevated at 248 IU (reference <192 IU). IgG4 level was 44.2 mg/dL (reference 4-86 mg/dL). Laparoscopic retroperitoneal mass biopsy revealed dense fibroadipose tissue with lymphocytic aggregates, focal scattered IgG4 positive plasma cells, and fibrin deposition without malignant cells.

Diagnoses. The diagnosis of idiopathic RPF was made. Kidney failure was thought to be due to severe bilateral ureteral encasement by RPF.

Clinical Follow-Up. Patient underwent bilateral nephrostomy placement with rapid improvement of serum creatinine. In addition, patient received a trial of prednisone 40 mg daily. At 4-month follow-up, kidney function normalized and CT revealed marked reduction in RPF size (Figure 3).

3. Discussion

Retroperitoneal fibrosis is thought to be a rare condition with an estimated incidence of 0.1-1.3 cases/100,000 persons/year and prevalence of 1.4 per 100,000 persons. It is plausible that the true incidence and prevalence of RPF may be higher due to the clinicians' generally low index of suspicion for the diagnosis as RPF is a condition with very nonspecific signs and symptoms. Reported cases have been generally observed in individuals between the ages of 40 and 60 with a male predominance of 2:1-3:1 [1–3].

RPF may be associated with various autoimmune diseases including small-vessel vasculitis, rheumatoid arthritis, Sjogren's disease, and thyroiditis [1–3, 5] or linked to a number of presumed etiologic factors including drugs, malignancy, infections, radiation, and trauma (Table 1) [2, 6–8]. In most cases, however, RPF is idiopathic where the inciting agent or event remains elusive [2]. The common pathway leading to RPF is not known but suggested to be via an exogenous antigen-driven or autoimmune process. Genetic polymorphisms (e.g., HLA-DRB1∗03, Δ32 polymorphism of the gene encoding CCR5, a chemokine receptor, and TTC-CAT haplotype of the gene encoding CCL11/eotaxin-1) and environmental exposures to tobacco smoking and asbestos are thought to be predisposing factors to the development of RPF [1, 9]. The underlying pathogenesis of RPF has been suggested to be antigen-driven, where antigen presenting cells activate CD4+ T-lymphocyte to produce interleukin-6 (IL-6), thereby leading to B-cell and fibroblast activation. The secretion of other interleukins including IL-4, IL-10, and IL-13 by activated CD4+ T-lymphocytes further lead to B-cell expansion and maturation into plasma cells, presumably with a preferential expansion of IgG4-producing plasma cells. Lymphoid cells may further secrete eotaxin-1, which effectively recruits eosinophils and mast cells to affected areas where they in turn produce cytokines to activate fibroblasts. Activated fibroblasts subsequently mature into myofibroblasts and secrete collagen to form fibrosing tissues (reviewed in [1]). As IgG4+ plasma cells are observed in both idiopathic RPF and IgG4-related disease (IgG4-RD), RPF has been recently suggested to be part of the spectrum of IgG4-RD [10–12].

Clinical manifestations reflect the underlying inflammatory process and dysfunction of affected structures, Table 1 [1–3, 6–9]. Most common manifestations appear to be flank and

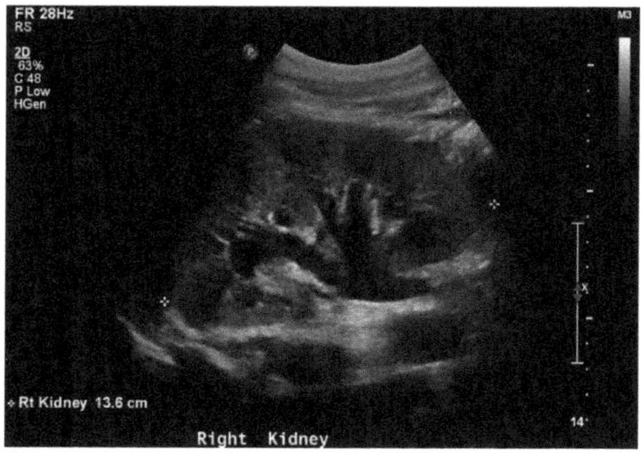

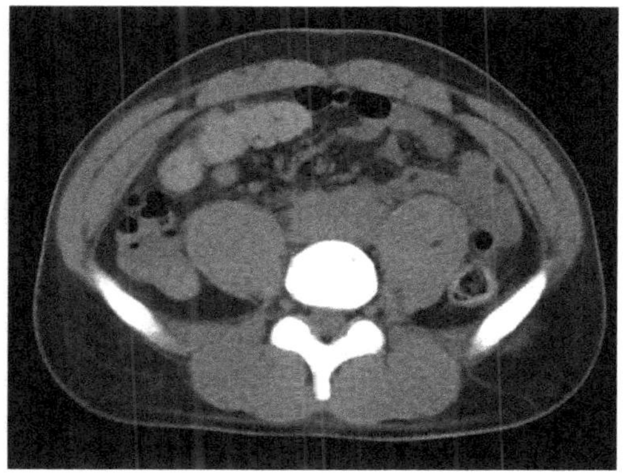

FIGURE 1: Initial imaging studies. Left: renal ultrasound at presentation revealed moderately enlarged kidneys with increased renal cortical echogenicity and mild bilateral hydronephrosis. Right: abdomen and pelvis computed tomogram without contrast revealed mild inflammatory changes without lymphadenopathy.

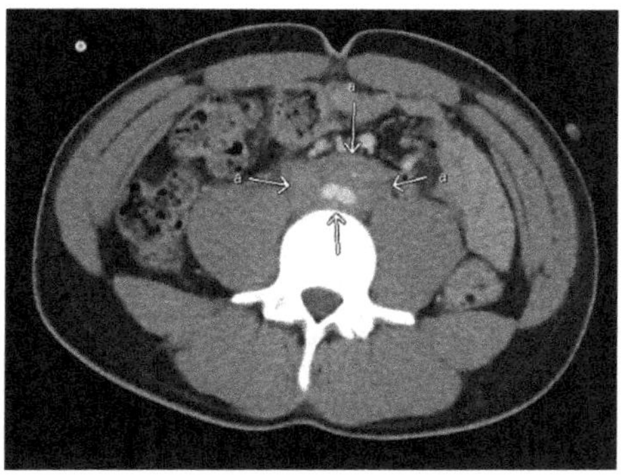

FIGURE 2: Abdomen and pelvis computed tomogram with intravenous contrast revealed mild bilateral hydroureteronephrosis with point of obstruction at the level of distal abdominal aorta and inferior vena cava. There was an ill-defined, infiltrative soft tissue mass encasing both aorta and IVC (approximately 7.2 cm). The mass appeared to infiltrate along the bilateral proximal common iliac vessels.

abdominal pain and lower extremity edema. Others include nonspecific abdominal distension, fatigue and sleepiness, nausea, low grade fevers, lower extremity and intestinal claudication, deep venous thrombosis, urinary symptoms such as frequency, dysuria, and hematuria, and hypertension. Although rare, intestinal infarction has been reported [13]. Testicular manifestations may occur in up to 50% of reported cases and may manifest as testicular pain, with or without hydrocele, varicocele, or both, presumably due to RPF encasement of the spermatic vein, retrograde ejaculation, and erectile dysfunction [1–3, 6–9]. It is plausible that male genitourinary manifestations may lead more male patients to seek medical care, thus higher diagnosis rate among males compared with that of females, rather than the disease having a predilection for males. Laboratory findings may reveal kidney injury in 40% to 70% and inflammatory markers including C-reactive protein and erythrocyte sedimentation rate in 50% to over 80% of cases [1–3, 6–8]. Serological markers including serum IgG4 and antinuclear antigen may be positive in over 25% of patients [8].

Histologically, RPF consists of inflammatory infiltrates, typically involving lymphocytes, plasma cells, and macrophages that are interspersed within collagen type I bundles or organized into nodular aggregates encircling small retroperitoneal vessels. RPF may be considered part of IgG4-related disease when plasma cells predominate inflammatory infiltrates, with IgG4+ to total IgG+ plasma cell ratio exceeding 40% [10–12].

The diagnosis of RPF, particularly in the setting of kidney injury, relies on the clinicians' prompt recognition of its classic symptomology as initial low-quality imaging studies (e.g., routine kidney ultrasound evaluation for acute kidney injury) may be unimpressive relative to the degree of kidney failure. Consideration for possible RPF should be given in cases of unexplained lower extremity edema or claudication, recurrent deep venous thrombosis, vague abdominal or flank pain, or even scrotal pain/edema, particularly in cases where a constellation of these symptoms are concurrently present. CT with intravenous contrast or magnetic resonance imaging may be used to diagnose RPF. RPF typically appears as a homogeneous mass encasing various retroperitoneal structures including the anterolateral sides of the abdominal aorta common iliac arteries, ureters, and inferior vena cava [1, 3, 7, 8]. The use of ^{18}F-fluorodeoxyglucose (^{18}F-FDG) positron emission tomography (PET) has recently been suggested to be a beneficial tool in monitoring RPF activity and guiding ongoing therapy. ^{18}F-FDG PET testing, however, is not specific for RPF and should not be used as a diagnostic tool [14]. Definitive diagnosis of the underlying etiology requires tissue biopsy and full evaluation for underlying malignancy, autoimmune diseases, and infectious etiology.

Management involves symptomatic relief for affected organs such as relief of urinary obstruction via nephrostomy placement as needed for kidney failure and anticoagulation therapy for deep venous thrombosis. Whenever applicable, treatment of the underlying etiology or withdrawal of offending agents and exacerbating factors should be considered. Once infectious and malignant sources have been ruled out, a trial of immunosuppressive therapy may be initiated. Corticosteroid is currently the mainstay of therapy. There

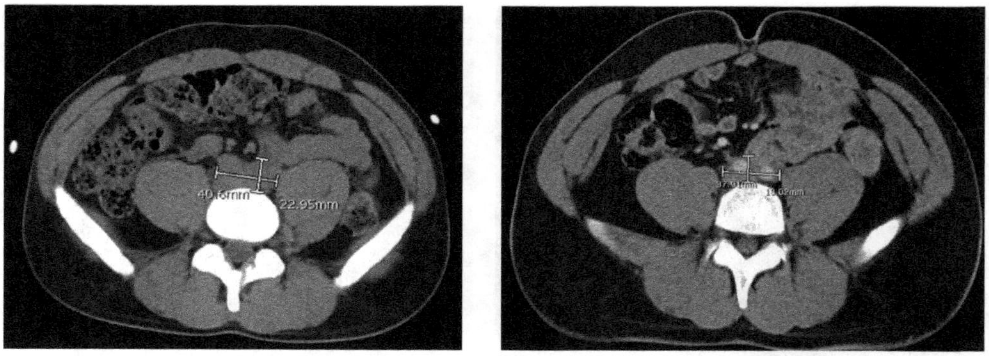

FIGURE 3: Follow-up abdomen and pelvis computed tomogram with and without intravenous contrast 4 months following a course of corticosteroid therapy revealed significant reduction in the soft tissue mass (approximately 4 cm in diameter compared with 7 cm at presentation).

TABLE 1: Etiologic factors and clinical manifestations of retroperitoneal fibrosis.

Etiologic factors	
Drugs	Methysergide and other ergot alkaloids, and less commonly, beta blockers, methyldopa, hydralazine, analgesics, etanercept, infliximab
Malignancy	Lymphoma, sarcoma, carcinoid, metastatic disease from primary cancers [e.g. gastrointestinal, breast, lung, genitourinary tract, thyroid])
Proliferative/infiltrative diseases	Erdheim-Chester disease, other histiocytosis, IgG4-related diseases
Infections	Mycobacterium tuberculosis, histoplasmosis, actinomycosis
Others	Radiation, asbestos exposure, trauma, idiopathic
Clinical manifestations	
Constitutional symptoms (as a result of underlying disease or consequences of any complications above)	Mild fevers, fatigue, sleepiness, anorexia, hypertension
Circulatory system	Aorta and its branches: Limb ischemia, claudication, testicular pain
	Inferior vena cava: Lower extremity deep venous thrombosis/phlebitis, lower extremity edema, varicocele
Gastrointestinal system	Pancreas: Pancreatitis (may be associated with underlying etiology of RPF, i.e. IgG4-related disease)
	Intestines (duodenum, ascending and descending colong): Abdominal pain (typically back, nonspecific to lower abdomen), abdominal distension, nausea, weight loss
Urinary tract	Adrenals: Fatigue, malaise
	Kidneys, ureters: Oliguria, anuria, kidney failure
Lymphatic system	Lumbar lymph nodes: Lower extremity edema, testicular hydrocele

is no consensus on the optimal corticosteroid regimen, but empirical therapy has been suggested to be prednisone 0.5-1.0 mg/kg/day with gradual taper to 5.0-7.5 mg/day within 6-9 months [8, 15]. Of note, however, relapse rates with corticosteroid monotherapy have been reported to be high and ranging from 9 up to 66% within a follow-up of 18 to 66 months [15]. Alternative therapeutic options including cyclophosphamide, tamoxifen, calcineurin inhibitors, azathioprine, among others for resistant or steroid-intolerant cases are listed in Table 2 [13, 16–23]. Given the reported high rate of relapse, close monitoring of disease activity is highly suggested.

4. Conclusions

In summary, RPF is presumably an uncommon and insidious disease that typically presents with nonspecific signs and symptoms. A strong clinical index of suspicion for RPF should be raised when patients present with an array of nonspecific signs and symptoms involving various structures from the abdomen and flank downward. Delayed diagnosis may lead to serious complications including kidney failure, deep venous thrombosis, bowel and extremity claudication, and even intestinal infarction. In patients with kidney involvement, the degree of kidney failure may be out of

TABLE 2: Alternative therapeutic options for retroperitoneal fibrosis.

Source	Study	n	Study Patients	Outcome
Vaglio et al., Lancet, 2011	Prednisone vs. tamoxifen (0.5 mg/kg/d) for 8 months	36	Patients in remission after 1 month of prednisone	Lower relapse rate in prednisone (17%) vs. tamoxifen (50%) group (p-value 0.04)
Van Bommel et al., Am J Kidney Dis, 2007	Prednisone (60 mg/d for 6 wks, tapered for 3 months to 10 mg/d for 1 y)	24	Patients with first presentation of idiopathic RPF	High initial success rate (75%) with high recurrence rate (72% of successes)
Van Bommel et al., Ann Intern Med, 2006	Tamoxifen (20 mg bid)	19	37% idiopathic RPF; 63% secondary to atherosclerosis	79% reported symptom improvement with 6% recurrence
Jois et al., Rheumatology, 2007	Cyclophosphamide (1 g/2 wks, 6 pulses) plus mycophenolate mofetil [MMF], 2.5 g/d) with reduced prednisolone	1	Relapsing RPF previously treated with reduced dose prednisolone and methotrexate	Asymptomatic No recurrence at 15 months
Scheel et al., Ann Intern Med, 2011	MMF (1g twice daily for 10-30 m) with prednisone(40 mg/d, tapered over 6 m)	7	1 patient had known RPF risk factor (external beam radiation)	Idiopathic RPF patients had 16%-62% mass regression; 10/11 ureters not obstructed after stent removal
Binder et al., Ann Rheum Dis, 2012	Cyclophosphamide plus low dose corticosteroid induction; long term azathioprine or methotrexate	35	All patients had chronic periaortitis	Significant reduction of transverse diameter of periaortic mantle Less time between insertion and removal of ureteral stents
Marcolongo et al., Am J Med, 2004	Prednisone plus either azathioprine or cyclophosphamide for 6 m	26	All patients had idiopathic RPF	Treatment failure rate of ~1 per 100 patient-years (95% CI: 0.02 to 5 per 100 patient-years)
Alberici et al., Ann Rheum Dis, 2012	Methotrexate (15-20 mg/wk) plus prednisone	14	All patients had relapsing idiopathic RPF	79% in remission, fewer relapses in patients continuing treatment; Significant CRP and ESR reduction, no significant mean mass reduction
Maritati et al., Ann Rheum Dis, 2012	Rituximab (375 mg/m^2/wk for 4 wks)	2	Both patients had chronic periaortitis. One relapsing; other administered rituximab plus low dose prednisone	Remission achieved in both patients

n, number of patients; RPF, retroperitoneal fibrosis; MMF, mycophenolate mofetil; CI, confidence interval; CRP, C-reactive protein; ESR, erythrocyte sedimentation rate.

proportion to the presenting hydronephrosis. Awareness of this disease entity among clinicians is necessary to ensure prompt diagnosis and optimal outcomes. The mainstay of therapy involves the empirical use of corticosteroids but relapse rates are high with monotherapy. Close follow-up and addition of a second immunosuppressive agent may be required.

Acknowledgments

We acknowledge our renal team for the care of current patient, especially Drs. Kathy Khaing, Raghu V. Konanur, Jimmy H. Pham, Anita Kamarzarian, and Golriz Jafari.

References

[1] A. Vaglio and F. Maritati, "Idiopathic retroperitoneal fibrosis," *Journal of the American Society of Nephrology*, vol. 27, no. 7, pp. 1880–1889, 2016.

[2] J. S. Engelsgjerd and C. A. LaGrange, "Retroperitoneal fibrosis," in *StatPearls [Internet]*, StatPearls Publishing, Treasure Island, Florida, 2018.

[3] E. F. H. Van Bommel, I. Jansen, T. R. Hendriksz, and A. L. H. J. Aarnoudse, "Idiopathic retroperitoneal fibrosis: Prospective evaluation of incidence and clinicoradiologic presentation," *Medicine*, vol. 88, no. 4, pp. 193–201, 2009.

[4] Y. Raissian, S. H. Nasr, and C. P. Larsen, "Diagnosis of IgG4-related tubulointerstitial nephritis," *Journal of the American Society of Nephrology*, vol. 22, no. 7, pp. 1343–1352, 2011.

[5] N. C. Droz and S. D. Mathew, "A case of idiopathic retroperitoneal fibrosis associated with Sjögren's Syndrome," *Military Medicine*, vol. 181, no. 10, pp. e1407–e1409, 2016.

[6] T. A. Kermani, C. S. Crowson, S. J. Achenbach, and H. S. Luthra, "Idiopathic retroperitoneal fibrosis: A retrospective review of clinical presentation, treatment, and outcomes," *Mayo Clinic Proceedings*, vol. 86, no. 4, pp. 297–303, 2011.

[7] P. J. Scheel and N. Feeley, "Retroperitoneal fibrosis: The clinical, laboratory, and radiographic presentation," *Medicine*, vol. 88, no. 4, pp. 202–207, 2009.

[8] H. Liu, G. Zhang, Y. Niu, N. Jiang, and W. Xiao, "Retroperitoneal fibrosis: a clinical and outcome analysis of 58 cases and review of literature," *Rheumatology International*, vol. 34, no. 12, pp. 1665–1670, 2014.

[9] A. S. Brandt, L. Kamper, S. Kukuk, P. Haage, and S. Roth, "Associated findings and complications of retroperitoneal fibrosis in 204 patients: Results of a urological registry," *The Journal of Urology*, vol. 185, no. 2, pp. 526–531, 2011.

[10] L. Lian, C. Wang, and J.-L. Tian, "IgG4-related retroperitoneal fibrosis: a newly characterized disease," *International Journal of Rheumatic Diseases*, vol. 19, no. 11, pp. 1049–1055, 2016.

[11] A. Khosroshahi, M. N. Carruthers, J. H. Stone et al., "Rethinking ormond's disease: "idiopathic" retroperitoneal fibrosis in the era of IgG4-related disease," *Medicine*, vol. 92, no. 2, pp. 82–91, 2013.

[12] Y. Zen, M. Onodera, D. Inoue et al., "Retroperitoneal fibrosis: A clinicopathologic study with respect to immunoglobulin G4," *The American Journal of Surgical Pathology*, vol. 33, no. 12, pp. 1833–1839, 2009.

[13] A. B. Crummy, W. B. Whittaker, J. F. Morrissey, and F. P. Cossman, "Intestinal infarction secondary to retroperitoneal fibrosis," *The New England Journal of Medicine*, vol. 285, no. 1, pp. 28-29, 1971.

[14] I. Jansen, T. R. Hendriksz, S. H. Han, A. W. L. C. Huiskes, and E. F. H. van Bommel, "18F-fluorodeoxyglucose position emission tomography (FDG-PET) for monitoring disease activity and treatment response in idiopathic retroperitoneal fibrosis," *European Journal of Internal Medicine*, vol. 21, no. 3, pp. 216–221, 2010.

[15] E. F. H. van Bommel, C. Siemes, L. E. Hak, S. J. van der Veer, and T. R. Hendriksz, "Long-term renal and patient outcome in idiopathic retroperitoneal fibrosis treated with prednisone," *American Journal of Kidney Diseases*, vol. 49, no. 5, pp. 615–625, 2007.

[16] A. Vaglio, A. Palmisano, F. Alberici et al., "Prednisone versus tamoxifen in patients with idiopathic retroperitoneal fibrosis: An open-label randomised controlled trial," *The Lancet*, vol. 378, no. 9788, pp. 338–346, 2011.

[17] E. F. H. Van Bommel, T. R. Hendriksz, A. W. L. C. Huiskes, and A. G. M. Zeegers, "Brief communication: Tamoxifen therapy for nonmalignant retroperitoneal fibrosis," *Annals of Internal Medicine*, vol. 144, no. 2, pp. 101–106, 2006.

[18] R. Jois, A. Gupta, and S. Krishnamurthy, "Ureteric vasculitis, an unusual presentation of polyarteritis nodosa: A case report," *International Journal of Rheumatic Diseases*, vol. 18, no. 5, pp. 577–579, 2015.

[19] P. J. Scheel Jr., N. Feeley, and S. M. Sozio, "Combined prednisone and mycophenolate mofetil treatment for retroperitoneal fibrosis: A case series," *Annals of Internal Medicine*, vol. 154, no. 1, pp. 31–36, 2011.

[20] M. Binder, M. Uhl, T. Wiech et al., "Cyclophosphamide is a highly effective and safe induction therapy in chronic periaortitis: A long-term follow-up of 35 patients with chronic periaortitis," *Annals of the Rheumatic Diseases*, vol. 71, no. 2, pp. 311-312, 2012.

[21] R. Marcolongo, I. M. Tavolini, F. Laveder et al., "Immunosuppressive therapy for idiopathic retroperitoneal fibrosis: A retrospective analysis of 26 cases," *American Journal of Medicine*, vol. 116, no. 3, pp. 194–197, 2004.

[22] F. Alberici, A. Palmisano, M. L. Urban et al., "Methotrexate plus prednisone in patients with relapsing idiopathic retroperitoneal fibrosis," *Annals of the Rheumatic Diseases*, vol. 72, no. 9, pp. 1584–1586, 2013.

[23] F. Maritati, D. Corradi, A. Versari et al., "Rituximab therapy for chronic periaortitis," *Annals of the Rheumatic Diseases*, vol. 71, no. 7, pp. 1262–1264, 2012.

15

Membranoproliferative Glomerulonephritis Associated with Nivolumab Therapy

Jessica Cruz-Whitley[1] **Nolan Giehl**[1] **Kuang-Yu Jen**[2] **and Brian Young**[3]

[1]*Department of Internal Medicine, University of California at Davis, Sacramento, CA, USA*
[2]*Department of Pathology, University of California at Davis, Sacramento, CA, USA*
[3]*Department of Internal Medicine, Division of Nephrology, University of California at Davis, Sacramento, CA, USA*

Correspondence should be addressed to Brian Young; byyoung@ucdavis.edu

Academic Editor: Raoul Bergner

Nivolumab is an immune checkpoint inhibitor that targets programmed death-1 on T cells and is designed to amplify an immunologic reaction against cancer cells. However, upregulation of the immune system with checkpoint inhibition is nonspecific, and it can be associated with certain renal side effects, the best documented of which is acute tubulointerstitial nephritis. We present a unique case of a patient with acute kidney injury associated with nephrotic syndrome shortly after starting nivolumab therapy for metastatic anal carcinoma. Subsequent renal biopsy revealed membranoproliferative glomerulonephritis (MPGN). We believe this represents the first reported direct case of nivolumab-associated MPGN. As immunotherapy becomes more widely used in cancer treatment, particular attention must be paid to possible consequences of immune checkpoint inhibitors.

1. Introduction

A common survival strategy employed by cancer cells is to activate immune checkpoints in order to evade immune surveillance. A new class of drugs known as immune checkpoint inhibitors counteracts this process, reactivating immunologic recognition and destruction of tumor cells. [1, 2] These drugs have revolutionized the field of oncology and are increasingly used to treat various types of malignancies.

Nivolumab is one of these immunotherapy agents and functions as an antagonistic antibody against the immune checkpoint cell surface receptor programmed death-1 (PD-1). Autoimmunity may be a consequence of immunotherapy, though renal side effects are fairly infrequent (1%) and when present are most often related to acute tubulointerstitial nephritis (AIN).[3, 4] Nephrotic syndrome as the major presenting adverse effect related to immunotherapy is exceedingly rare, with cases of minimal change disease and focal segmental glomerulosclerosis only recently being reported. [5–8] With more experience and widespread use of immune checkpoint inhibitors, there appears to be increasing recognition that a broader spectrum of immune-related kidney injury may be experienced.

In this report, we present a patient who developed acute kidney injury and nephrotic syndrome shortly after starting nivolumab for anal carcinoma. Renal biopsy revealed features of membranoproliferative glomerulonephritis (MPGN). Given that her renal clinical course closely followed the timing of nivolumab initiation and subsequent discontinuation, her MPGN was thought to be most likely due to nivolumab exposure. To our knowledge, this is the first reported case of MPGN directly related to nivolumab therapy.

2. Case Report

2.1. Clinical History and Initial Laboratory Data. A 75-year-old female with a history of non-Hodgkin lymphoma, status-post allogenic bone marrow transplant 10 years ago, and heart failure from restrictive cardiomyopathy was diagnosed with metastatic squamous cell anal carcinoma. She underwent laparoscopic loop diverting colostomy with combined 5-fluororuacil and mitomycin C with radiation. Recurrence was noted several months after initial therapy. She was then treated with nivolumab (2.4 mg/kg) monotherapy. The patient had relatively preserved renal function with the serum creatinine (SCr) level of 1.07 mg/dL prior to starting nivolumab. Over the course of five cycles of nivolumab received over a two month period, she developed acute kidney injury with SCr rise that peaked at 1.63 mg/dL. She had no other identifiable nephrotoxic exposures or medications at that time. Nivolumab was held, and she was empirically started on prednisone 40 mg daily by her oncologist for presumed acute tubulointerstitial nephritis.

Physical exam revealed bilateral lower extremity edema and an ostomy bag. The patient had chronic anemia and thrombocytopenia, as well as variable hypoalbuminemia (as low as 2.6 g/dL). Urine dipstick was notable for proteinuria and hematuria, but without significant pyuria. She had an estimated 12.7 grams of protein on spot urine protein-creatinine ratio (UPCR). Urine microscopy showed <15 nondysmorphic red cells per high power field. Workup included antinuclear, antidouble-stranded DNA, proteinase 3, and myeloperoxidase antibodies, which were all negative. C3 and C4 were low at 76 mg/dL and 10 mg/dL, respectively. There was no evidence for monoclonal gammopathy, and tests for active hepatitis B and C were negative. Kidney ultrasound was overall unremarkable. After four weeks of prednisone, her kidney function was largely unchanged.

2.2. Renal Biopsy Findings. To assess the cause of the patient's persistent proteinuria, a kidney biopsy was performed. Light microscopy revealed mild to moderate mesangial widening, mild mesangial hypercellularity, and minimal endocapillary proliferation (Figure 1(a)). Segmental double contours of the glomerular basement membrane were identified, but no large subendothelial deposits or hyaline thrombi were seen (Figure 1(b)). Mild, patchy interstitial inflammation consisting of mononuclear leukocytes was present along with acute tubular injury, but the degree of interstitial inflammation was relatively trivial. On immunofluorescence microscopy, there was C3-dominant staining (2+) with less-intense IgM staining (1+) in the mesangium and scattered along the glomerular capillary loops (Figure 1(c)). Ultrastructural analysis revealed scattered subendothelial and mesangial electron-dense immune deposits with associated glomerular basement membrane reduplication and mesangial cell interposition (Figure 1(d)). The majority of the podocyte foot processes were effaced. The combination of these findings in the context of the patient's laboratory values supported the diagnosis of MPGN.

2.3. Treatment and Clinical Course. Due persistent acute kidney injury and nephrotic syndrome, nivolumab was held for approximately eight weeks, while prednisone was continued. Her course was complicated by Klebsiella urosepsis requiring a rapid tapering of her prednisone. As the next treatment course was being discussed, she was admitted once more to the hospital with altered mental status and hypercalcemia, at which point her cancer was discovered to be progressive. She ultimately chose to be discharged on hospice, passing away shortly after. Around that time, SCr was 1.17 mg/dl, and spot UPCR was 1.1 g/g, both approximately 4 months after her kidney biopsy.

3. Discussion

Immunotherapy is a revolutionary approach to cancer management, particularly in advanced malignancies that have progressed despite traditional chemotherapy. One approach targets the interaction between programmed cell death-1 (PD-1), a transmembrane receptor protein expressed on immune cells and its ligand (PD-L1). PD-L1 is found on many native cell types, and induces self-tolerance by preventing T-cell-mediated apoptosis and down-regulating T-effector cell activity. Cancer cells can take advantage of these checkpoint mechanisms by also expressing PD-L1, thus avoiding detection by the host immune system. Novel checkpoint inhibitors such as nivolumab, an anti-PD-1 monoclonal antibody, facilitate host immune response to cancer cells by eliminating tumor cell PD-L1 binding to PD-1 on T cells. [1].

Immune-related adverse events can occur as a consequence of checkpoint inhibitor due to impaired self-tolerance from the loss of T-cell inhibition. Adverse events are common in several large organ systems, including colitis, pneumonitis, hepatitis, skin toxicities, and endocrinopathies. [9] Kidney adverse effects are rare, accounting for approximately 1% of all immune-related adverse events. [10] AIN is the most common kidney pathology associated with checkpoint inhibitors, including nivolumab. [3–5] In clinical trials of nivolumab, kidney dysfunction occurred in 1.2% of patients receiving nivolumab as a single agent with a median time to onset of 4.6 months. [11] In case reports, the onset to acute kidney injury (AKI) from AIN varied from 21 days to 18 months. Discontinuation of the drug was the mainstay of treatment, followed by prednisone administration in most cases with partial to full recovery of renal function. [2].

Our patient had AKI approximately 2 months into her nivolumab treatment. Atypical for AIN, the patient had nephrotic syndrome with proteinuria estimated by the spot ratio of over 12 grams at the time of consultation. Although there was no formal assessment of proteinuria prior to her nephrology visit, urine dipsticks done the year before were only significant for trace to 1+ proteinuria, suggesting the nephrotic syndrome was of recent and rapid onset. Because of this unusual finding, the patient underwent kidney biopsy.

The kidney biopsy showed MPGN as the primary cause of her AKI and nephrotic syndrome. Nivolumab has only previously been associated with nephrotic syndrome from focal segmental glomerulosclerosis. [6–8] Nephrotic syndrome from minimal change disease has also been reported with other checkpoint inhibitors such as pembrolizumab, another PD-1 antibody, and ipilimumab, an anti-CTLA4 antibody. Other patterns of glomerular disease have been documented with checkpoint inhibitors, including IgA

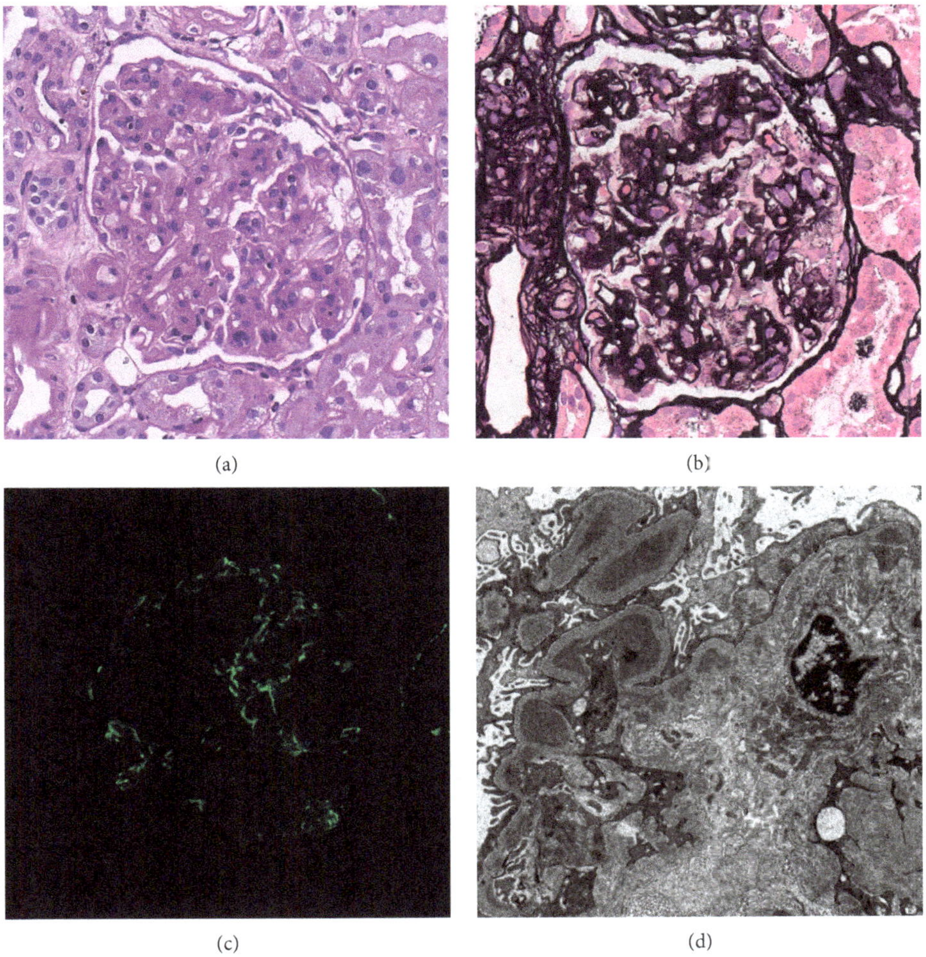

FIGURE 1: Kidney biopsy findings. (a) Periodic acid-Schiff and (b) Jones methenamine silver-stained sections demonstrate mild-to-moderate mesangial widening and minimal endocapillary proliferation with associated segmental double contours of the glomerular basement membrane. (c) C3-dominant staining is present in the mesangium and peripheral glomerular capillary loops. (d) Electron microscopy reveals subendothelial immune deposits with evidence of glomerular basement membrane reduplication.

dominant glomerulonephritis and lupus-like glomerulonephritis. [12–15] The mechanism by which nivolumab may cause glomerular disease remains to be elucidated. It is possible that loss of T-cell inhibition and thus self-tolerance may result in autoantibodies which form immune complexes with either circulating self-antigens or native antigen already within the glomerulus.

However, an alternative and thought-provoking possibility is that autoimmunity may result in excessive activation of the alternative complement cascade. Our biopsy showed moderate C3 staining and only weak IgM staining on immunofluorescence microscopy. It remains classified as immune complex-mediated MPGN based on current diagnostic criteria, given that the intensity of staining of C3 was only one grade level above IgM. Yet, the possibility of complement-mediated MPGN (i.e., C3 glomerulonephritis) must be considered given that IgM may also result from nonspecific trapping, especially when the staining is weak. A recent report by Ashour et al. showed similar C3-dominant subepithelial and mesangial deposits with sequential exposure to pembrolizumab and nivolumab, though in their case it was IgG predominant deposition [16]. Our case hints more to the potential of complement-mediated disease. If checkpoint inhibitors can activate the complement cascade should be a topic of study in the future. We believe our case adds to the growing body of literature that checkpoint inhibitors can cause a wide spectrum of immune-mediated kidney pathology, spanning the gamut of both interstitial and glomerular disease.

We acknowledge that given our patient's bone marrow transplant history and prior mitomycin C exposure, there is potential that the MPGN pattern could be secondary to thrombotic microangiopathy (TMA) from either chronic graft-versus-host disease or drug-induced TMA. However, there were no glomerular or vascular lesions suggestive of active or prior TMA. Moreover, the kidney injury temporally and rapidly occurred after nivolumab initiation with biopsy immunofluorescence showing subendothelial immune deposits, a finding not seen with TMA. The deposits suggest an immune-mediated injury from checkpoint inhibition. Finally, the patient's AKI and nephrotic syndrome resolved upon withdrawal of nivolumab and provision of a prolonged steroid course.

Checkpoint inhibitor-associated AKI is most commonly associated with AIN. Here, we report the first case of MPGN directly due to nivolumab therapy. Given the increasing popularity of cancer immunotherapy, recognition that checkpoint inhibitors may cause glomerular disease is paramount to management of AKI in our oncology patients.

References

[1] R. Wanchoo, S. Karam, N. N. Uppal et al., "Adverse renal effects of immune checkpoint inhibitors: a narrative review," *American Journal of Nephrology*, vol. 45, no. 2, pp. 160–169, 2017.

[2] M. A. Perazella and A. C. Shirali, "Nephrotoxicity of cancer immunotherapies: past, present and future," *Journal of the American Society of Nephrology*, vol. 29, no. 8, pp. 2039–2052, 2018.

[3] A. C. Shirali, M. A. Perazella, and S. Gettinger, "Association of acute interstitial nephritis with programmed cell death 1 inhibitor therapy in lung cancer patients," *American Journal of Kidney Diseases*, vol. 68, no. 2, pp. 287–291, 2016.

[4] F. B. Cortazar, K. A. Marrone, M. L. Troxell et al., "Clinicopathological features of acute kidney injury associated with immune checkpoint inhibitors," *Kidney International*, vol. 90, no. 3, pp. 638–647, 2016.

[5] N. Murakami, S. Motwani, and L. V. Riella, "Renal complications of immune checkpoint blockade," *Current Problems in Cancer*, vol. 41, no. 2, pp. 100–110, 2017.

[6] A. Kitchlu, W. Fingrut, C. Avila-Casado et al., "Nephrotic syndrome with cancer immunotherapies: a report of 2 cases," *American Journal of Kidney Diseases*, vol. 70, no. 4, pp. 581–585, 2017.

[7] J. M. Kidd and A. B. Gizaw, "Ipilimumab-associated minimal-change disease," *Kidney International*, vol. 89, no. 3, p. 720, 2016.

[8] R. A. Daanen, R. J. H. Maas, R. H. T. Koornstra, E. J. Steenbergen, C. M. L. van Herpen, and A. E. C. A. B. Willemsen, "Nivolumab-associated nephrotic syndrome in a patient with renal cell carcinoma," *Journal of Immunotherapy*, vol. 40, no. 9, pp. 345–348, 2017.

[9] C. J. Voskens, S. M. Goldinger, C. Loquai et al., "The price of tumor control: an analysis of rare side effects of anti-CTLA-4 therapy in metastatic melanoma from the ipilimumab network," *PLoS One*, vol. 8, no. 1, Article ID e53745, 2013.

[10] L. Spain, S. Diem, and J. Larkin, "Management of toxicities of immune checkpoint inhibitors," *Cancer Treatment Reviews*, vol. 44, pp. 51–60, 2016.

[11] FDA, *Highlights of prescribing information*, FDA, Silver Spring, MD, USA, 2018.

[12] H. Izzedine, C. Mateus, C. Boutros et al., "Renal effects of immune checkpoint inhibitors," *Nephrology Dialysis Transplantation*, vol. 32, no. 6, pp. 936–942, 2017.

[13] K. Jung, X. Zeng, and M. Bilusic, "Nivolumab-associated acute glomerulonephritis: a case report and literature review," *BMC Nephrology*, vol. 17, no. 1, p. 188, 2016.

[14] F. Fadel, K. E. Karoui, and B. Knebelmann, "Anti-CTLA4 antibody-induced lupus nephritis," *New England Journal of Medicine*, vol. 361, no. 2, pp. 211-212, 2009.

[15] J. Belliere, N. Meyer, J. Mazieres et al., "Acute interstitial nephritis related to immune checkpoint inhibitors," *British Journal of Cancer*, vol. 115, no. 12, pp. 1457–1461, 2016.

[16] T. Ashour, G. Nakhoul, P. Patil, P. Funchain, and L. Herlitz, "Immune check point inhibitor-associated glomerulonephritis," *Kidney International Reports*, vol. 4, no. 2, pp. 355–359, 2019.

A Case of Paediatric Anti-Glomerular Basement Membrane Disease Associated with Thrombotic Thrombocytopenic Purpura

Joseph McAllister, Pradeep Nagisetty, and Kay Tyerman

Paediatric Nephrology, Leeds Childrens Hospital, Leeds LS2 9NS, West Yorkshire, UK

Correspondence should be addressed to Joseph McAllister; joseph.mcallister@nhs.net

Academic Editor: Kouichi Hirayama

Anti-GBM disease is a rare vasculitis that causes rapid progressive glomerulonephritis and pulmonary haemorrhage. It is usually an adult diagnosis with isolated paediatric cases reported. Thrombotic thrombocytopenic purpura (TTP) is a rare thrombotic microangiopathy mainly affecting adults that causes multiorgan ischaemia, microangiopathic haemolytic anaemia, and thrombocytopenia. We present the first paediatric case of concurrent anti-GBM disease and TTP. A 14-year-old boy presented with acute kidney failure and severe pulmonary haemorrhage due to anti-GBM disease confirmed on auto-antibody testing. There was thrombocytopenia and moderately low ADAMTS13 activity suggestive of TTP. The renal prognosis was poor with a need for dialysis. He was severely unwell with pulmonary haemorrhages requiring the use of extracorporeal membrane oxygenation (ECMO). His disease was treated with corticosteroids, plasma exchange (PEX), rituximab, and cyclophosphamide, resulting in remission. Anti-GBM disease is rare in children but should be considered in those presenting with acute kidney injury, particularly where there has been exposure to pulmonary irritants. An aggressive presentation warrants aggressive treatment with methylprednisolone, PEX, and cyclophosphamide. Rituximab may benefit patients that have concurrent TTP. TTP may exacerbate pulmonary disease, but complete respiratory recovery is possible. Disease relapse is rare in the paediatric age group, and these patients are candidates for kidney transplantation.

1. Introduction

Our case report describes a paediatric patient with anti-GBM disease and concurrent anaemia and thrombocytopenia attributed to thrombocytopenic thrombotic purpura (TTP). Anti-GBM disease is a serious and very rare small vessel vasculitis that occurs in 1–2 per million people per year [1]. It is seen more frequent in white Caucasians, females, and people in their third and sixth decades [2]. It is an extremely rare disease in paediatric patients, with data limited to case reports. In our tertiary paediatric nephrology center no cases of anti-GBM disease had been recorded over the previous two decades.

The aetiology of the anti-GBM disease has not been fully determined [3]. Cigarette smoking correlates positively with the incidence of pulmonary haemorrhage in anti-GBM disease and has been hypothesised as a potential trigger [4, 5]. Hydrocarbon inhalation appears to be another important environmental factor [5, 6]. Infectious triggers may also play a role, and Goodpasture's has been reported following cases of influenza A [7] and Burkholderia infection [8]. In patients presenting with Goodpasture's disease and pyrexia, infection was found in 78% of patients [9]. Genetic susceptibility is important and anti-GBM disease is frequently associated with HLA-DRB1 alleles [10]. The key clinical features of the anti-GBM disease are rapidly progressive glomerulonephritis and pulmonary haemorrhage. However, association with thrombotic thrombocytopenic purpura (TTP) and microangiopathic haemolytic anaemia has been described in adult patients [11, 12].

TTP is a rare thrombotic microangiopathy that annually affects 10 per million people. In paediatrics, the diagnosis is even rarer, and childhood TTP accounts for just 10% of cases [13]. The underlying pathology is a severe deficiency in ADAMTS13 activity caused by autoantibodies to ADAMTS13 or, rarely, recessively inherited genetic mutations of ADAMTS13 (Upshaw–Schulman syndrome). ADAMTS13 cleaves the A2 subunit of the von Willebrand factor (VWF) [14], and deficiency of ADAMTS13 results in abnormally large prothrombotic VWF polymers [23]. This results in TTP and the findings of multiorgan ischaemia, microangiopathic haemolytic anaemia, and severe thrombocytopenia [15]. It is a serious and life-threatening disease in its own right, with a mortality rate of 10–20% [13].

2. Case Presentation

A 14-year-old boy presented to his local emergency department with a three-week history of illness. His symptoms were diarrhoea, vomiting, lethargy, epistaxis, haematuria, and oliguria for two days. At presentation, he had a cardiovascular shock and an intravenous bolus of 20 ml/kg of 0.9% sodium chloride was administered. He was treated for sepsis with intravenous cefotaxime and metronidazole. Urgent blood testing revealed metabolic acidosis and severe acute kidney injury (AKI) with hyperkalaemia (urea 151 mmol/L, creatinine 4120 umol/L, K 8.7 mmol/L). Electrocardiogram changes of hyperkalaemia were evident. The full blood count showed anaemia (Hb 85 g/L, platelets 181 10 ∗ 9/L, WCC 19.7 10 ∗ 9/L).

Emergency management of hyperkalaemia was administered and he commenced haemodiafiltration via a femoral simple central venous dialysis catheter. He was transferred to a tertiary paediatric intensive care unit (PICU) for continuous venovenous haemodialysis (CVVHD). Renal ultrasound was unremarkable and further workup of his kidney injury was undertaken.

He was transferred to the regional paediatric nephrology unit after two days. At this point, he appeared alert and well, was normotensive at 118/70 mmHg, and self-ventilating in air. Repeat bloods on the ward showed anaemia and thrombocytopenia (Hb 65 g/L, Plt 43 10 ∗ 9/L). He continued on intermittent haemodialysis, pending the results of a nephritis screen and an investigation of possible haemolytic uraemic syndrome. Over the next 24 hours, he experienced respiratory deterioration requiring intubation and ventilation. This was initially attributed to pulmonary oedema, but during intubation there was evidence of massive pulmonary haemorrhage (shown in Figure 1). He was resuscitated with blood products (6 units of red cells, 3 units of fresh frozen plasma, 2 units of cryoprecipitate, and 2 units of platelets). His coagulation screen was normal (PT 12s, APTT 25.7s, INR 1.0, fibrinogen 3.4 g/L). The diagnosis of anti-GBM disease was suspected with clinical evidence of nephritis and pulmonary haemorrhage and he commenced intravenous methylprednisolone and plasma exchange (PEX).

Oxygenation was challenging despite high-frequency oscillatory ventilation (HFOV). His stay was also complicated by hypertension. Extracorporeal membrane oxygenation (ECMO) was commenced and continued for 55 hours at a quaternary ECMO center. His anti-GBM titer returned at >8 antibody index (AI) (reference range <0.99 AI) confirming the diagnosis of anti-GBM disease.

After repatriation to the PICU, he was noted to have persistent anaemia and thrombocytopenia despite transfusions of red cells and platelets. There had been no further pulmonary haemorrhage and examination did not reveal any other bleeding. There was no splenomegaly. Anaemia was attributed to haemolysis, and this was supported by raised serum bilirubin and LDH peaking at 155umol/L (2–21) and 1929 iu/L (120–246), respectively, and low serum haptoglobin of 0.07 g/L (0.50-2-00). Red cell fragments were detected on the blood film. Heparin-induced thrombocytopenia (HIT) secondary to heparin administration during plasma exchange was considered and excluded following a negative IgG platelet factor 4/heparin test. Atypical haemolytic ureamic syndrome was considered, and genetic testing was later found to be negative. ADAMTS13 activity was low at 26.7 IU/dL (reference range 52.0–149.0 IU/dL) and the ADAMTS13 inhibitor was negative. This raised the suspicion of concurrent TTP.

In planning further therapy, the kidneys were not expected to recover and we hoped to avoid cyclophosphamide and its side effects. Rituximab was initiated to treat both anti-GBM disease and TTP. During his first rituximab infusion, the patient developed high pyrexia, tachycardia, and testicular pain, and the treatment was abandoned. On the day of rituximab treatment, he received a platelet transfusion for a platelet count was 9 10 ∗ 9/L. Over the following three weeks, there was a gradual increment in platelet count to greater than 150 10 ∗ 9/L.

Our patient had a third PICU admission after his 16th session of PEX, secondary to a pulmonary haemorrhage and a generalised tonic-clonic seizure attributed to posterior reversible encephalopathy syndrome. He required intubation, paralysis, sedation, and high-frequency oscillatory ventilation with nitric oxide. Initially, he was extremely unstable, with episodes of bradycardia requiring chest compressions, and hypoxaemia prompting serious consideration of his risk of death. Intravenous cyclophosphamide was commenced whilst in PICU and the anti-GBM levels improved (Regimen: 500 mg/m2 on day 0; 750 mg/m2 on days 16, 47, and 77) providing hope that his respiratory status would improve. After 28 days of ventilation, he was successfully extubated and moved to high dependency. He appeared neurologically intact but with significant loss of lean tissue mass, weighing 32.3 kg, down from 44.4 kg at admission.

PEX was continued for a total of 33 sessions. Prednisolone was gradually reduced (by 5 mg every two weeks to 10 mg daily, then 10 mg alternate days, 5 mg alternate days, and then stopped) and then stopped over a four-month period. The anti-GBM antibody and the ADAMTS13 levels normalised within 3 months of diagnosis, at 0.80AI and 59.9 IU/dL, respectively (shown in Figure 2). The patient has defied all expectations and made a full respiratory recovery. One year after his presentation, he continues on in-centre haemodialysis three times a week and is progressing toward renal transplantation. Anti-GBM levels remain within the normal range.

3. Discussion

This was a very challenging case of anti-GBM disease and TTP. The association between anti-GBM disease and microangiopathic haemolytic anaemia or TTP is increasingly

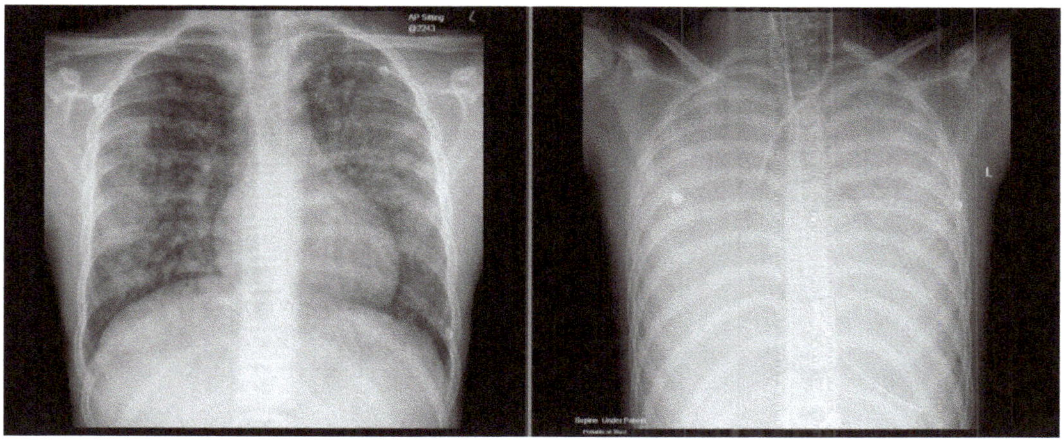

FIGURE 1: Early and late chest radiograph's demonstrating pulmonary haemorrhage.

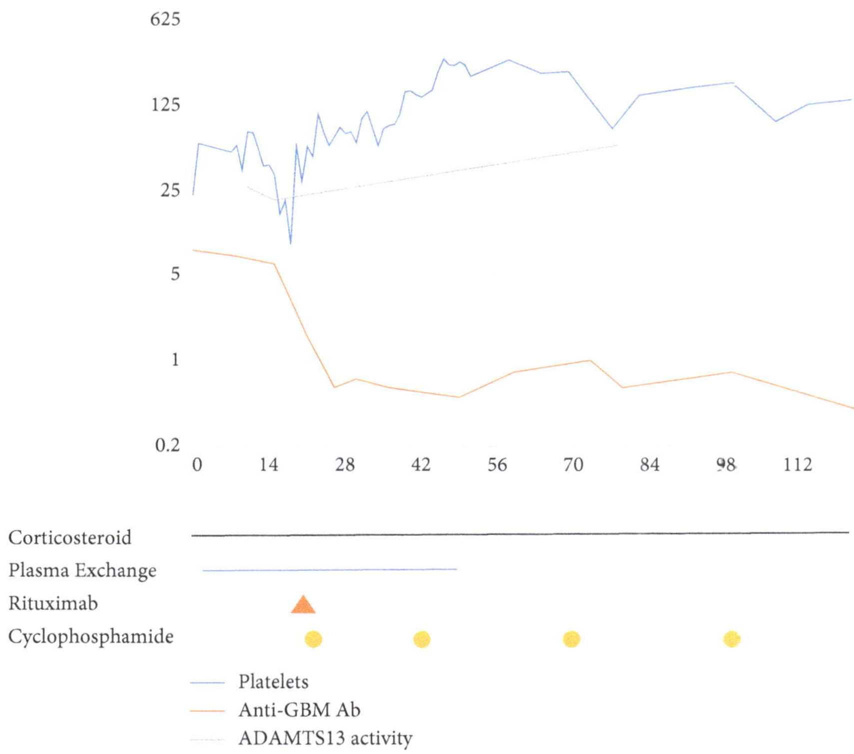

FIGURE 2: Logarithmic graph demonstrating platelet levels, anti-GBM antibody levels, ADAMTS13 activity alongside immunosuppressive therapy.

recognised after being reported by Stave et al. (1984) [11]. Our literature review identified a further eight case reports of thrombotic microangiopathy in adult patients with anti-GBM disease (shown in Table 1). Our case appears to be the first reported incidence of TTP and anti-GBM disease in a paediatric patient. Our case also stands out because of the extreme severity of nephritis and pulmonary disease.

40–60% of patients with anti-GBM disease present with both rapidly progressive glomerulonephritis and pulmonary haemorrhage [3]. Patients who smoke, as in this case, are at an increased risk of pulmonary haemorrhage [4]. The combination of TTP with anti-GBM-associated pulmonary haemorrhage may have potentiated our patients' pulmonary haemorrhage via deranged coagulation, already disrupted by plasma exchange therapy. Despite this, complete pulmonary recovery was achieved once remission was achieved.

Patients who require dialysis have a minimal prospect of renal recovery with 8% renal survival at 1 year [3]. Avoiding cytotoxic medication may be appropriate in these circumstances, and consideration of reproductive health and malignancy risk in teenagers is important. However, our experience suggests that in patients with severe and life-threatening pulmonary haemorrhage cyclophosphamide may induce disease remission more readily than rituximab.

Table 1: Summary of reports of concurrent anti-GBM disease and thrombotic microangiopathy.

First author	Year	Cohort size	Age	Sex	Hb (g/L)	Schistocytes	Platelet count (10 * 9/L)	Biopsy confirmed TMA	ADAMTS13	ADAMTS13 inhibitor	Treatment	Outcome
Stave [11]	1984	6						Yes				
Stallworthy [16]	2006	1	64	Male	65	Present	42	No			PEX	Spontaneous remission over 3 months
Terryn [12]	2007	1	37	Male	77	Present	87	No			PEX Corticosteroids	Partial remission
Gowrishankar [17]	2009	1	38	Male	68	Present		Yes			PEX 9 sessions Corticosteroids	
Torok [18]	2010	1	43	Male	60	Present	35	No	Low (17)	Negative	PEX Corticosteroids Cyclophosphamide	Remission after 10 weeks
Vega-Carbrera [19]	2013	1	27	Male	100	Present	60	Yes	Low (<1%)	Present	PEX Corticosteroids Cyclophosphamide Rituximab Immunoglobulin	Remission within 5 weeks
Yu [20]	2017	1	41	Female	55	Present	28	Yes	Normal		PEX Corticosteroids	Remission
Alirezaei [21]	2018	1	25	Male	62	Present	44	Yes	Normal		PEX Corticosteroids Cyclophosphamide Rituximab	Remission within 1 month
Micarelli [22]	2020	1	71	Female	95	Present	13	No	Low (64)	Negative	PEX Corticosteroids Cyclophosphamide	Improvement in platelet count after 5 days

* PEX = Plasma exchange. Empty cells represent unreported data.

The diagnosis of TTP was made with input from the tertiary paediatric haematology service. Our patient's ADAMTS13 was 26.7 IU/dL and he was ADAMTS13 inhibitor-negative. Although this was a modestly low ADAMTS13 level for TTP, the test was performed ten days after the commencement of steroids and PEX. PEX is known to increase ADAMTS13 activity in patients with inhibitor negative idiopathic TTP [23]. It is possible that the absence of the ADAMTS13 inhibitor is also attributable to PEX. The normalisation of the ADAMTS13 level to 59.9 IU/dL following treatment is suggestive of acquired TTP, as patients with the recessive Upshaw-Schulman syndrome continue to have severely reduced ADAMTS13 activity when well [15].

Following recovery, the patient has not relapsed during follow-up for over one-year allowing renal transplantation to be considered. Relapse in the anti-GBM disease is very rare (<3%) but may be associated with ongoing exposure to pulmonary irritants and ANCA positivity [3]. At least 40% of patients with autoimmune TTP experience at least one relapse [23]. Without the ADAMTS13 inhibitors, patients rarely relapse [13].

In conclusion, although rare in the paediatric age group, anti-GBM disease should be considered in children and young people presenting with acute kidney injury, particularly where there is a history of known risk factors. An aggressive presentation warrants aggressive treatment with methylprednisolone, PEX, and cyclophosphamide. Rituximab may have a beneficial therapeutic effect in patients with features suggesting associated TTP. Despite requiring ECMO support and prolonged periods of ventilation, a full pulmonary recovery is possible and disease remission achievable, allowing future kidney transplantation.

Acknowledgments

The cost of publication was funded by the Leeds Hospital Charity.

References

[1] M. Canney, P. V. O'Hara, C. M. McEvoy et al., "Spatial and temporal clustering of anti-glomerular basement membrane disease," *Clinical Journal of the American Society of Nephrology*, vol. 11, no. 8, pp. 1392–1399, 2016.

[2] N. Kambham, "Crescentic glomerulonephritis: an update on pauci-immune and anti-GBM diseases," *Advances in Anatomic Pathology*, vol. 19, no. 2, pp. 111–124, 2012.

[3] S. P. McAdoo and C. D. Pusey, "Anti-Glomerular basement membrane disease," *Clinical Journal of the American Society of Nephrology*, vol. 12, no. 7, pp. 1162–1172, 2017.

[4] M. Donaghy and A. J. Rees, "Cigarette smoking and lung haemorrhage in glomerulonephritis caused by autoantibodies to glomerular basement membrane," *The Lancet*, vol. 322, no. 8364, pp. 1390–1393, 1983.

[5] A. Sessa, F. Conte, M. Meroni, and G. Battini, "Cigarette smoking and the kidney," in *Contributions to Nephrology*, G. M. Berlyne and C. Ronco, Eds., vol. 130, pp. 94–102, Karger, Basel, NY, USA, 2000.

[6] G. J. Bombassei and A. A. Kaplan, "The association between hydrocarbon exposure and anti-glomerular basement membrane antibody-mediated disease (Goodpasture's syndrome)," *American Journal of Industrial Medicine*, vol. 21, no. 2, pp. 141–153, 1992.

[7] C. B. Wilson and R. C. Smith, "Goodpasture's syndrome associated with influenza A2 virus infection," *Annals of Internal Medicine*, vol. 76, no. 1, pp. 91–94, 1972.

[8] D. Mackintosh, M. Mantha, and K. Oliver, "Goodpasture disease as a consequence of melioidosis," *Internal Medicine Journal*, vol. 46, no. 12, pp. 1446–1449, 2016.

[9] Q. H. Gu, L. J. Xie, X. Y. Jia et al., "Fever and prodromal infections in anti-glomerular basement membrane disease," *Nephrology*, vol. 23, no. 5, pp. 476–482, 2018.

[10] R. G. Phelps and A. J. Rees, "The HLA complex in Goodpasture's disease: a model for analyzing susceptibility to autoimmunity," *Kidney International*, vol. 56, no. 5, pp. 1638–1653, 1999.

[11] G. M. Stave and B. P. Croker, "Thrombotic microangiopathy in anti-glomerular basement membrane glomerulonephritis," *Archives of Pathology and Laboratory Medicine*, vol. 108, no. 9, pp. 747–751, 1984 Sep.

[12] W. Terryn, D. Benoit, A. Van Loo et al., "Goodpasture's syndrome associated with autoimmune thrombotic thrombocytopenic purpura an unusual case," *Nephrology Dialysis Transplantation*, vol. 22, no. 12, pp. 3672-3673, 2007.

[13] J. E. Sadler, "What's new in the diagnosis and pathophysiology of thrombotic thrombocytopenic purpura," *Hematology*, vol. 2015, no. 1, pp. 631–636, 2015.

[14] B. S. Joly, P. Coppo, and A. Veyradier, "Thrombotic thrombocytopenic purpura," *Blood*, vol. 129, no. 21, pp. 2836–2846, 2017.

[15] J. A. Kremer Hovinga and J. N. George, "Hereditary thrombotic thrombocytopenic purpura," *New England Journal of Medicine*, vol. 381, no. 17, pp. 1653–1662, 2019.

[16] E. Stallworthy and M. Yehia, "Thrombotic microangiopathy in a patient with anti-glomerular basement membrane antibody disease," *Nephrology*, vol. 11, no. 4, pp. 375-376, 2006.

[17] S. Gowrishankar, A. Patro, and S. Maitra, "Anti-GBM antibody disease sans crescents with thrombotic microangiopathy," *Clinical Kidney Journal*, vol. 2, no. 4, pp. 282–284, 2009.

[18] N. Torok, M. Niazi, Y. Al Ahwel, M. Taleb, J. Taji, and R. Assaly, "Thrombotic thrombocytopenic purpura associated with anti-glomerular basement membrane disease," *Nephrology Dialysis Transplantation*, vol. 25, no. 10, pp. 3446–3449, 2010.

[19] C. Vega-Cabrera, G. Del Peso, A. Bajo et al., "Goodpasture's syndrome associated with thrombotic thrombocytopenic purpura secondary to an ADAMTS-13 deficit," *International Urology and Nephrology*, vol. 45, no. 6, pp. 1785–1789, 2013.

[20] X. J. Yu, S. S. Han, S. X. Wang et al., "Anti-glomerular basement membrane glomerulonephritis with thrombotic microangiopathy: a case report," *Immunologic Research*, vol. 65, no. 4, pp. 769–773, 2017.

[21] A. Alirezaei, M. Bakhtiyari, and E. Zare, "Anti-Glomerular basement membrane disease with thrombotic thrombocytopenic purpura," *CRCP*, vol. 3, no. 4, pp. 106–112, 2019.

[22] D. Micarelli, T. V. Ranalli, A. R. Taddei, A. Solazzo, F. Moccia, and S. Feriozzi, "Rapid progressive anti-GBM glomerulonephritis with multiple auto-antibodies," *Journal of Nephropathology*, vol. 9, no. 3, p. e30, 2020.

[23] X. L. Zheng, R. M. Kaufman, L. T. Goodnough, and J. E. Sadler, "Effect of plasma exchange on plasma ADAMTS13 metalloprotease activity, inhibitor level, and clinical outcome in patients with idiopathic and non-idiopathic thrombotic thrombocytopenic purpura," *Blood*, vol. 103, no. 11, pp. 4043–4049, 2004.

Successful Subsequent Pregnancy in a Woman Receiving Eculizumab for Pregnancy-Associated Atypical Haemolytic Uraemic Syndrome

Samantha Bateman,[1] **Maleeka Ladhani**,[1,2] **and Shilpanjali Jesudason**[1,3]

[1]*Central and Northern Adelaide Renal and Transplantation Service (CNARTS), Royal Adelaide Hospital, Adelaide, Australia*
[2]*Sydney School of Public Health, University of Sydney, Australia*
[3]*School of Medicine, University of Adelaide, South Australia, Australia*

Correspondence should be addressed to Samantha Bateman; samantha.bateman@sa.gov.au

Academic Editor: Władysław Sułowicz

Atypical haemolytic uraemic syndrome (aHUS) is a form of thrombotic microangiopathy precipitated by unopposed complement activation, the treatment of which has been revolutionised by the availability of the monoclonal anti-complement (C5) antibody, eculizumab. Historically, women with aHUS would be unable to achieve a successful pregnancy due to the severity of their renal disease and for the few who could conceive, recurrence of aHUS was a significant risk. In spite of this, parenthood remains a priority for many. Experience with eculizumab use in the management of aHUS during pregnancy is growing and with it comes a significant change in the course of the disease. We present the case of a 28-year-old woman diagnosed with severe aHUS in the first trimester of her first pregnancy. She received rescue therapy with eculizumab and had a return to normal renal function. While this pregnancy was lost, she strongly desired a family. We managed her through a subsequent pregnancy while receiving eculizumab. This pregnancy was uncomplicated and carried to term and she birthed a healthy 2500 g baby girl. The complexities of managing a pregnancy in a woman with a history of aHUS are vast but not insurmountable, as demonstrated by this case.

1. Introduction

Atypical haemolytic uraemic syndrome (aHUS) is a form of thrombotic microangiopathy (TMA) precipitated by unopposed complement activation. Until 2009 aHUS was managed similarly to thrombotic thrombocytopenic purpura (TTP) with plasma infusion and/or exchange, the efficacy of which was poor [1]. Over the last decade the treatment of aHUS has been revolutionised by the recognition of the underlying pathophysiology and the availability of the monoclonal anti-complement (C5) antibody, eculizumab. This treatment has improved outcomes for those with aHUS to the extent that return to normal or near normal renal function is a common, if not expected, outcome of treatment [1].

Women with a history of aHUS historically would be rendered unable to achieve a successful pregnancy due to the severity of their renal disease and for the few who could conceive, recurrence of aHUS during the pregnancy and peri-partum period remained a significant risk [2]. Parenthood remains a goal and priority for a woman with all forms of chronic kidney disease (CKD) [3] including aHUS. aHUS that occurs during or immediately post pregnancy, known as 'Pregnancy associated aHUS' (P-aHUS) is associated with high maternal and foetal morbidity and mortality with more than 50% of woman progressing to end-stage kidney disease (ESKD) [2]. The complexities of managing a pregnancy in a woman with a history of P-aHUS, are vast but not insurmountable, as demonstrated by this case.

2. Case

This report describes the case of a 28-year-old woman with no past comorbidity or relevant family history. Her first pregnancy (G1P0) was conceived via in-vitro fertilization with ongoing oestradiol therapy in the first trimester and suspected

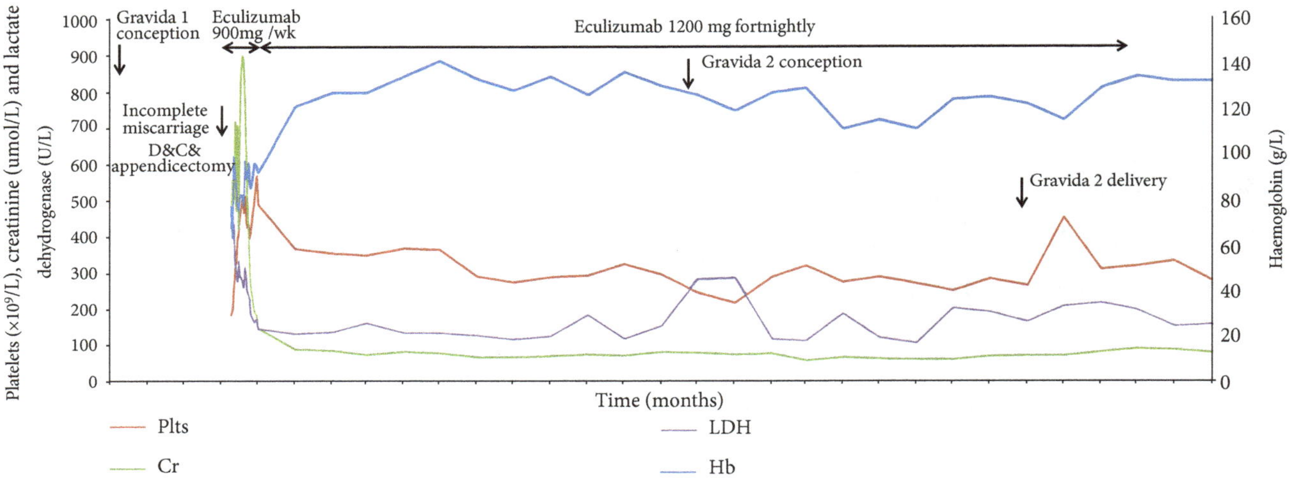

FIGURE 1: Trends of haemoglobin (Hb), platelets (Plts), creatinine (Cr), and lactate dehydrogenase (LDH) over time.

ovarian hyper-stimulation syndrome. Her baseline blood pressure was within normal limits. She presented with abdominal pain and per vaginal bleeding at 10-weeks gestation. She proceeded to have a dilation and curettage of an incomplete miscarriage, and also underwent a laparoscopic appendectomy for presumed appendicitis. On the first post-operative day she developed rapidly progressive, severe haemolytic anaemia with thrombocytopenia, liver function abnormalities, dialysis-requiring acute kidney injury (Figure 1), pancreatitis and pulmonary oedema requiring a brief period of ventilatory support. aHUS was diagnosed based on the clinical scenario and ADAMTS13 activity >70%. The patient was initially treated with plasmapheresis, but ultimately stabilized with urgent eculizumab therapy of 900 mg weekly for four weeks, with antibiotic coverage for meningococcal disease and subsequent vaccination. She made a rapid clinical recovery, with return to normal renal function within 2 weeks. She was Shiga-toxin negative. Subsequent genetic sequencing for C3, CD46, CFB, CFH, CFHR1-3 & 5, CFI, DGKE, MMACHC, PIGA, and THBD did not reveal any complement-related mutations or genetic variants associated with aHUS. Secondary forms of aHUS were considered but given the degree of clinical uncertainty and the severity of her presentation, eculizumab therapy was continued. She transitioned to a maintenance dose of 1.2 g fortnightly, with no evidence of further haemolysis and normal kidney function. In the context of her ongoing remission, the patient made it clear that she wished to pursue a further pregnancy. There was extensive counselling with obstetric nephrology and reproductive medicine experts regarding family planning including the uncertainties of IVF and pregnancy whilst receiving eculizumab.

Fourteen months after her initial diagnosis, while still receiving eculizumab and in clinical remission with a serum creatinine of 80 μmol/L, the patient underwent a successful low-oestrogen in-vitro fertilization process and live embryo implantation resulting in a successful pregnancy. The pregnancy was uncomplicated with no infection, haemolysis or renal dysfunction (Figure 1). Her urine remained bland without any detectable blood or protein and her blood pressure within normal range without the need for treatment. Haptoglobin, C3, and C4 were measured in each trimester and remained normal throughout the pregnancy. Fortnightly blood films were reviewed and did not show any schistocytes. C5 and free eculizumab levels were not available at our institution. She had close monitoring of foetal growth with involvement of maternal-foetal medicine and an expert multidisciplinary team (Figure 2). She was delivered at 37 weeks via elective caesarean section, due to patient preference. The healthy female infant had a birthweight of 2500 g, on the 14th centile. The patient remained well and received eculizumab throughout the pregnancy and post-partum period. As per Australian government access scheme guidelines she ceased eculizumab therapy 2 years after initiation, which was 8 weeks post-partum. At the time of writing, six months post-cessation of therapy there has been no sign of relapse. She is not planning a further pregnancy.

3. Discussion

The treatment of aHUS has been revolutionised by the availability of eculizumab. Pregnancy, which was once considered relatively contraindicated for women with history of aHUS, is now achievable. This case highlights a number of the complexities in managing women who have experienced P-aHUS and wish to have a subsequent pregnancy.

In 2010, Fakhouri et al. [2] identified and implicated alternative complement pathway dysregulation as the underlying pathophysiological aetiology of P-aHUS. Prior to this time, P-aHUS had been considered a secondary cause of aHUS which should, in turn resolve with resolution of the pregnancy. In that study of 100 women with a history of aHUS, they identified that 21% of cases were associated with pregnancy: 18 were de-novo and 3 were cases of relapsed aHUS during a subsequent pregnancy. The prevalence of complement abnormalities in P-aHUS was 86%, which is in fact higher than the rate of complement abnormalities (76%) in woman with non-pregnancy aHUS. This finding has been confirmed in several

17

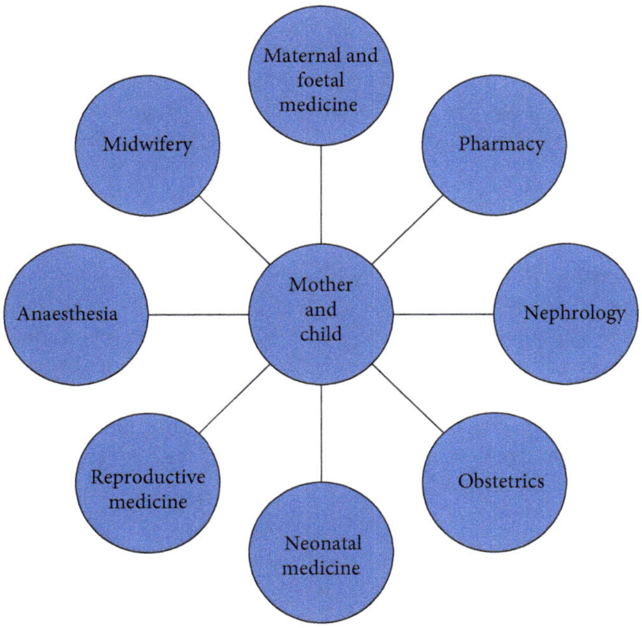

FIGURE 2: The integrated, multidisciplinary team involved in the provision of co-ordinated care of this high-risk pregnancy.

subsequent studies [4–6] which report rates of genetic complement abnormalities in woman with P-aHUS within the expected prevalent range of 27–59% of adults with nonpregnancy associated aHUS [1]. The importance of this recognition of the underlying pathophysiology of P-aHUS is magnified by the availability of a specific anti-complement therapy in eculizumab.

P-aHUS most commonly presents in the post-partum period, typically in the first week post-delivery [2]. Less frequently it may occur during the pregnancy, a tendency that has been noted to be more common in women with a personal history of aHUS [4], this is typically in the third trimester with only rare cases seen in early pregnancy [2]. The timing of P-aHUS is in contrast to other forms of TMA that may complicate pregnancy such as TTP and haemolysis with elevated liver enzymes and low platelets (HELLP), which more commonly occur earlier in the pregnancy; in the first and third trimesters respectively [7].

The mechanism by which pregnancy precipitates unopposed complement activation remains unclear. In normal pregnancy the placenta plays an important role in complement activation but is tightly regulated by two specific inhibitory proteins, CD59 and Decay Accelerating Factor, neither of which have been implicated in genetic pathophysiological mechanisms that lead to aHUS [4]. When the placenta is removed and these factors are no longer expressed this balance may be disrupted and unopposed activation triggered, which in part explains the predilection of P-aHUS to post-partum presentation. The timing in this case, at 10-weeks gestation, was unusual but may be explained by alterative triggers of complement activation namely the oestrogen hyper-stimulation, incomplete miscarriage and surgical intervention with dilation and curettage.

Mrs FG does not have a currently identifiable complement gene variant to explain her P-aHUS. The science around genetic testing for pathologically relevant variants in aHUS continues to evolve. Simplistically, missense variants in complement factor H, complement factor I and membrane cofactor protein result in impaired function of these inhibitory proteins, while pathogenic variants of C3 and complement factor B result in gain-of-function mutations, which in turn result in unregulated activation [1]. Novel and rare mutations have been identified but their pathological significance remains unclear including some variations that are more common in P-aHUS [1].

Given the historically devastating prognosis of aHUS there is very little evidence around the risk of relapse, maternal and foetal outcomes of women with a history of aHUS who proceed with pregnancy. Two recent studies [4, 8] have followed women with a history of aHUS through subsequent pregnancies and have reported variable outcomes. Servais et al. [8] followed three patients with a history of aHUS through five pregnancies, four of which were treated with eculizumab. They found increased rates of pre-term birth, growth retardation and pre-eclampsia but no recurrence of aHUS. It must however, be noted that all of these women had at least moderate CKD and hypertension, both of which are known risk factors for the above-mentioned complications.

In contrast, Gaggl et al. [5] followed 14 patients with a history of aHUS through 27 pregnancies, 7 of which were complicated by TMA. When extrapolated through the cohort this gives a rate of 6.94 episodes per 1000 weeks-at-risk for those with a known or unknown predilection to aHUS [5]. Three of the seven pregnancies complicated by recurrent aHUS appeared to be provoked by an additional known trigger; infection, bleeding and spontaneous abortion necessitating curettage. Seven of the 14 woman had a history specific for P-aHUS. Together they had 14 pregnancies, six of which were managed prospectively. Pregnancy outcomes within this sub-cohort, none of whom received prophylactic eculizumab, varied significantly. Rates of adverse foetal outcomes were 22 per 100 pregnancies where the woman had a history of aHUS, this increased to 70 per 100 pregnancies in those pregnancies that were complicated by P-aHUS. Term birth occurred in 70% of these pregnancies; 15% had spontaneous abortion before the 21st week and 15% resulted in pre-term birth, half of which were still-births, with adverse foetal outcomes more common in those with pre-pregnancy renal impairment.

Given its relative rarity, the optimal management of P-aHUS remains unclear. Plasma exchange (PEX) is not effective with high rates (up to 50%) of progression to ESKD, similar to those who did not receive PEX [4]. Eculizumab however, has been shown to be similar in its efficacy in treating P-aHUS as nonpregnancy related aHUS. A Spanish registry study by Huerta et al. [6] found that the use of eculizumab in the management of P-aHUS improved renal survival at 24 months from 50% to 100% ($p < 0.05$), independent of the presence of a known genetic complement variation. The required duration of treatment remains unclear. Eculizumab was discontinued in 7 of 10 patients after a median of 10 months, subsequently 2 (29%) patients relapsed at 5 and 7 months post discontinuation and required further treatment [6].

The safety of eculizumab during pregnancy remains unknown but experience is growing and it is important to continue reporting cases. Pregnant women were excluded from the prospective HUS trials with eculizumab [4], however; studies of women with paroxysmal nocturnal haemoglobinuria treated with eculizumab during pregnancy have been encouraging with no increase in foetal adverse effects in this group. Eculizumab has been shown to cross the placenta but even when at therapeutic levels in the mother does not affect complement activation in the newborn, it is not known to be excreted in breast milk [9].

Given the paucity of experience with eculizumab in P-aHUS, an optimal dosing regimen is yet to be established. The efficacy of standard dosed eculizumab is thought to fall in pregnancy, demonstrated by an increase in CH50 levels [8]. This is hypothesised to be due to an increase in its metabolism in addition to the physiological changes of pregnancy causing an increased volume of distribution and effective dilution of the active drug, a phenomena which is most apparent in the later stages of pregnancy. Despite this relative dose reduction, in what is to our knowledge, the largest study of eculizumab use in P-aHUS [8], Servais et al. did not see any associated clinical manifestations of the residual complement activation at standard dosing. C5 inhibition in this same cohort remained inadequate despite increases in both dose and administration frequency of eculizumab and is thought to potentially be due to increased C5 production during pregnancy [8].

Monitoring of complement blockade during pregnancy, by way of C5 and free eculizumab levels with a dose increase in those women with incomplete C5 inhibition (from the recommended 1200 mg) to 1500 mg fortnightly has been trialled [8]. However, the dose–response curve of eculizumab is known to be nonlinear, which means to achieve saturation of complement blockade a very high dose of eculizumab may be required. What is not known is the degree of complement blockade required to prevent clinical manifestations of unopposed complement activation, particularly in the pregnant state in order to prevent a relapse of aHUS [8].

Despite the risks and the relative unknowns, pregnancy remains a priority for many women with all forms of CKD, including those with aHUS. Feelings of fear, grief, and anxiety for woman surrounding the failure to fulfil social norms and forgoing parenthood are contrasted by those related to disease exacerbation, birth defects and even death [3]. Pre-pregnancy counselling with shared decision-making regarding family planning that specifically takes into consideration the woman's experiences, values and priorities is a vital part of holistic medical care. Furthermore, multidisciplinary pregnancy care with a patient-specific team has been shown to optimise the management of pregnancies in woman with CKD [3].

4. Conclusion

This case describes a successful pregnancy outcome in a woman with a history of foetal loss and P-aHUS, with the use of prophylactic eculizumab before, during and after pregnancy. Eculizumab appears to be safe and effective in pregnancy however the pharmacokinetics and long-term sequelae of its use remain unknown. Pre-pregnancy counselling with shared decision-making along with integrated multidisciplinary pregnancy care is essential in the management of women with aHUS who wish to, or successfully become pregnant in order to achieve the best outcomes for both mother and child.

Additional Points

Teaching Points: Women with a history of aHUS, including P-aHUS are able to achieve a successful pregnancy. Eculizumab appears to be safe and effective in pregnancy however the long-term sequelae of its use remain unknown. Pre-pregnancy counselling for women with a history of aHUS is essential. Integrated care, through a multidisciplinary team approach, works to achieve best outcomes for high risk pregnancies including those with aHUS.

References

[1] F. Fakhouri, J. Zuber, V. Frémeaux-Bacchi, and C. Loirat, "Haemolytic uraemic syndrome," *The Lancet*, vol. 390, no. 10095, pp. 681–696, 2017.

[2] F. Fakhouri, L. Roumenina, F. Provot et al., "Pregnancy-associated hemolytic uremic syndrome revisited in the era of complement gene mutations," *Journal of the American Society of Nephrology*, vol. 21, no. 5, pp. 859–867, 2010.

[3] S. Jesudason and A. Tong, "The patient experience of kidney disease and pregnancy," *Best Practice & Research Clinical Obstetrics & Gynaecology*, vol. 57, pp. 77–88, 2018.

[4] A. Bruel, D. Kavanagh, M. Noris et al., "Hemolytic uremic syndrome in pregnancy and postpartum," *Clinical Journal of the American Society of Nephrology*, vol. 12, no. 8, pp. 1237–1247, 2017.

[5] M. Gaggl, C. Aigner, D. Csuka et al., "Maternal and fetal outcomes of pregnancies in women with atypical hemolytic uremic syndrome," *Journal of the American Society of Nephrology*, vol. 29, no. 3, pp. 1020–1029, 2018.

[6] A. Huerta, E. Arjona, J. Portoles et al., "A retrospective study of pregnancy-associated atypical hemolytic uremic syndrome," *Kidney International*, vol. 93, no. 2, pp. 450–459, 2018.

[7] M. Gupta, B. Feinberg, and R. Burwick, "Thrombotic microangiopathies of pregnancy: differential diagnosis," *Pregnancy Hypertension*, vol. 12, pp. 29–34, 2018.

[8] A. Servais, N. Devillard, V. Frémeaux-Bacchi et al., "Atypical haemolytic uraemic syndrome and pregnancy: outcome with ongoing eculizumab," *Nephrology Dialysis Transplantation*, vol. 31, no. 12, pp. 2122–2130, 2016.

[9] R. J. Kelly, B. Höchsmann, J. Szer et al., "Eculizumab in pregnant patients with paroxysmal nocturnal hemoglobinuria," *New England Journal of Medicine Medicine*, vol. 373, no. 11, pp. 1032–1039, 2015.

18

Late Onset Graft Plasmacytoma-Like PTLD Presenting as Acute Hyperglycemia in a Kidney-Pancreas Transplant Recipient

P. Ventura-Aguiar,[1] M. T. Cibeira,[2] A. Martinez,[3] M. Cuatrecasas,[3] M. Aymerich,[2] J. Ferrer,[4] J. Blade,[2] F. Diekmann,[1] and M. J. Ricart[1]

[1] *Department of Nephrology and Renal Transplant, Hospital Clínic, Barcelona, Spain*
[2] *Department of Hematology, Hospital Clínic, Barcelona, Spain*
[3] *Department of Pathology, Hospital Clínic, Barcelona, Spain*
[4] *Department of Hepatobiliopancreatic Surgery, Hospital Clínic, Barcelona, Spain*

Correspondence should be addressed to P. Ventura-Aguiar; pventura@clinic.cat

Academic Editor: Phuong Chi Pham

Allograft infiltration has been described in up to 20% of all patients with posttransplant lymphoproliferative disorder (PTLD), most representing EBV-positive B-cell lymphomas. Plasma cells are often observed in humoral rejection biopsies, but graft infiltration by plasmacytoma-like PTLD is rare. We report the case of a 54-year-old simultaneous pancreas-kidney transplant recipient (immunosuppression: OKT3, methylprednisolone, cyclosporine, and azathioprine), diagnosed with an IgG-kappa monoclonal gammopathy of undetermined significance eighteen years after transplant. Nine months later, pancreas allograft biopsy performed due to new-onset hyperglycemia (HgA1C 8.6%, C-peptide 6.15ng/mL and anti-GAD 0.9UI/mL) revealed a monotypic plasma cell infiltrate, CD19, CD79a, CD138 positive, with IgG-kappa light chain restriction, and EBV negative. PET-scan FDG uptake was limited to pancreas allograft. Tumor origin could not be established (using DNA microsatellite analysis). Despite treatment with bortezomib and dexamethasone, patient eventually died one month later. This is the first report of a late onset extramedullary plasmacytoma involving a pancreas allograft.

1. Introduction

Posttransplant lymphoproliferative disorder (PTLD) is a frequent complication among solid organ transplant (SOT) recipients, with an incidence up to 5.72% [1]. Several factors have been associated with PTLD risk, such as induction therapy, recipient age, HLA mismatching, transplant era, or type of transplanted organ [1].

The vast majority of PTLDs' corresponds to EBV-associated monotypic B-cell lymphomas, with graft involvement in up to 20% of all cases [2].

Polyclonal allograft infiltrating plasma cells have been described during rejection episodes [3]. Continuous antigen exposure leading to localized lymphoid proliferation of donor-specific antibody-producing plasma cells [4] may promote a switch towards monoclonal immunoglobulin production and finally overtly malignant monomorphic plasmacytoma-like graft infiltration [5].

Herein we report the case of an extramedullary plasmacytoma-like PTLD localized to the pancreas allograft in a recipient of a simultaneous kidney-pancreas transplant diagnosed on a biopsy performed due to new-onset hyperglycemia.

2. Case Report

A 54-year-old male with a history of type 1 diabetes mellitus and biopsy confirmed IgA nephropathy and received a simultaneous pancreas-kidney (SPK) transplant in 1996. He received induction immunosuppression with OKT3, methylprednisolone (MPN), cyclosporine A (CyA), and azathioprine (AZA). The immediate posttransplant period was complicated with acute cellular grade Ia kidney rejection (treated with three bolus of MPN), and a biopsy confirmed Herpes simplex virus (HSV) and cytomegalovirus (CMV) esophagitis (treated with acyclovir and ganciclovir, respectively). At six months, seroconversion of hepatitis C virus (HCV) was diagnosed following transient elevation of transaminases and cholestasis. HCV infection route could not be determined, since donor was HCV negative (ELISA), and HCV detection (ELISA) was standard protocol at hospital blood bank previous to blood transfusions. Azathioprine was withdrawn due to the hepatotoxicity risk. Follow-up from month 6 onwards was uneventful while on maintenance immunosuppression with CSA and prednisone 5mg and with functioning allografts (serum creatinine 0.9mg/dL, HbA1c <6% and normal serum amylase and lipase). Despite positive HCV viremia (latest RNA determination with 1.637.000 copies/mL), a conservative management was decided due to the increased treatment induced rejection risk.

In October 2014, patient was diagnosed with an IgG-kappa monoclonal gammopathy of undetermined significance (serum M protein of 24 g/L, serum κ/λ ratio of 5.2, proteinuria of 249 mg/24h with the presence of monoclonal IgG-kappa by immunofixation in urine, and <10% plasma cells in the bone marrow aspirate), without end-organ damage that could be attributed to the gammopathy. Both grafts presented normal function (HgA1C 5.9%, serum creatinine 1.5mg/dL).

Nine months later (19 years after transplant) patient presents a new-onset hyperglycemia (HgA1C 8.6%, C-peptide 6.15ng/mL, anti-GAD 0.9U/mL). Ultrasound revealed a globular and heterogeneous pancreas allograft, with biopsy evidencing a diffuse monotypic plasma cell infiltrate, with scarce normal parenchyma observed. Plasma cells were CD19, CD79a, CD138, and IgG-κ positive, with a cell proliferation index (Ki-67) under 3% (Figure 1). In situ hybridization for EBV (EBER) was negative. Serum calcium and hemoglobin remained normal, and kidney function was stable (serum creatinine 1.4mg/dL). Serum M protein had increased up to 34 g/L (Figure 2(c)), serum κ/λ ratio was 8.2, urinary protein excretion was normal, and 7% plasma cells were with abnormal phenotype identified on a bone marrow aspirate. Solid-phase Luminex® bead array was negative for HLA class I and class II antibodies. Positron emission tomography (PET) scan revealed a fludeoxyglucose (FDG) uptake limited to pancreas allograft (Figures 2(a) and 2(b)). Serum EBV and HHV-6 PCR were negative.

Tumor origin determination was attempted using DNA extracted from a highly infiltrated section of the paraffin block. HLA phenotyping revealed a mixed chimerism (Figures 2(d)–2(f)). Sex mismatching was unsuitable for determination of tumor origin (male donor).

Diagnosis of extramedullary plasmacytoma localized to the pancreas allograft was established and treatment with bortezomib and dexamethasone initiated, following CSA withdrawal. Patient eventually died one month following the beginning of treatment due to spontaneous cerebral hemorrhage, secondary to a hypertensive emergency.

3. Discussion

Extramedullary plasmacytoma is a rare disease, representing less than 5% of all plasma cell dyscrasias [6]. Contrary to mixed cryoglobulinemia, in which a correlation is well established, no clear association between hepatitis C and multiple myeloma has been established to date [7]. Despite the absence of a known cause-effect of hepatitis C in plasma cell dyscrasias, several cases of extramedullary plasmacytoma in patients with hepatitis C infection, such as the one herein presented, have been reported in the literature [6, 8–11].

B- and T-cell lymphomas are a common form of PTLD, most of which are EBV-related [2]. Plasma cell dyscrasias are a rare form of PTLD [2], with extramedullar plasmacytoma accounting for less than 4% of all cases [12]. A late onset, as in the case herein reported (19 years after transplant), is frequent. In two retrospective analysis [5, 12], plasmacytoma was diagnosed more than 10 years after SOT in up to 59% of cases. These studies also highlight the variability between clinical presentation, treatment options, and outcomes.

Allograft involvement as a manifestation of plasmacytoma-like PTLD has been previously described in SOT, infiltrating liver [5, 12], kidney [13], and heart [14] transplants. Pancreas graft infiltration by an EBV-positive B-cell lymphoma was described by Rehbinder et al. [15]. To our knowledge, this is the first report of an isolated pancreas allograft plasmacytoma-like PTLD.

A common feature of allograft restricted plasmacytoma-like involvement is the absence of the systemic features of plasma cell dyscrasias. Lytic bone lesions and elevated serum calcium are often absent, and the bone marrow plasma cells infiltration is low [5, 12]. Therefore, in the presence of monoclonal gammopathy of undetermined significance and allograft dysfunction, a plasmacytoma-like diagnosis should be suspected. The case herein presented suggests a potential role of the PET-scan to increase diagnostic accuracy in those cases where biopsy cannot be performed [13, 16].

The pathophysiology of plasmacytoma-like PTLD with isolated graft involvement is yet to be established. Chronic antigen exposure and consequent B-cell stimulus in the germinal center of lymph nodes, leading to an immunoglobulin switch and clonal expansion, may explain allograft restricted pathology [5]. Two premises support this hypothesis.

First, it has been suggested that chronic antigen exposure increases the risk of plasma cell dyscrasias. In Gaucher's disease, Nair et al. [17] identified an association between lyso-glucosylceramide (LGL1) continuous antigen exposure and the increased risk of multiple myeloma in this population. In a SOT setting, a similar pathogenesis is likely to exist, with the frequent late onset of the disease supporting this hypothesis [5, 18]. Moreover, allograft plasma cell infiltration is a well-documented histopathology finding and has been associated with antibody-mediated rejection (and worse response to treatment) [3]. The importance of local allograft lymphoid tissue in the development of immune responses has been recently highlighted in heart transplant [19].

Multiple myeloma is a clonal B-cell neoplasm of fully differentiated B cells. It has been proposed that, following the switch of immunoglobulin class, plasma cells migrate to bone

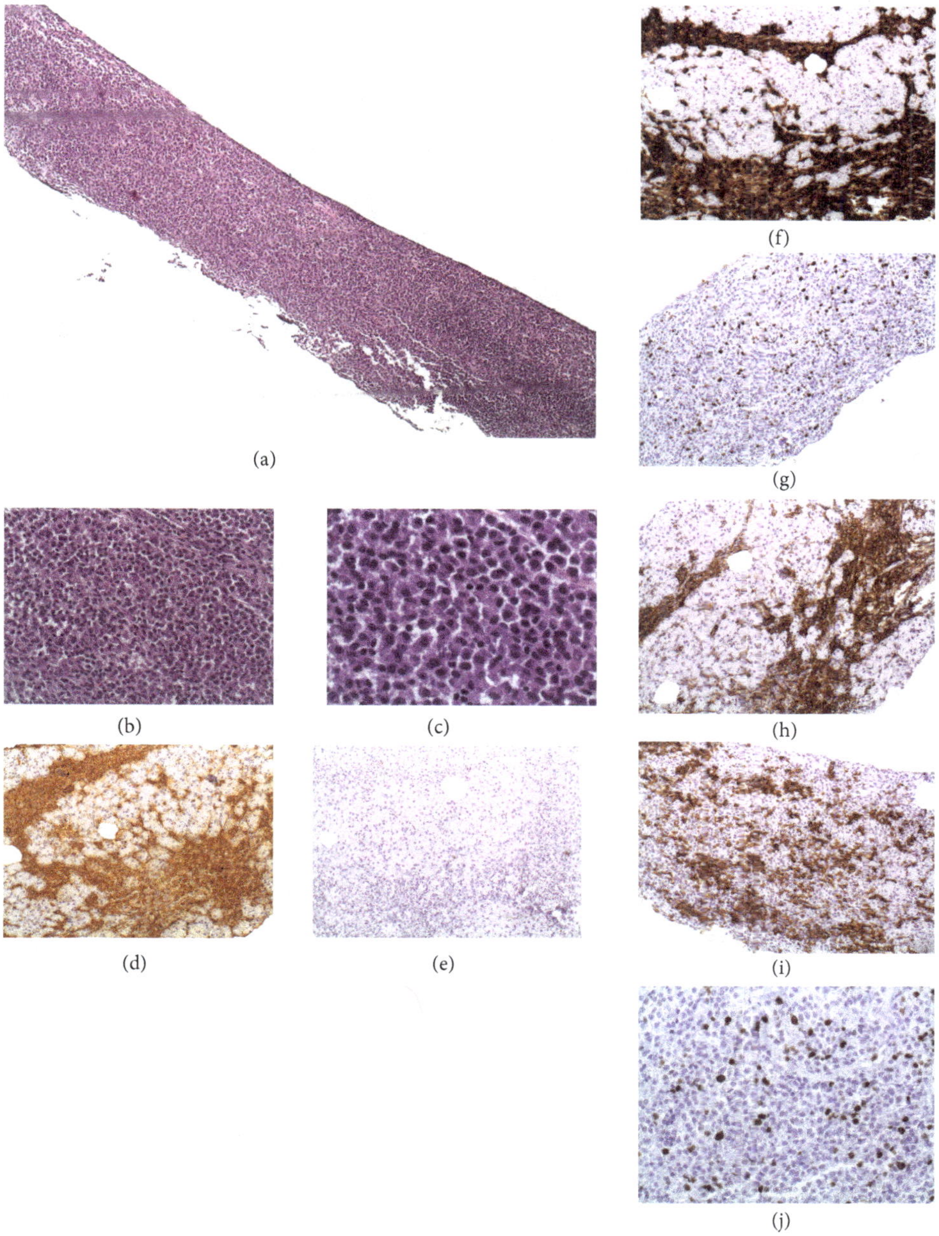

Figure 1: *Plasma cells infiltration of pancreas allograft on indication biopsy due to elevation of amylase and lipase.* (a–c) Extensive diffuse infiltration and pancreatic tissue replacement with plasma cells observed on H&E ((a): X40; (b): x200; (c): x400). (d) Extensive immunostaining for IgG-kappa chains, x100; (e) absence of lambda staining, x100; (f) immunohistochemical staining were positive for CD79 plasma cells, x100; (g) negative for CD20, x100; and (h) extensively positive for CD138, x100; (i) and (j) Ki67 proliferation index was under 3%.

marrow, where they find the microenvironment that enables them to mature and expand [20]. Hubier et al. have recently identified mature donor-specific antibody-producing plasma cells localized to allograft ectopic lymphoid structures [4].

In our case, single antigen assay was not performed, but solid-phase single bead Luminex® screening was negative the day of pancreas biopsy, being therefore unlikely to present a donor-specific antibody (DSA). Recently, Hamada et al. described a case series of kidney transplant recipients with plasma cell rich acute rejection (PCAR) [21]. Of the 6 patients, only two were characterized as presenting an acute rejection, and all the remaining four cases did not present DSAs. In the setting of immunosuppression, these could undergo a local clonal expansion without the need of the bone marrow microenvironment. Molecular analysis to graft biopsies has been expanding the understanding of the interplay between immune cells in SOT. The molecular microscope has been

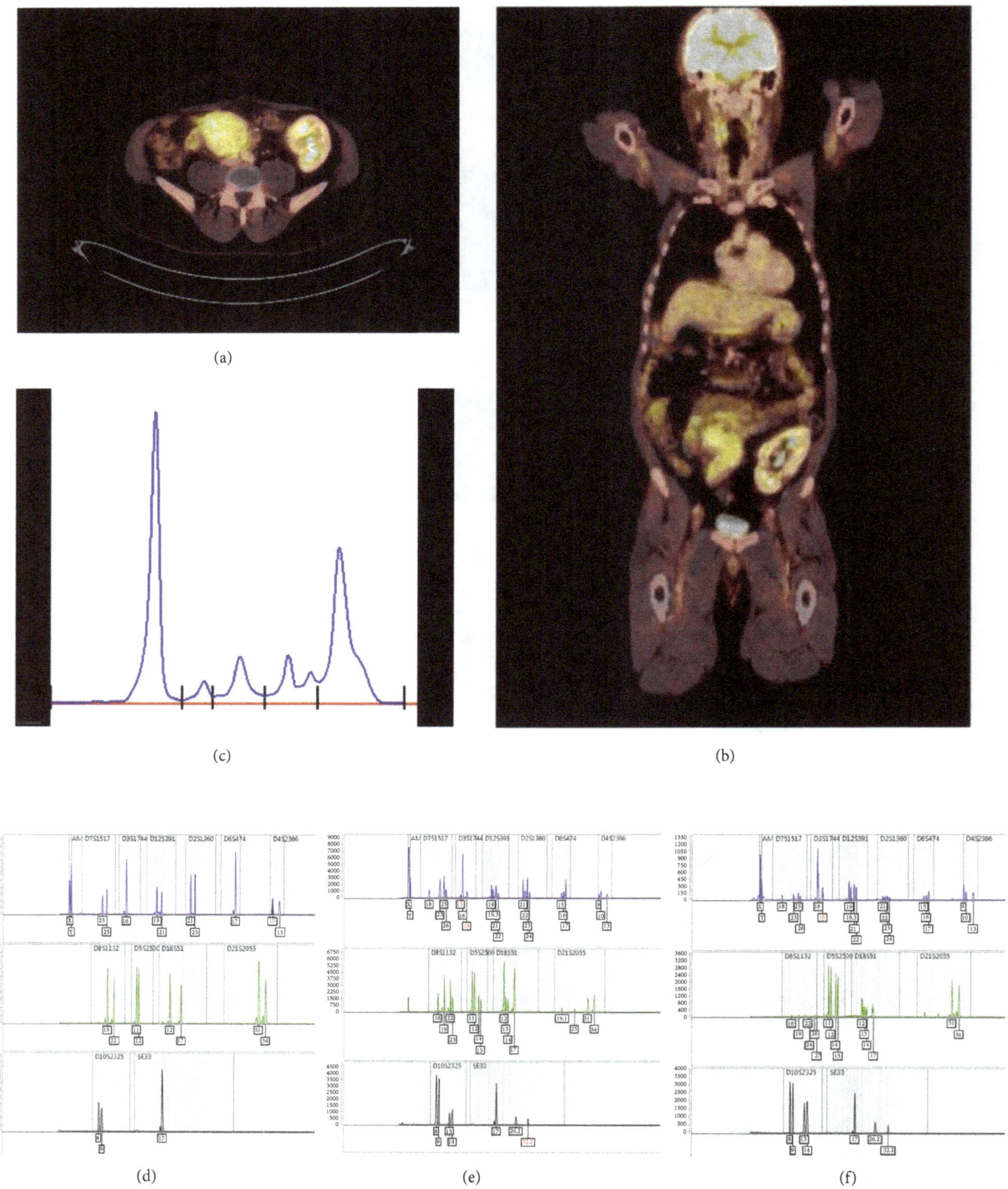

Figure 2: *PET/CT scan (a) and (b)*: diffuse uptake of FDG and enlargement of pancreas allograft (arrow), without focal lesions. Normal captions of bone marrow, brain, and kidney (arrow heads); (c) *serum proteinogram*: typical M protein gamma peak; (d) *microsatellite analysis* (Mentype® Chimera®): DNA from recipient peripheral blood (leukocytes). (e-f) Mixed donor and recipient microsatellite analysis was observed in the DNA extracted from the paraffin block obtained from selected areas with a high infiltration of plasma cells.

exposing some yet unknown mechanisms occurring during episodes of acute rejection. Through a transcriptomic analysis, expression of molecules associated with antibody-mediated rejection (AMR) in the absence of DSAs and/or incomplete histopathological features of AMR is thought to increase diagnosis accuracy [22–24]. These results highlight the fact that antigen exposure leading localized plasma cell stimulation may be present despite the absence of DSAs.

Tumor origin in PTLD is often difficult to establish. Olagne et al. [25] identified tumor origin of 43 cases using a variety of analysis (FISH hybridization for sex mismatched cases, HLA immunostaining, and microsatellite analysis). Similarly, we have performed a microsatellite analysis using DNA extracted from an area with >80% of plasma cell infiltration (as previously described [25]) but were still unable to determine tumor origin due to the presence of a mixed chimerism. FISH hybridization was unsuitable for this case (no sex mismatching). Since patient autopsy was performed in another hospital, microsatellite analysis could only be performed using DNA extracted from the pancreas graft biopsy paraffin block. Nevertheless, the observed mixed chimerism suggests a recipient tumor origin, donor DNA being representative of pancreas acinar tissue and recipient from plasma cells. Shall the tumor have been donor-derived, recipient DNA expression in such a highly infiltrated area would be expected to be marginal (or absent). Additionally, and based on the French analysis [25] in which PTLD of donor origin presented significantly earlier than those of recipient origin (64% versus 22% <12 months after transplant, average time to PTLD 20 ± 28 versus 69 ± 68 months, respectively), the 228 months elapsed from pancreas transplant to disease diagnosis support the hypothesis of recipient origin.

Treatment of extramedullary plasmacytomas is not consensual and several different approaches have been reported, including surgery, chemotherapy, radiation, or surveillance [16]. PTLD allograft infiltration has been described in up to 20% of all cases and is usually associated with a better prognosis [1, 18]. In the setting of graft infiltrating plasmacytoma, surgical approach with transplantectomy, with or without adjuvant chemotherapy, may be attempted as a curative approach. The psychological burden it represents (patient return to dialysis or to insulin therapy if kidney or pancreas graft affected, respectively) is not to be underrated. Chemotherapy with protocols similar to those used to multiple myeloma, with melphalan, bortezomib, thalidomide, and plus steroids, have been described with conflicting outcomes [16]. As proposed by Caillard et al., an early diagnosis due to organ dysfunction prompts a timely institution of chemotherapy, immunosuppression withdrawal, and even transplantectomy, leading to better long-term outcomes [5, 18]. In the case herein reported, treatment with steroids and bortezomib was attempted, but patient premature death precludes conclusions regarding its efficiency.

In conclusion, we report the first case of an extramedullary plasmacytoma involving a pancreas allograft, presenting as new-onset hyperglycemia 19 years after transplant. Tumor origin could not be established, but long transplant vintage and current evidence for plasmacytoma pathophysiology suggest a recipient origin.

Abbreviations

Anti-GAD:	Glutamic Acid Decarboxylase Autoantibodies
AZA:	Azathioprine
CMV:	Cytomegalovirus
CSA:	Cyclosporine A
EBV:	Epstein-Barr Virus
ELISA:	Enzyme-linked immunosorbent assay
FDG:	Fludeoxyglucose
HCV:	Hepatitis C Virus
HHV-6:	Human Herpesvirus 6
HSV:	Herpes Simplex Virus
LGL1:	Lyso-glucosylceramide
MPN:	Methylprednisolone
PET:	Positron emission tomography
PTLD:	Posttransplant lymphoproliferative disorder
SOT:	Solid organ transplant
SPK:	Simultaneous pancreas-kidney.

Disclosure

This case report was presented at the 6th EPITA Winter Symposium & 35th AIDPIT Workshop in Igls/Innsbruck, Austria, in January 2016.

References

[1] S. Caillard, F. X. Lamy, C. Quelen et al., "Epidemiology of posttransplant lymphoproliferative disorders in adult kidney and kidney pancreas recipients: report of the French registry and analysis of subgroups of lymphomas," *American Journal of Transplantation*, vol. 12, no. 3, pp. 682–693, 2012.

[2] S. Caillard, C. Lelong, F. Pessione, and B. Moulin, "Post-transplant lymphoproliferative disorders occurring after renal transplantation in adults report of 230 cases from the French registry," *American Journal of Transplantation*, vol. 6, no. 11, pp. 2735–2742, 2006.

[3] J. Alexander, W. Chu, F. E. Swanson, and M. M. Yeh, "The significance of plasma cell infiltrate in acute cellular rejection of liver allografts," *Human Pathology*, vol. 43, no. 10, pp. 1645–1650, 2012.

[4] M. M. H. Huibers, A. J. Gareau, J. M. T. Beerthuijzen et al., "Donor-specific antibodies are produced locally in ectopic lymphoid structures in cardiac allografts," *American Journal of Transplantation*, vol. 17, no. 1, pp. 246–254, 2017.

[5] M. Karuturi, N. Shah, D. Frank et al., "Plasmacytic post-transplant lymphoproliferative disorder: a case series of nine patients," *Transplant International*, vol. 26, no. 6, pp. 616–622, 2013.

[6] L. Cormio, V. Mancini, B. Calò, O. Selvaggio, T. Mazzilli, F. Sanguedolce et al., "Asymptomatic solitary bladder plasmocytoma," *Medicine (Baltimore)*, vol. 96, no. 50, Article ID e9347, 2017.

[7] A. L. Zignego, C. Giannini, and C. Ferri, "Hepatitis C virus-related lymphoproliferative disorders: an overview," *World Journal of Gastroenterology*, vol. 13, no. 17, pp. 2467–2478, 2007.

[8] E. Bigot-Corbel, M. Gassin, I. Corre, D. L. Carrer, O. Delaroche, and S. Hermouet, "Hepatitis C virus (HCV) infection, monoclonal immunoglobulin specific for HCV core protein, and plasma-cell malignancy," *Blood*, vol. 112, no. 10, pp. 4357-4358, 2008.

[9] P. Di Micco, A. Niglio, R. Torella, and B. Di Micco, "Solitary plasmacytoma of the jaw occurring in an elderly woman affected by hepatitis C virus infection: a case report," *Tumori*, vol. 88, no. 5, pp. 420–423, 2002.

[10] K. Ueda, H. Matsui, T. Watanabe et al., "Spontaneous rupture of liver plasmacytoma mimicking hepatocellular carcinoma," *Internal Medicine*, vol. 49, no. 7, pp. 653–657, 2010.

[11] P. A. Brannan, A. Cetinkaya, A. S. Kim, and E. M. Palkovacs, "Solitary orbital plasmacytoma associated with chronic hepatitis C: a case report," *Orbit*, vol. 28, no. 1, pp. 71–73, 2009.

[12] R. Trappe, H. Zimmermann, S. Fink et al., "Plasmacytoma-like post-transplant lymphoproliferative disorder, a rare subtype of monomorphic B-cell post-transplant lymphoproliferation, is associated with a favorable outcome in localized as well as in advanced disease: a prospective analysis of 8 cases," *Haematologica*, vol. 96, no. 7, pp. 1067–1071, 2011.

[13] S. Kuppachi, H. V. Naina, S. Self, and R. Fenning, "Plasmacytoma-like post-transplantation lymphoproliferative disorder confined to the renal allograft: a case report," *Transplantation Proceedings*, vol. 45, no. 7, pp. 2791–2794, 2013.

[14] S. R. P. Short, S. L. Cook, A. S. Kim, J. M. Lamour, E. J. Lowe, and W. C. Petersen, "Plasmacytoma-like posttransplant lymphoproliferative disorder in a pediatric heart transplant recipient," *Journal of Pediatric Hematology/Oncology*, vol. 38, no. 2, pp. e71–e74, 2016.

[15] B. Rehbinder, C. Wullstein, W. O. Bechstein et al., "Epstein-barr virus-associated posttransplant lymphoproliferative disorder of donor origin after simultaneous pancreas-kidney transplantation limited to pancreas allograft," *American Journal of Transplantation*, vol. 6, no. 10, pp. 2506–2511, 2006.

[16] A. Pham and A. Mahindra, "Solitary plasmacytoma: a review of diagnosis and management," *Current Hematologic Malignancy Reports*, 2019.

[17] S. Nair, A. R. Branagan, J. Liu, C. S. Boddupalli, P. K. Mistry, and M. V. Dhodapkar, "Clonal immunoglobulin against lysolipids in the origin of myeloma," *The New England Journal of Medicine*, vol. 374, no. 6, pp. 555–561, 2016.

[18] M. T. Cibeira, A. Lopez-Guillermo, D. Colomer et al., "Diffuse large B-cell lymphoma arising from donor lymphoid cells after renal and pancreatic transplantation," *Annals of Hematology*, vol. 82, no. 2, pp. 131–135, 2003.

[19] M. M. H. Huibers, A. J. Gareau, A. Vink et al., "The composition of ectopic lymphoid structures suggests involvement of a local immune response in cardiac allograft vasculopathy," *The Journal of Heart and Lung Transplantation*, vol. 34, no. 5, pp. 734–745, 2015.

[20] G. Tricot, "New insights into role of microenvironment in multiple myeloma," *The Lancet*, vol. 355, no. 9200, pp. 248–250, 2000.

[21] A. M. Hamada, I. Yamamoto, M. Kawabe et al., "Clinicopathological features and outcomes of kidney allografts in plasma cell-rich acute rejection: a case series," *Nephrology*, vol. 23, pp. 22–26, 2018.

[22] O. Aubert, A. Loupy, L. Hidalgo et al., "Antibody-mediated rejection due to preexisting versus de Novo donor-specific antibodies in kidney allograft recipients," *Journal of the American Society of Nephrology*, vol. 28, no. 6, pp. 1912–1923, 2017.

[23] L. G. Hidalgo, G. Einecke, K. Allanach et al., "The transcriptome of human cytotoxic T cells: MeasurIng the Burden of CTL-associated transcripts in human kidney transplants," *American Journal of Transplantation*, vol. 8, no. 3, pp. 637–646, 2008.

[24] L. G. Hidalgo, B. Sis, J. Sellares et al., "NK cell transcripts and NK cells in kidney biopsies from patients with donor-specific antibodies: dvidence for NK cell involvement in antibody-mediated rejection," *American Journal of Transplantation*, vol. 10, no. 8, pp. 1812–1822, 2010.

[25] J. Olagne, S. Caillard, M. P. Gaub, M. P. Chenard, and B. Moulin, "Post-transplant lymphoproliferative disorders: Determination of donor/recipient origin in a large cohort of kidney recipients," *American Journal of Transplantation*, vol. 11, no. 6, pp. 1260–1269, 2011.

19

Intravitreal Injection of Anti-VEGF Antibody Induces Glomerular Endothelial Cells Injury

F. Touzani [1,2] **C. Geers,** [3] **and A. Pozdzik** [1,2]

[1]*Department of Nephrology and Dialysis, Centre Hospitalier Universitaire, Hospital Brugmann, Brussels, Belgium*
[2]*Faculty of Medicine, Université Libre de Bruxelles (ULB), Brussels, Belgium*
[3]*Department of Pathology, Centre Hospitalier Universitaire, Hospital Brugmann, Brussels, Belgium*

Correspondence should be addressed to F. Touzani; fahd.touzani@ulb.be

Academic Editor: Ze'ev Korzets

Introduction. Antiangiogenic agents that inhibit vascular endothelial growth factor have emerged as important tools in cancer therapy and ocular diseases. Their systemic use can induce renal limited microangiopathy. Local use of anti-VEGF agent is supposed to be safe. We report here a unique case of early endothelial cells injury induced by intravitreal injection of bevacizumab. *Case Presentation.* A 72-year-old man was addressed for acute kidney injury with proteinuria. He was under treatment with intravitreal injections of bevacizumab for glaucoma. Kidney biopsy was performed and electron microscopy showed signs of early stages of glomerular microangiopathy. Bevacizumab was discontinued resulting in the improvement of renal function and albuminuria. *Discussion.* Bevacizumab, a humanized monoclonal antibody to VEGF is an approved therapy for metastatic cancer. Systemic adverse events including thrombotic microangiopathy have been mainly reported after its systemic injection. Podocytes produce VEGF that interacts with endothelial cells VEGF receptor-2 maintaining glomerular basement membrane integrity. Bevacizumab induce the detachment of endothelial cells from glomerular basement membrane leading to the proteinuria and renal function decline. Intravitreal bevacizumab is generally supposed to be safe. However, glomerular injury with microangiopathy features, even after intravitreal injection is possible. *Conclusion.* We report the electron microscopy evidence that intravitreal injection of anti-VEGF induces glomerular endothelial cells injury. Nephrologists and ophthalmologists should be aware of this complication.

1. Introduction

Antiangiogenic agents that inhibit vascular endothelial growth factor (VEGF) have emerged as important tools to treat metastatic cancer and various ocular diseases [1, 2]. Their systemic use can induce nephrotoxicity, mainly glomerular injury characterized by minimal change disease, or most frequently features of renal limited microangiopathy, leading to proteinuria, nephrotic syndrome, and hypertension [3, 4]. This anti-VEGF induced renal microangiopathy is rarely associated to the classical hematologic abnormalities found in acute thrombotic microangiopathy (TMA), as it occurs among other things in typical, atypical haemolytic uremic syndrome, or malignant hypertension [4]. Intravitreal injection of anti-VEGF agent is supposed to be safe. However, systemic absorption may occur. We report here an exceptional case of kidney injury related to glomerular microangiopathy after intravitreal injection of bevacizumab, an anti-VEGF humanized antibody.

2. Case Presentation

A 72-year-old man was addressed to the nephrology department for acute kidney injury with increased creatininemia at 2.2 mg/dL (*N*: 0.72–1.17) corresponding to an estimated glomerular filtration rate (eGFR) of 30 mL/min/1.73 m^2 according to the CKD-EPI formula. He was asymptomatic. He had no personal or family history of kidney disease. He did not travel, had no allergies, and had no known contact with ill patients. He was not taking any nonsteroidal anti-inflammatory drugs. His medical history comprised of pleural tuberculosis treated 20 years before, well controlled hypertension under treatment with calcium antagonists and glaucoma treated by monthly

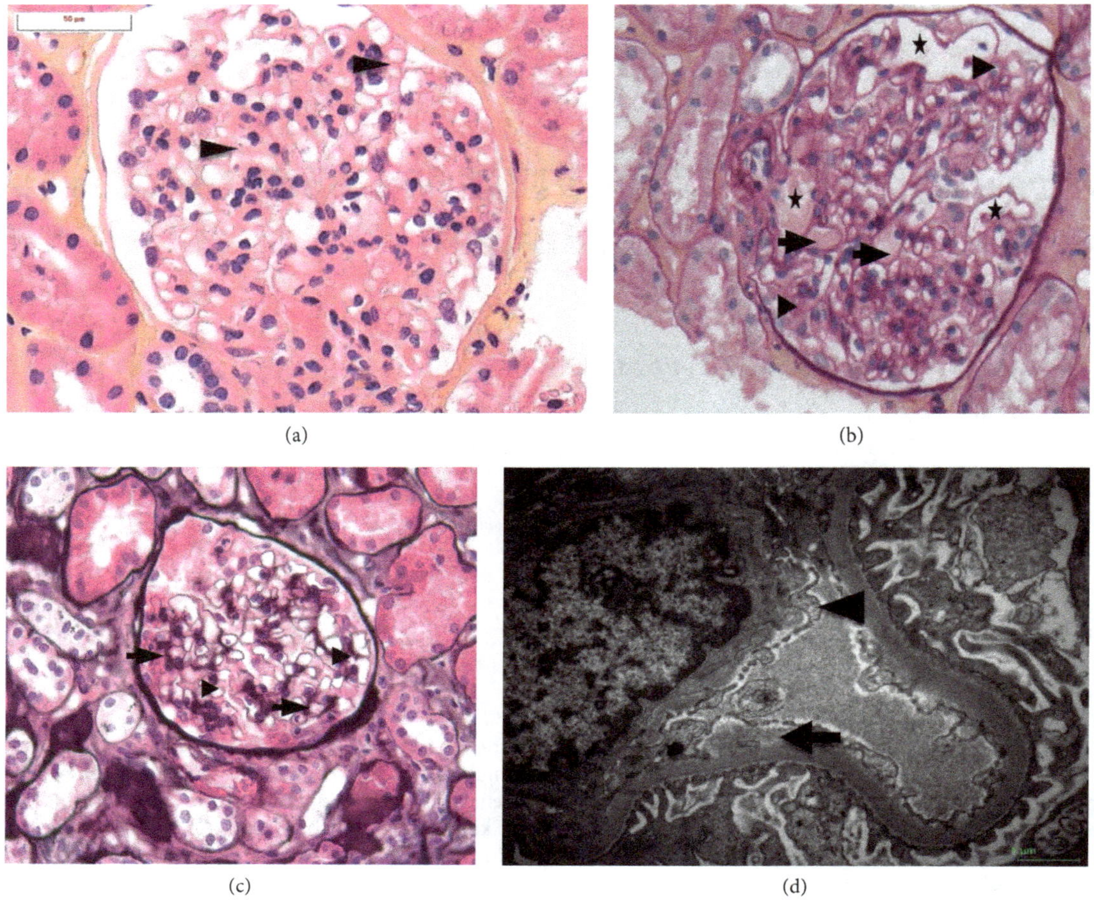

(a) (b) (c) (d)

FIGURE 1: (a) Hematoxylin eosin stained sections show minimal thickening of capillary wall (arrowheads). Arterioles were normal (magnification ×400). (b) PAS stained slide showing a hyaline pseudothrombi (arrows) and segmental microaneurysms filled with pale material (stars). Double contours are visible (arrowheads) (magnification ×400). (c) Jones silver staining showing thickening of the capillary wall (arrows) and double contours (arrowheads). (d) Electron microscopy show focal loss of fenestrations of endothelial cells (arrowheads) and subendothelial space expansion by electron-lucent material (arrow) (magnification ×7000).

intravitreal injections of bevacizumab in the past 6 months. Physical examination and blood pressure were normal. There was no swelling. Laboratory investigations did not show any sign of TMA, with normal haemoglobin and platelet count. Immunological testing was positive only for antiphospholipid antibodies. Infectious serology was negative. The urinalysis showed no haematuria but increase of albuminuria from 2.9 to 226 mg/g of creatinine (*N*: <30). Urine cultures were negative. Kidney ultrasound was normal. A renal biopsy performed two weeks after showed ten glomeruli. Two of them were obsolescent glomeruli with complete glomerulosclerosis. The other glomeruli demonstrated thickening of capillary wall (Figure 1(a)). There were segmental glomerular capillary microaneurysms, filled with pale material, and segmental hyaline thickening of the glomerular basement membrane (Figure 1(b)). Silver staining showed some double contours (Figure 1(c)). Mild focal interstitial fibrosis and tubular atrophy with a mononuclear cells infiltrate were seen. Immunofluorescence for IgA, IgG, IgM, C1q, kappa, and lambda was negative. However, C3 immunofluorescence showed a sparse endothelial positivity in arterioles (not shown). On electron microscopy, the endothelial cells showed irregularities, and focal loss of fenestrations. Subendothelial space expansion by electron-lucent material was visible (Figure 1(d)). This was consistent with signs of endothelial injury. Intravitreal injections of anti-VEGF were suspended. Four months after withdrawal, serum creatinine was of 1.20 mg/dL, and albuminuria normalized, supporting our hypothesis of intravitreal anti-VEGF induced renal microangiopathy. One year after bevacizumab was stopped, serum creatinine was of 0.95 mg/dL, and urinary albumin-creatinine ratio was of 3.3 mg/g. The patient did not present any thromboembolic event.

3. Discussion

Bevacizumab is a humanized monoclonal antibody to VEGF approved for the treatment of metastatic cancer, mainly colorectal, breast, and renal cell carcinoma [5]. By preventing the binding of VEGF-A to the endothelial cell surface receptors, it inhibits neovascularization, and then tumour growth [6]. The use of intravitreal bevacizumab has been successful in various ocular diseases with neovascularization, including exudative age-related macular degeneration (AMD), retinal neovascularization in proliferative diabetic retinopathy, or neovascular glaucoma as in our case [7].

Systemic adverse events are reported with the intravenous use of anti-VEGF therapy, including kidney injury with hypertension, proteinuria (even nephrotic syndrome), and features of TMA [8–11]. However, intravitreal anti-VEGF antibody injection is generally supposed to be safe. Within 1.173 patients treated with intravitreal bevacizumab and followed during one year, systemic side effects mainly hypertension, and cerebrovascular disease have been reported in 1.5% of cases. The most frequent complications were local, dominated by subconjunctival haemorrhage observed in 838 patients. No glomerular disease has been reported [12].

Kidney toxicity after intravitreal use of anti-VEGF is exceptional. This complication was first reported in a 77-year-old patient treated by intravitreal injections of ranibizumab (a Fab fragment of the bevacizumab humanized monoclonal antibody) for AMD. He presented nonimmune haemolytic anaemia associated with acute kidney injury and impure nephrotic syndrome. Kidney biopsy showed glomerular basement membranes duplications, endothelial swelling, and arteriolar thrombi compatible with TMA diagnosis. Electron microscopy study was not available. After discontinuation of ranibizumab injections, kidney function normalized [13]. Cheungpasitporn et al. described a 67-year-old man with polycystic kidney disease who underwent kidney transplantation and was treated by intravitreal injections of bevacizumab followed by aflibercept (another anti-VEGF-therapy) for AMD. He developed glomerular proteinuria that worsened during the follow-up. One year after transplantation, kidney allograft biopsy showed phospholipase A 2 receptor—negative membranous nephropathy but no TMA. The second case was a 52-year-old patient who underwent kidney transplantation for tuberous sclerosis. Sixteen years after transplantation, kidney biopsy was performed after progressive increase in proteinuria, and revealed acute, and chronic antibody-mediated rejection with glomerular thrombi. The patient had been started on intravitreal anti-VEGF therapy for AMD six months before. In these two cases, the temporal link of local anti-VEGF injections and allograft dysfunction has only been suggested but not demonstrated [14].

Our patient had positive antiphospholipid antibodies. He might present antiphospholipid antibody syndrome, a multisystem disorder that can induce TMA. We considered this diagnostic less likely as our patient improved his renal function and albuminuria after withdrawal of bevacizumab. Furthermore, glomerular anti-VEGF therapy induced microangiopathy display a histologic pattern that differs from other causes of TMA lesions, among other things the absence of fibrin thrombi, platelet thrombi, or fragmented erythrocytes [15]. Instead, segmental glomerular capillary microaneurysms filled with pale material are usually found as in our case. After local injection, bevacizumab has been detected in a very low serum concentration as compared to intraocular concentration (0.413 μg/mL *vs* 406.25 μg/mL) in experimental rabbit model [16]. In glomeruli, podocytes produce VEGF that binds to VEGF receptor-2 expressed on endothelial cells. This interaction is necessary to the normal function of the glomerular filtration barrier and for recovery of renal microvascular injury [17]. Ultrastructure study in a murine model of doxycycline induced VEGF deletion in podocytes showed swelling of the endothelial cells. This indicate the crucial role of VEGF in maintaining glomerular endothelium integrity [10]. The endothelial cells injury in our patient after intravitreal bevacizumab injections, indicate that even very low systemic concentrations of anti-VEGF could significantly impair interaction between VEGF derived from podocytes, and VEGF receptor on the endothelial cells.

As far as we know, we report for the first time the electron microscopy evidence that intravitreal injection of anti-VEGF induces glomerular endothelial cells injury. As the use of anti-VEGF therapy is increasing, particularly in ocular diseases with local injections, ophthalmologists, and nephrologists should be aware of this complication. A regular monitoring of renal function and proteinuria after introducing anti-VEGF antibodies is advised.

References

[1] R. Ronca, M. Benkheil, S. Mitola, S. Struyf, and S. Liekens, "Tumor angiogenesis revisited: regulators and clinical implications," *Medicinal Research Reviews*, vol. 37, no. 6, pp. 1231–1274, 2017.

[2] M. W. Stewart, "Treatment of diabetic retinopathy: recent advances and unresolved challenges," *World Journal of Diabetes*, vol. 7, no. 16, pp. 333–341, 2016.

[3] H. Izzedine, B. Escudier, C. Lhomme et al., "Kidney diseases associated with anti-vascular endothelial growth factor (VEGF)," *Medicine*, vol. 93, no. 24, pp. 333–339, 2014.

[4] F. Person, M. M. Rinschen, S. R. Brix et al., "Bevacizumab-associated glomerular microangiopathy," *Modern Pathology*, vol. 32, no. 5, pp. 684–700, 2019.

[5] G. M. Keating, "Bevacizumab: a review of its use in advanced cancer," *Drugs*, vol. 74, no. 16, pp. 1891–1925, 2014.

[6] N. Ferrara, K. J. Hillan, H.-P. Gerber, and W. Novotny, "Discovery and development of bevacizumab, an anti-VEGF antibody for treating cancer," *Nature Reviews Drug Discovery*, vol. 3, no. 5, pp. 391–400, 2004.

[7] J. B. Gunther and M. M. Altaweel, "Bevacizumab (avastin) for the treatment of ocular disease," *Survey of Ophthalmology*, vol. 54, no. 3, pp. 372–400, 2009.

[8] F. Gurevich and M. A. Perazella, "Renal effects of anti-angiogenesis therapy: update for the internist," *The American Journal of Medicine*, vol. 122, no. 4, pp. 322–328, 2009.

[9] S. Yılmaz, Z. B. Özçakar, A. Taktak et al., "Anti-VEGF-related thrombotic microangiopathy in a child presenting with nephrotic syndrome," *Pediatric Nephrology*, vol. 31, no. 6, pp. 1029–1032, 2016.

[10] V. Eremina, J. A. Jefferson, J. Kowalewska et al., "VEGF inhibition and renal thrombotic microangiopathy," *New England Journal of Medicine*, vol. 358, no. 11, pp. 1129–1136, 2008.

[11] N. Toriu, A. Sekine, H. Mizuno et al., "Renal-limited thrombotic microangiopathy due to bevacizumab therapy for metastatic colorectal cancer: a case report," *Case Reports in Oncology*, vol. 12, no. 2, pp. 391–400, 2019.

[12] L. Wu, M. A. Martínez-Castellanos, H. Quiroz-Mercado et al., "Twelve-month safety of intravitreal injections of bevacizumab

(Avastin): results of the Pan-American Collaborative Retina Study Group (PACORES)," *Graefe's Archive for Clinical and Experimental Ophthalmology*, vol. 246, no. 1, pp. 81–87, 2007.

[13] G. Pellé, N. Shweke, J. P. Duong Van Huyen et al., "Systemic and kidney toxicity of intravitreal administration of vascular endothelial growth factor inhibitors," *American Journal of Kidney Diseases*, vol. 57, no. 5, pp. 756–759, 2011.

[14] W. Cheungpasitporn, F. T. Chebib, L. D. Cornell et al., "Intravitreal antivascular endothelial growth factor therapy may induce proteinuria and antibody mediated injury in renal allografts," *Transplantation*, vol. 99, no. 11, pp. 2382–2386, 2015.

[15] F. Pfister, K. Amann, C. Daniel, M. Klewer, A. Büttner, and M. Büttner-Herold, "Characteristic morphological changes in anti-VEGF therapy-induced glomerular microangiopathy," *Histopathology*, vol. 73, no. 6, pp. 990–1001, 2018.

[16] S. J. Bakri, M. R. Snyder, J. M. Reid, J. S. Pulido, and R. J. Singh, "Pharmacokinetics of intravitreal bevacizumab (Avastin)," *Ophthalmology*, vol. 114, no. 5, pp. 855–859, 2007.

[17] S. I. Suga, Y. G. Kim, A. Joly et al., "Vascular endothelial growth factor (VEGF121) protects rats from renal infarction in thrombotic microangiopathy," *Kidney International*, vol. 60, no. 4, pp. 1297–1308, 2001.

20

Reversible Nephropathy Associated with Jet Fuel Exposure

Latif A. Salam,[1] Khabbab Amin,[1] Regina Cheng,[1] Noriyuki Murakami,[1] Clinton Brown,[2] and Lawrence Kwon[3]

[1]*Department of Internal Medicine, Section of Hospital Medicine, State University of New York (SUNY) Downstate Health Sciences University, 450 Clarkson Avenue, Brooklyn, NY 11203, USA*
[2]*Brooklyn Health Disparities Center, Division of Nephrology, State University of New York (SUNY) Downstate Health Sciences University, 450 Clarkson Avenue, Brooklyn, NY 11203, USA*
[3]*Department of Internal Medicine, Division of Nephrology, State University of New York (SUNY) Downstate Health Sciences University, 450 Clarkson Avenue, Brooklyn, NY 11203, USA*

Correspondence should be addressed to Latif A. Salam; latif.salam@downstate.edu

Academic Editor: Mahzuz Karim

Acute kidney injury (AKI) with progression to oliguric or anuric acute renal failure (ARF) is often related to use of well-known nephrotoxic agents including medications such as nonsteroidal anti-inflammatory drugs (NSAIDs), angiotensin-converting enzyme inhibitors (ACEis)/angiotensin II receptor blockers (ARBs), and certain classes of antibiotics. Hyperosmolar IV contrast is also a well-known nephrotoxic agent. Severe sepsis with subsequent hypotension, marked hyperglycemia, and those with difficulty accessing water or with poor oral intake can also present with acute kidney injury related to kidney hypoperfusion, dehydration, and volume depletion. In this case report, we discover and discuss the possible effects of regular and daily occupational exposure of jet fuel (a mixture of hydrocarbons) on renal function. Jet fuel is an underdescribed and not well-known nephrotoxic agent; however, its direct toxicity on kidney function appears to be reversible with removal of exposure and aggressive fluid hydration.

1. Introduction

Jet fuel is a common exposure amongst those working in airports and military bases. Jet fuel is composed of a mix of hydrocarbons including mostly isoparaffins, cycloparaffins, and aromatics, as well as certain additives such as alkylated phenols, dinonylnaphthylsulfonic acid, fuel system icing inhibitor (FSII) agents, biocides, and metal deactivators [1–3]. Hydrocarbon exposure has well-documented clinical effects through inhalation, ingestion, and dermal contact [4]. Hydrocarbons undergo biotransformation primarily through the liver and accumulate in lipid-rich tissues [5]. Detoxification of organic solvents within the liver produces water-soluble compounds, which are then excreted through urine or bile, making the kidneys a potential site of injury in the metabolism of hydrocarbons found in jet fuels [6]. Few studies have been conducted on the exposure of hydrocarbons and jet fuel and their potential effect on the kidney. Experimental animal studies have demonstrated jet fuel dose-related nephropathy, with histopathologic changes seen in subchronic exposures to fuel vapors most notably in male rats [7]. In humans, the renal effects associated with acute and chronic exposure is not well defined. There are reports of glomerulonephritis among subjects with chronic exposure to hydrocarbons [8]. In Saudi Arabia, there has been a case report of a young patient (without history suggestive of connective tissue disease) with work-related exposure to jet fuel by both inhalation and direct skin contact with an initial presentation of nausea, fatigue, and bilateral flank pain. He was found to have acute renal failure with electrolyte levels within normal range, hepatitis (B and C) and HIV negative serology, ANCA/ANA negative, and normal C3/C4 [9]. Histopathologic changes have been reported in humans in association with exposure to hydrocarbons. The two histopathologic changes that have been reported are acute tubular necrosis and rapidly progressive glomerulonephritis [8]. The kidney failure reported in humans was noted at acute, as well as high levels, and appears to reversible [9].

2. Case Report

A 50-year-old man presented to the emergency department (ED) at SUNY Downstate Medical Center with complaint of intermittent epigastric pain that began a few days prior. The patient was slightly confused at time of presentation but was able to provide some history. Collateral history was collected from his daughter who lives with the patient and was also present at time of the patient's presentation to the ED. The patient reported that his epigastric pain was nonradiating, associated with nausea along with multiple episodes of nonbilious, nonbloody emesis. The patient also reported subjective fevers, chills, and cough for one week. He denied any flank pain, changes in bowel habits, appetite, or amount of oral intake. He also denied any changes in his weight. His daughter, however, noted that over the past week, she observed a decrease in the patient's appetite and oral intake. Patient's medical history was significant for hypertension, for which he did not take any medication, and hepatitis B (Hep B), for which he was hospitalized in 1983. He was unable to recall the cause of the hepatitis. He denied any history of tobacco, alcohol, illicit drug, or recent NSAID use. He does not take any prescribed or over-the-counter medications. His family history was unremarkable.

A thorough occupational history collected later in the course of hospitalization revealed that the patient has worked in the aviation industry as an aircraft refueler at a local airport, where he refuels up to nine aircrafts per day for the past three and half years. At work, the patient reports wearing a uniform and "long medical gloves," which he described as being approximately five times the thickness of standard hospital gloves. He also stated that he wears a respirator mask about 60% of the time during refueling. The patient reported direct skin contact with jet fuel when it spills onto his arms at least three times per day on average, despite wearing a uniform and gloves. He mentioned one instance, where he was completely covered in jet fuel. He also noted that he could often smell fuel on his hands for several days after a spill. At time of admission, the patient was oliguric and in acute renal failure (ARF) as his serum chemistry showed a strikingly elevated blood urea nitrogen (BUN) and creatinine that were each about 20 times over the normal limits. He was normotensive, and his physical exam was only revealing of dry mucous membranes, clear lungs, and a cardiac exam that was within normal limits. He had no edema of his lower extremities bilaterally. The cause of his ARF was unknown at this time.

The patient's hospital course included extensive medical and diagnostic testing to investigate the etiology of his acute renal failure. His baseline renal function was unknown. The patient's initial serum chemistry showed a BUN level of 215 mg/dL and creatinine level of 20.41 mg/dL with an estimated glomerular filtration rate (eGFR) of 3 mL/min/1.73 m^2. Electrolytes showed slight hyponatremia with a serum sodium level of 126 mmol/L, normal serum potassium level of 4.6 mmol/L, blood glucose level of 130 mg/dL, normal magnesium level of 2.3 mg/dL, modest hyperphosphatemia level of 5.3 mg/dL, calcium level of 9.1 mg/dL, and a mild metabolic acidosis with a serum bicarbonate level of 17 mmol/L. The patient was seen by the Nephrology consultation service who recommended continuing aggressive intravenous fluid (IVF) hydration and strict urine output monitoring and deferred on initiating renal replacement therapy at the time. The patient had placement of an indwelling Foley catheter for strict urine output measurement. His urinalysis was mainly unrevealing showing no glucosuria, no proteinuria, 11 white blood cells, 6 red blood cells per high-power field, and a specific gravity of 1.010. His calculated fractional extraction of sodium (FeNa) was 6% indicating an intrinsic renal or post-obstructive cause. As we continued aggressive IVF hydration, patient's urine output improved and so did his mental status. He became more awake and alert and was able to provide better history. Other workups during hospital course included a negative HIV and negative hepatitis C serology. He had a known history of hepatitis B, and his serology demonstrated prior exposure with developed immunity (positive Hep B core antibody, positive Hep B surface antibody, and a negative Hep B surface antigen). The patient also had normal C3 and C4 levels. C-ANCA and P-ANCA testings were also negative. The creatinine phosphokinase (CPK) level was only modestly elevated to 493 u/L, which is insufficient to explain the degree of renal impairment in the patient. As we continued aggressive hydration, his renal function continued to improve with a quicker fall in the serum creatinine compared to the BUN. Other laboratory testings included an elevated iPTH level of 275.4 pg/mL. The patient also underwent a computed tomography (CAT) scan of the abdomen and pelvis without intravenous contrast that showed no acute pathology in the abdomen, and a renal ultrasound did not show any evidence of obstruction bilaterally but, however, did report mildly echogenic kidneys consistent with medical renal disease. After 11 days of hospitalization, the patient had fully returned to his baseline mental status and was stable for discharge to home. His chemistry on the final day of hospitalization showed a BUN level of 39, serum creatinine level of 1.8 mg/dL, and serum bicarbonate level of 23 mmol/L.

3. Discussion

Although the patient's renal function had not returned to normal limits at time of discharge, there was substantial improvement in his serum BUN and Cr from time of admission in comparison to the day of discharge as shown in Figure 1. There was also marked improvement in his clinical and mental status throughout his hospitalization. It is very likely that our patient has underlying chronic kidney disease stage II or III and the BUN/Cr values at discharge are his baseline renal function. His baseline chronic kidney disease diagnosis is suggested by his elevated iPTH and a normal serum calcium, indicative of some bone mineral disease often seen with chronic kidney disease. His renal ultrasounds also showed evidence of underlying medical renal

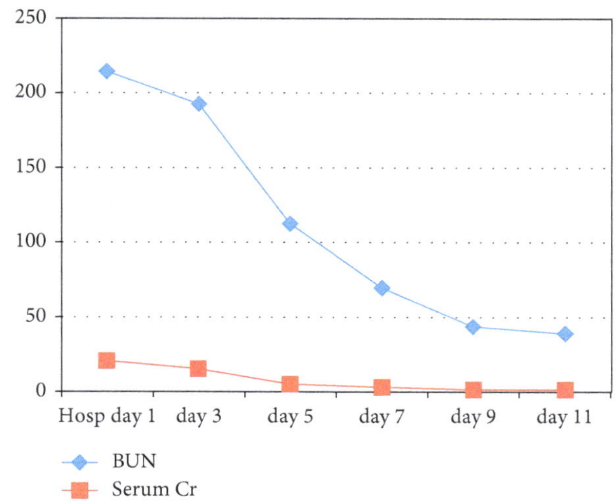

FIGURE 1: Table showing relationship between patient's renal functional markers (BUN/Cr in mg/dL) over days during the course of hospitalization.

disease, which supports this notion. The patient's baseline chronic kidney disease is likely the result of his untreated longstanding hypertension. We believe that an acute insult led to his ARF and uremia. Through extensive diagnostic testing and careful history taking, we concluded that it is most likely the patient's occupational exposure to jet fuel is implicated in causing his acute nephropathy. Fortunately, we were able to reverse the majority of the damage with aggressive intravenous and then oral fluid hydration. A kidney biopsy would have been helpful in establishing the exact renal pathology and diagnosis but was not pursued in this case because of resolution of the acute renal failure.

To conclude, the assessment of a patient with acute kidney injury should involve a comprehensive history, including an inquiry of potential environmental or occupational exposures. History of either potential toxin exposure or suggestion of Mesoamerican nephropathy may redirect management of kidney injury from other potential pathologies. Further investigation is necessary to establish a relationship between jet fuels and kidney injury.

Acknowledgments

The authors thank the Brooklyn Health Disparities Center and Dr. Moro O. Salifu, MD, MBA, MPH, MACP, Professor and Chairman of Medicine at SUNY Downstate University Hospital.

References

[1] Components of conventional jet fuel," https://www.icao.int/environmental-protection/Pages/AltFuels-Paraffins.aspx.

[2] Turbine Fuel, Aviation Kerosine Type, Jet A-1 Archived 2010-08-14 at the UK Government Web Archive. Ministry of Defence (UK), 2008.

[3] ASTM D1655-09a, *Standard Specification for Aviation Turbine Fuels*, ASTM International, West Conshohocken, PA, USA, 2010.

[4] L. M. Tormoehler, K. J. Tekulve, and K. A. Nañagas, "Hydrocarbon toxicity a review," *Clinical Toxicology*, vol. 52, no. 5, pp. 479–489, 2014.

[5] National Research Council (US), *Subcommittee on Permissible Exposure Levels for Military Fuels. Permissible Exposure Levels for Selected Military Fuel Vapors*, National Academies Press, Washington DC, USA, 1996, https://www.ncbi.nlm.nih.gov/books/NBK231243/.

[6] N. Brautbar, "Industrial solvents and kidney disease," *International Journal of Occupational and Environmental Health*, vol. 10, no. 1, pp. 79–83, 2004.

[7] Abdulkareem Alsuwaida Saudi University, "Jet fuel intoxication and acute renal failure," *Saudi Journal of Kidney Diseases and Transplantation*, vol. 21, no. 1, pp. 150–152, 2010.

[8] K. Bergman and L.-E. Appelgren, "Application and results of whole-body autoradiography in distribution studies of organic solvents," *CRC Critical Reviews in Toxicology*, vol. 12, no. 1, pp. 59–118, 1983.

[9] R. Toftgård and J.-Å. Gustafsson, "Biotransformation of organic solvents. a review," *Scandinavian Journal of Work, Environment & Health*, vol. 6, no. 1, pp. 1–18, 1980.

21

Severe Hypocalcemia and Dramatic Increase in Parathyroid Hormone after Denosumab in a Dialysis Patient: A Case Report and Review of the Literature

Ravinder D. Bhanot[1,2] **Jasleen Kaur**[2] **and Zeenat Bhat**[2,3]

[1]*Division of Pulmonary and Critical Care, St. Mary's of Michigan Medical Center, Saginaw, MI, USA*
[2]*Department of Internal Medicine, Wayne State University, Detroit, MI, USA*
[3]*Division of Nephrology, Department of Internal Medicine, Wayne State University, Detroit, MI, USA*

Correspondence should be addressed to Ravinder D. Bhanot; ravinder.bhanot@ascension.org

Academic Editor: Rumeyza Kazancioglu

Chronic kidney disease-mineral and bone disorder (CKD-MBD) is frequently present in advanced stages of chronic kidney disease (CKD) patients with high risk of fracture and elevated socioeconomic burden. Denosumab, an injectable human monoclonal antibody with affinity for nuclear factor-kappa ligand (RANKL), is an effective treatment for osteoporosis in postmenopausal women and men. Unlike the bisphosphonates, the pharmacokinetics and pharmacodynamics of denosumab are not influenced by the renal function and are being increasingly used for patients having CKD-MBD with low bone mineral density (BMD) to reduce the risk of fragility fractures. Hypocalcemia is a known side effect of this drug along with compensatory increase in parathyroid hormone (PTH). However, limited information is available in the literature regarding this potentially life-threatening side effect with denosumab in end-stage renal disease (ESRD) patients on dialysis. We present a patient with ESRD on peritoneal dialysis who developed severe symptomatic hypocalcemia and dramatic increase in PTH following denosumab therapy. She was conservatively managed with calcium supplementation and appropriate adjustment in calcium dialysate. We have also reviewed the literature on the use of denosumab in dialysis patients and looked at additional factors that may precipitate severe hypocalcemia in these patients. We believe that denosumab should be used with caution in dialysis patients since it may lead to profound hypocalcemia. Clinicians should ensure special attention in recognizing patients at risk of developing this serious adverse effect, so that prompt treatment and preventive strategies can be implemented.

1. Introduction

Disorders of mineral and bone metabolism are common sequelae of chronic kidney disease (CKD) that are collectively termed as chronic kidney disease-mineral and bone disorder (CKD-MBD). It often leads to increased bone fragility and fractures, due to varying combinations of low bone mineral content and abnormal bone quality. More severe stages of CKD (stages 4–5D) are associated with progressively reduced bone mineral density (BMD), a higher prevalence of fracture [1], and a mortality rate after fracture about twice as high as that compared to those without severe CKD [2].

Denosumab is a fully human monoclonal antibody that specifically binds to the receptor activator of nuclear factor-κB ligand (RANKL) [3] leading to reduced osteoclast activity and bone resorption. When compared with bisphosphonates, it has greater effectiveness in increasing bone mineral density (BMD) [4] and better pharmacologic profile especially in CKD patients and is being increasingly used for patients having CKD-MBD with low BMD to reduce the risk of fragility fractures. It is known to cause severe hypocalcemia in certain high-risk individuals along with compensatory increase in parathyroid hormone (PTH); however, there have been few reported cases in peritoneal dialysis patients [5]. We present a patient with ESRD on peritoneal dialysis who developed severe symptomatic hypocalcemia and dramatic increase in PTH following denosumab therapy. We also reviewed the literature on the use of denosumab in dialysis

TABLE 1: Laboratory data at baseline and after denosumab therapy.

Laboratory parameters	Before treatment	After denosumab therapy			Reference range
		Day 10	Day 15	Day 30	
Corrected Calcium (mg/dL)	9.9	6.9	8.7	9.3	8.4 – 10.2
Phosphorus (mg/dl)	3.8	3.1	3.6	3.6	2.5 – 5.0
Intact PTH (pg/ml)	442	2601	799	349	150 – 300 (Caucasian Dialysis patients)
Alkaline phosphatase (U/L)	96	84	54	49	34- 104
25-OH Vitamin D (ng/ml)	35	-	-	-	30 - 100

patients and looked at additional factors that may precipitate severe hypocalcemia in them.

2. Case Report

A 55-year-old Caucasian woman on peritoneal dialysis for the last three years due to lupus nephritis was seen in the dialysis clinic for a routine follow-up. Her medical problems included hypertension, secondary hyperparathyroidism, and documented osteoporosis on DEXA scan (Dual energy X-ray absorptiometry) with left femoral neck BMD at 0.637 g/cm^2; 2.9 standard deviation below peak BMD. Her medications included Amlodipine 5mg, Cinacalcet 60 mg, and Epoetin weekly injections.

She complained of fatigue, muscle cramps, and paresthesias of the hands and feet for the past week. Vital signs were stable. Physical exam was unremarkable with negative Chvostek's and Trousseau's signs. Laboratory work-up showed profound hypocalcemia with a total calcium level of 6.4 mg/dL with corrected calcium level of 6.9mg/dL (serum albumin level of 3.4 g/dL) and markedly increased serum intact PTH level (iPTH) of 2601 pg/mL (Table 1). Serum phosphate and serum alkaline phosphatase level was within normal reference range at 3.1 mg/dl and 84 U/L, respectively. Upon history taking, she was found to have received a new medication, denosumab 60mg subcutaneously, prescribed by her rheumatologist 10 days prior to the current presentation.

Before the administration of denosumab, the patient had normal serum values of calcium (9.5 mg/dL), phosphorus (3.8 mg/dL), alkaline phosphatases (96 U/L), and 25 vitamin D with slightly elevated iPTH level at 442 pg/mL. The patient was supplemented with 3,000 mg/dL of oral calcium along with oral Calcitriol 0.5mcg daily and Cinacalcet was held. The peritoneal dialysis solution was also changed from low calcium to regular calcium. All these measures resolved her symptoms with serum calcium normalizing (corrected calcium, 8.7 mg/dL) 5 days later whereas iPTH took almost 4 weeks to come back to baseline level (Table 1). Subsequently, she was managed as an out-patient with close monitoring of calcium homeostasis.

3. Discussion

CKD is characterized by spectrum of mineral and bone disorders (CKD-MBD) that worsen with progressive loss of kidney function and is associated with an increased risk of fragility (low trauma) fractures. Presently, there is no established effective therapy for patients having CKD-MBD with low BMD (stage 4-5D) or fragility fractures [2, 5]. Bisphosphonates, which are the longest established and most widely prescribed osteoporosis treatment class, are not recommended in patients with severe renal impairment due to their direct nephrotoxic effect, risks of adynamic bone disease, and prolonged retention in the bone [2].

Denosumab is an anti-resorptive drug which has been FDA approved since 2010 for the treatment of post-menopausal osteoporosis and recently for the prevention of skeletal-related events in patients with bone metastases [6, 7]. It is a fully human monoclonal antibody directed against the receptor activator of nuclear factor-$\kappa\beta$ (RANK) ligand. Normally, binding of RANK ligand to its receptor results in activation of osteoclasts, and thus inactivating the RANK ligand with denosumab reduces osteoclasts activity and bone resorption. It is cleared by the reticuloendothelial system and treatment efficacy of denosumab is neither affected by kidney function nor it affects the kidney function [8]. When compared with bisphosphonates, it offers improved efficacy, better tolerability, and convenient administration via subcutaneous injection making it a preferable choice in patients with advanced kidney disease [9].

However, despite these benefits, denosumab has been associated with severe hypocalcemia which is usually asymptomatic but can also present in certain high-risk patients with serious manifestations, including cardiac arrhythmia and death [5, 10]. The generally recognized risk factors for hypocalcemia include osteoblastic metastases, high bone turnover states, elevated alkaline phosphatase, vitamin D deficiency, concomitant bisphosphonates use, and renal dysfunction with creatinine clearance (CrCl) of less than 30 mL/min and/or dialysis dependence [10]. A recently published meta-analysis of six observational studies [11] assessing the incidence of denosumab-associated hypocalcemia in 84 ESRD patients found that the pooled estimated incidence of hypocalcemia was as high as 42% (95% CI 29–55%, $I^2 = 0\%$). The authors cautioned against the use of this medication in ESRD patients even though there was significant increase in BMD proving its efficacy in these patients. In another study of the 85 women with postmenopausal osteoporosis treated with denosumab, 22 (25.9%) developed hypocalcemia who had significantly higher bone turnover markers at baseline (e.g., total N-terminal propeptide of type 1 procollagen, tartrate-resistant acid phosphatase 5b, etc.) suggesting that high bone turnover is potentially a risk factor in denosumab-induced hypocalcemia [12]. Our patient had ESRD, secondary hyperparathyroidism that is associated with a high bone turnover status, and was on Cinacalcet, thus posing a high cumulative risk for development of hypocalcemia on receiving denosumab.

The transient increase in PTH is expected after the drug administration which helps to maintain calcium homeostasis. This is mostly seen in patients with severe renal impairment (CrCl<30 mL/min) or on dialysis, in whom secondary hyperparathyroidism is also common, making it an expected finding. In a retrospective study performed in 14 patients with CKD stages 4–5 treated with denosumab [5], a 3.1-fold rise in the mean PTH level was observed at the time of the corrected calcium nadir (defined as the lowest observed corrected calcium level occurring in the first 90 days after receiving the medication). However, our patient had a dramatic increase in her iPTH which has been sporadically reported before. Torregrosa [13] published intense prolonged hypocalcemia and hyperparathyroidism after denosumab in a kidney transplanted patient while Martin-Gomez and colleagues [14] recently reported similar results in a hemodialysis patient. Consistent with these reported cases, this finding is likely the result of profound hypocalcemia in our patient who already had severe secondary hyperparathyroidism necessitating Cinacalcet therapy at baseline.

Denosumab-induced hypocalcemia usually lasts for few weeks and the risk has been found to be highest in the first 2 weeks [15]. However, certain case reports indicate that it can be more prolonged lasting up to 5-6 months [16]. Hyperparathyroidism correction appears to lag behind in most of the reported patients similar to our case. Treatment usually includes calcium and vitamin D supplementation, dose reduction or stoppage of hypocalcemic agents such as Cinacalcet, and dialysis using high calcium dialysate in severe, resistant cases [5, 9].

To conclude, the usage of denosumab has increased for osteoporosis. However, its use in patients with advanced chronic kidney disease requires caution since it may lead to profound hypocalcemia. There appears to be lack of widespread awareness among prescribing practitioners and communication gap with the nephrology team that may be contributing to this side effect being still prevalent. Having said that, recent meta-analysis does suggest an efficacy of denosumab in the improvement in BMD among ESRD patients on dialysis and the benefit of the drug is prevailing. We advocate careful consideration before using denosumab in dialysis patients and notifying patient's nephrologist when initiating the treatment so that close biochemical monitoring can be arranged. Certain preventive strategies including appropriate adjustment in calcium dialysate, adequate calcium and vitamin D supplementation, and avoiding concomitant use of hypocalcemic agents such as Cinacalcet can help to potentially prevent symptomatic hypocalcemia in ESRD patients treated with denosumab.

References

[1] S. Klawansky, E. Komaroff, P. F. Cavanaugh Jr. et al., "Relationship between age, renal function and bone mineral density in the US population," *Osteoporosis International*, vol. 14, no. 7, pp. 570–576, 2003.

[2] Kidney Disease: Improving Global Outcomes (KDIGO) CKD-MBD Work Group, "KDIGO clinical practice guideline for the diagnosis, evaluation, prevention, and treatment of Chronic Kidney Disease-Mineral and Bone Disorder (CKD-MBD)," *Kidney International*, vol. 76, pp. S1–S130, 2009.

[3] S. R. Cummings, J. S. Martin, M. R. McClung et al., "Denosumab for prevention of fractures in postmenopausal women with osteoporosis," *The New England Journal of Medicine*, vol. 361, no. 8, pp. 756–765, 2009.

[4] C. Beaudoin, S. Jean, L. Bessette, L.-G. Ste-Marie, L. Moore, and J. P. Brown, "Denosumab compared to other treatments to prevent or treat osteoporosis in individuals at risk of fracture: a systematic review and meta-analysis," *Osteoporosis International*, vol. 27, no. 9, pp. 2835–2844, 2016.

[5] V. Dave, C. Y. Chiang, J. Booth, and P. F. Mount, "Hypocalcemia post denosumab in patients with chronic kidney disease stage 4-5," *American Journal of Nephrology*, vol. 41, no. 2, pp. 129–137, 2015.

[6] B. B. McCormick, J. Davis, and K. D. Burns, "Severe hypocalcemia following denosumab injection in a hemodialysis patient," *American Journal of Kidney Diseases*, vol. 60, no. 4, pp. 626–628, 2012.

[7] U. Brown-Glaberman and A. T. Stopeck, "Role of denosumab in the management ofskeletal complications in patients with bone metastases from solid tumors," *Biologics*, vol. 6, pp. 89–99, 2012.

[8] M. A. Tabrizi, C.-M. L. Tseng, and L. K. Roskos, "Elimination mechanisms of therapeutic monoclonal antibodies," *Drug Discovery Therapy*, vol. 11, no. 1-2, pp. 81–88, 2006.

[9] S. Saleem, S. Patel, A. Ahmed, and N. Saleem, "Denosumab causing severe, refractory hypocalcaemia in a patient with chronic kidney disease," *BMJ Case Reports*, 2018.

[10] K. A. Autio, A. Farooki, I. G. Glezerman et al., "Severe hypocalcemia associated with denosumab in metastatic castration-resistant prostate cancer: risk factors and precautions for treating physicians," *Clinical Genitourinary Cancer*, vol. 13, no. 4, pp. 305–319, 2019.

[11] C. Thongprayoon, P. Acharya, C. Acharya et al., "Hypocalcemia and bone mineral density changes following denosumab treatment in end-stage renal disease patients: a meta-analysis of observational studies," *Osteoporosis International*, vol. 29, no. 8, pp. 1737–1745, 2018.

[12] K. Ishikawa, T. Nagai, K. Sakamoto et al., "High bone turnover elevates the risk of denosumab-induced hypocalcemia in women with postmenopausal osteoporosis," *Therapeutics and Clinical Risk Management*, vol. 12, pp. 1831–1840, 2016.

[13] J.-V. Torregrosa, "Dramatic increase in parathyroid hormone and hypocalcemia after denosumab in a kidney transplanted patient," *Clinical Kidney Journal*, vol. 6, no. 1, p. 122, 2013.

[14] M. A. Martin-Gomez, P. E. Martinez, M. A. Hidalgo Rico et al., "Intense prolonged hypocalcemia and hyperparathyroidism after denosumab in hemodialysis patients in response to the published article," *Clinical Practice*, vol. 12, no. 1, pp. 5–7, 2015.

[15] H. Ikesue, T. Tsuji, K. Hata et al., "Time course of calcium concentrations and risk factors for hypocalcemia in patients receiving denosumab for the treatment of bone metastases from

cancer," *Annals of Pharmacotherapy*, vol. 48, no. 9, pp. 1159–1165, 2014.

[16] P. Ivanov and M. Khedr, "Prolonged hypocalcaemia following single doses of 60 mg denosumab in two patients with CKD 4/5 on Cinacalcet treatment for tertiary hyperparathyroidism," *Clinical Kidney Journal*, vol. 6, no. 2, p. 245, 2013.

22

Portal Vein Thrombosis in a 21-Year-Old Man with Membranoproliferative Glomerulonephritis and Nephrotic Syndrome

Ilya Seleznev,[1] Dinara Jumadilova,[1] Assiya Naushabayeva,[2] Kairat Kabulbayev,[2] Gulaiym Karashasheva,[3] and Francesca Cainelli[1]

[1] *Department of Medicine, Nazarbayev University School of Medicine, Nur-Sultan, Kazakhstan*
[2] *Research Institute of Cardiology and Medicine, Almaty, Kazakhstan*
[3] *National Scientific Center for Oncology and Transplantation, Nur-Sultan, Kazakhstan*

Correspondence should be addressed to Francesca Cainelli; francescacainelli@yahoo.it

Academic Editor: Sophia Lionaki

Membranoproliferative glomerulonephritis, one of the main causes of nephrotic syndrome, is associated with a state of hypercoagulability that leads to increased risk of thrombotic events. Portosystemic collaterals may reopen due to reversal of the flow within the existing veins and be a presenting feature of thrombosis. We describe a patient who presented with large portosystemic collaterals and signs of portal hypertension and was subsequently found to be affected by membranous proliferative glomerulonephritis. Proteinuria and microscopic haematuria in a patient with signs of portal hypertension and no pre-existing liver disease should raise the suspicion of an underlying kidney disease.

1. Introduction

Membranoproliferative glomerulonephritis is one of the main causes of nephrotic syndrome in adults and can cause renal failure [1]. Renal vein and deep vein thrombosis may be associated with the nephrotic syndrome [2–5], and the risk appears to depend on the duration and severity of the syndrome and to correlate with very low albumin levels. Portal vein thrombosis has been rarely reported [6–8].

2. Case Presentation

A 21-year-old Kazakh man was referred to the National Research Center for Oncology and Transplantation in Astana, Kazakhstan, in October 2017 because of portosystemic shunts secondary to portal vein thrombosis. The past medical history did not reveal abdominal trauma, previous surgery, omphalitis, gastrointestinal bleeding, or hepatitis. The patient had been healthy until March 2017, when he developed lumbar pain, malaise, peripheral oedema, and nausea and began to lose weight. In May 2017, he felt right upper quadrant discomfort and developed abdominal distension; an abdominal ultrasound revealed splenomegaly and ascites. Liver cirrhosis was suspected. Alanine aminotransferase and aspartate aminotransferase levels were within the normal range; HBsAg, anti-HCV, and tumour markers (CEA, Ca19-9, and alpha- fetoprotein) were negative, total protein and albumin levels were reduced (49.2 g/L and 22.6 g/L, respectively), and total cholesterol increased (6.6 mmol/L; normal 3.1-5.2). Urea, creatinine, and electrolyte levels were normal. An EGDS showed superficial distal gastritis; oesophageal or gastric varices were not detected.

In June 2017, an abdominal CT scan confirmed the presence of splenomegaly and mild ascites and detected voluminous paraoesophageal varices, left splenorenal shunts, and hepatomegaly. A Doppler ultrasound of the liver showed no flow in the portal vein and its branches and enlarged splenic vein (diameter 1.7 cm) with laminar blood flow. The patient received a provisional diagnosis of portal vein thrombosis and was started on IV heparin, which was stopped

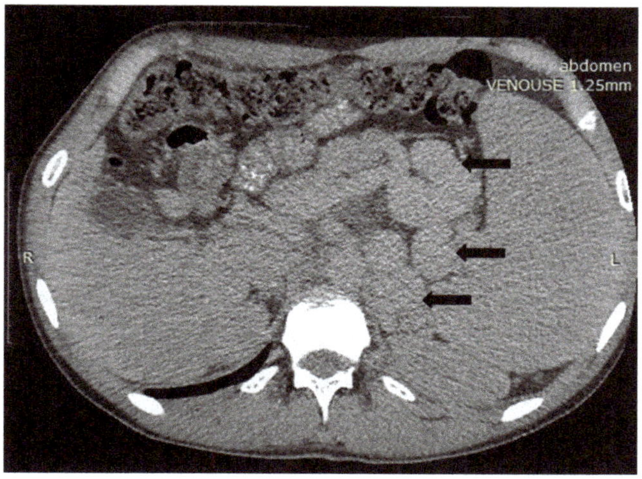

FIGURE 1: Axial postcontrast CT shows voluminous splenorenal collaterals (arrows).

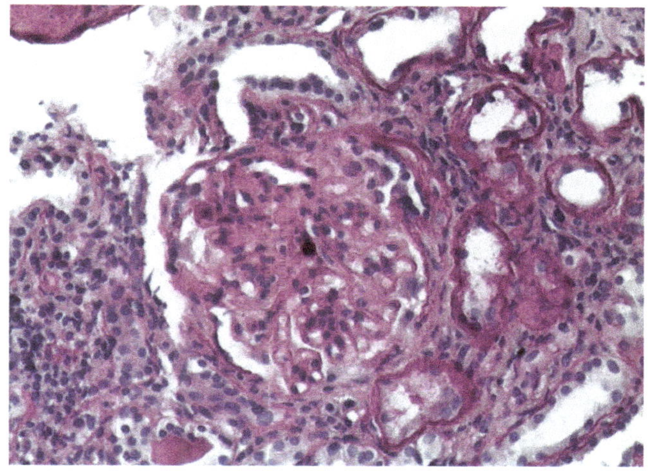

FIGURE 2: PAS x 300 Glomerulus with lobular presentation, widened mesangium, and thickened capillary walls.

four days later because of worsening thrombocytopenia. Further serologic tests revealed subclinical hypothyroidism and hypergammaglobulinemia (25.8%); ANA and AMA were negative. A urine test showed proteinuria (1.3 to 2.0 g/L) and microscopic haematuria (18-22 RBC/high power field). The patient was started on spironolactone 100 mg/day and torasemide 5 mg/day.

In October 2017, he was admitted to the National Research Center for Oncology and Transplantation and underwent mesentericoportography, which showed hepatic arterial buffer response, an indirect sign of reduced or absent blood flow in the portal vein. An abdominal ultrasound did not visualise the portal vein and showed an enlarged spleen. Lab tests revealed mild leukopenia (3.6 WBC/μL), normocytic normochromic anaemia (Hb 9.8 g/dL), thrombocytopenia (80,000 platelets/μL), proteinuria (2.1 g/L), and microscopic haematuria. Further tests revealed that the patient was heterozygous for both factor V Leiden (FV) and methylenetetrahydrofolate reductase (MTHFR) genes; methionine synthase (MTR) A2756G mutation was not detected. IgM and IgG anticardiolipin antibodies and antiphospholipid antibodies were negative, and homocysteine levels were normal.

A revision of the images of the CT scan performed in June 2017 revealed voluminous collaterals between the left renal and the splenic veins, paraoesophageal varices, dilatation of the superior mesenteric vein with lack of visualization of the intrahepatic portal branches, dilatation of the left renal vein with a possible filling defect, and enlarged left kidney (Figure 1).

In May 2018, the patient was admitted to another hospital where an echocardiography showed global enlargement of the cardiac chambers and hypertrophy of the posterior wall of the left ventricle (1.3 cm) with normal ejection fraction, II degree mitral valve regurgitation, I degree aortic regurgitation, and no signs of pulmonary hypertension. Arterial blood pressure monitoring revealed Max BP – 173/86 mm Hg, Average BP - 145/73 mm Hg, max BP (night) 141/70 mm Hg, and average BP (night) – 122/57 mm Hg. Indices of average BP were elevated during night and day, being 92% and 58%, respectively. A kidney biopsy showed moderate to severe mesangial hyper cellularity, dilation of mesangial matrix with focal lymphocytic stasis in the capillary space, basal membrane thickening of capillary loops with well-defined fuchsinophilic granules and focal total glomerulosclerosis (16%), grade II epithelial renal tubular dysplasia, diffused moderate fibrosis of the interstitium, tubular atrophy, intimal fibrosis, and hypertrophy of the arterial muscle layer of middle calibre with narrowing of one artery to 1/3 (Figures 2 and 3). A diagnosis of membranoproliferative glomerulonephritis was made and the patient was started on methylprednisolone (64 mg/day, tapering down to 16 mg/day maintenance dose) and perindopril 10 mg/day. Unfortunately the response to treatment was not optimal, leakage of ascitic fluid from the umbilicus developed, and further deterioration of the renal function led to haemodialysis. No episodes of bleeding or clinically symptomatic thrombosis occurred after the diagnosis.

3. Discussion

The portal vein thrombosis in our patient, who was not cirrhotic, was most likely due to the nephrotic state, a condition where depletion of intravascular volume, high fibrinogen levels and deposition as fibrin, increased platelet aggregation, urinary loss of anticoagulant factors (free Protein S, antithrombin III), and loss of fluid from the intravascular compartment with ensuing haemoconcentration contribute to a heightened thrombosis risk [9]. The few reported cases of portal vein thrombosis in nephrotic patients have indeed all occurred in males [6–8].

In our case the diagnosis of membranoproliferative glomerulonephritis was delayed as the patient presented with established signs of portal hypertension, and the presence of proteinuria and microhaematuria was not given due attention. The factor V Leiden heterozygous state might have

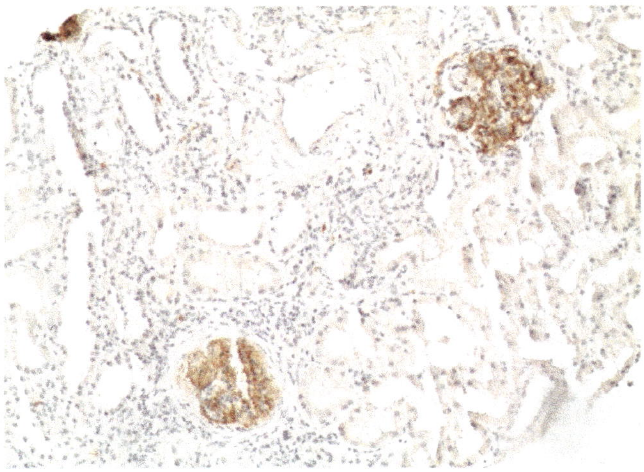

Figure 3: C4d x150.

contributed to the development of thrombosis in our patient but contrasting data have been reported in the literature with the risk being increased [10, 11] or not [12] in nephrotic patients heterozygous for FV mutation.

4. Conclusion

The possibility of a nephrotic syndrome should be considered when assessing a patient with unexplained portal vein thrombosis/portosystemic shunts.

Authors' Contributions

All authors were involved in the intellectual content, interpretation, and writing of the manuscript.

References

[1] S. Sethi and F. C. Fervenza, "Membranoproliferative glomerulonephritis — a new look at an old entity," *The New England Journal of Medicine*, vol. 366, no. 12, pp. 1119–1131, 2012.

[2] F. Llach, "Hypercoagulability, renal vein thrombosis, and other thrombotic complications of nephrotic syndrome," *Kidney International*, vol. 28, no. 3, pp. 429–439, 1985.

[3] R. J. Crew, J. Radhakrishnan, and G. Appel, "Complications of the nephrotic syndrome and their treatment," *Clinical Nephrology*, vol. 62, no. 4, pp. 245–259, 2004.

[4] R. Singhal and K. S. Brimble, "Thromboembolic complications in the nephrotic syndrome: pathophysiology and clinical management," *Thrombosis Research*, vol. 118, no. 3, pp. 397–407, 2006.

[5] B. Barbano, A. Gigante, A. Amoroso, and R. Cianci, "Thrombosis in nephrotic syndrome," *Seminars in Thrombosis and Hemostasis*, vol. 39, no. 5, pp. 469–476, 2013.

[6] V. Unni, J. Varghese, A. Mathew, N. Seethalekshmy, and G. Kurian, "Isolated portal vein thrombosis in nephrotic syndrome," *Indian Journal of Nephrology*, vol. 17, no. 1, pp. 26–28, 2007.

[7] B. S. Park, S. Park, K. Jin et al., "Nephrotic syndrome complicated with portal, splenic, and superior mesenteric vein thrombosis," *Kidney Research and Clinical Practice*, vol. 33, no. 3, pp. 161–164, 2014.

[8] E. M. Plaisier, B. Legallicier, J. M. Faintuch, and P. M. Ronco, "Acute portal vein thrombosis at the onset of a nephrotic syndrome," *Nephrology Dialysis Transplantation* , vol. 11, no. 4, pp. 696–698, 1996.

[9] F. Llach, "Thromboembolic complications in nephrotic syndrome. coagulation abnormalities, renal vein thrombosis and other conditions," *Postgraduate Medical Journal*, vol. 76, no. 6, pp. 111–123, 1984.

[10] J. Martínez Ara, R. Gómez Rioja, C. Riñón, M. S. García Muñoz, M. L. Ruiz Caravaca, and J. L. Miguel, "Prevalence of genetic prothrombotic factors (factor V Leiden and II20210 prothrombin mutation) in glomerular nephropathies with or without thrombosis," *Nefrología*, vol. 20, no. 2, pp. 139–144, 2000.

[11] M. Sahin, S. Ozkurt, N. A. Degirmenci, A. Musmul, G. Temiz, and M. Soydan, "Assessment of genetic risk factors for thromboembolic complications in adults with idiopathic nephrotic syndrome," *Clinical Nephrology*, vol. 79, no. 6, pp. 454–462, 2013.

[12] A. B. Irish, "The factor V Leiden mutation and risk of renal vein thrombosis in patients with nephrotic syndrome," *Nephrology Dialysis Transplantation* , vol. 12, no. 8, pp. 1680–1683, 1997.

Renal Mucormycosis: Post-COVID-19 Infection Presenting as Unilateral Hydronephrosis in a Young Immunocompetent Male

Rabin Nepali[1] **Shreya Shrivastav,**[2] **and Dibya Singh Shah**[1]

[1]*Department of Nephrology and Transplant Medicine, Tribhuvan University Teaching Hospital, Kathmandu, Nepal*
[2]*Department of Pathology, Tribhuvan University Teaching Hospital, Kathmandu, Nepal*

Correspondence should be addressed to Rabin Nepali; rabinnepali@gmail.com

Academic Editor: David Mudge

Mucormycosis is a rare invasive fungal infection with a high mortality rate caused by members of the family Mucoraceae. It mainly affects immunocompromised hosts such as poorly controlled diabetes mellitus, previous solid organ transplant, high-dose steroids, and hematologic malignancy. The most common sites of the disease are rhinocerebral, the skin, the lungs, and the gastrointestinal tract. In this era of COVID-19 infection, there has been a significant rise in invasive mucormycosis predominantly reported from southeast. We present a case of isolated renal mucormycosis in an apparently healthy individual with post-COVID-19 infection presenting as unilateral hydronephrosis. Timely identifying at-risk populations and having a high degree of suspicion with involvement of multidisciplinary teams are of utmost importance to diagnose and treat a rare and fatal infection. Even if there is a long history, antifungal drugs and removal of the source can result in a good outcome.

1. Background

Mucormycosis is an invasive fungal infection caused by members of the family Mucoraceae [1]. The disease is known to affect patients with immunocompromised status from a variety of causes such as diabetes mellitus, hematologic malignancy, and HIV infection. The most common form of presentation is rhinocerebral infection although primary infections of the skin, the lungs, and the gastrointestinal tract have been reported [2]; however, isolated presentation of renal mucormycosis is rare [3].

With the ongoing COVID-19 pandemic and the use of high-dose steroids and antibiotics, there have been increasing reports of bacterial and fungal coinfections in the COVID-19 positive group of patients [4]. We report a rare case of isolated renal mucormycosis, post-COVID-19 infection, in an apparently healthy individual presenting as unilateral hydronephrosis.

2. Case Presentation

A previously healthy 39 years old male presented to us with complaints of burning micturition and a weak stream of urine for 1 month. He did not give a history of diabetes mellitus, hypertension, or other chronic illness. However, 5 months ago, he gave a history of being diagnosed with COVID-19 infection after developing fever and shortness of breath for 3 days. He was admitted at first to a private hospital for shortness of breath where he received IV dexamethasone along with other supportive treatment during which he developed high blood sugar and was shifted to the intensive care unit of another private hospital. During the treatment in the intensive care unit, he developed left-sided hemopneumothorax with bronchopleural fistula which was managed with chest tube insertion with negative suction. His sputum culture showed *Citrobacter koseri* and *Coagulase-negative staphylococcus* along with *Pseudomonas aeruginosa* in his blood culture for which he received multiple broad-spectrum antibiotics. After 6 weeks of treatment, he started having burning micturition and a weak urinary stream during micturition. He was again referred to another centre for further treatment where he underwent abdominal ultrasound which showed a polypoidal urinary bladder mass involving the right vesicoureteric junction and right hydroureteronephrosis. For this finding, he was referred to our centre. On evaluation, his hemoglobin was 10.6 gm/dl, total count of 7500/cmm, and platelets of 363000/cmm. His renal function test and liver function test were within normal limits with random blood sugar of 12 mmol/L. His urine routine and microscopy examination showed plenty of pus cells per high-power field, but his urine culture was sterile.

His contrast CT abdomen showed thickening and enhancement of the right distal ureter and the adjacent vesicoureteric junction (VUJ) region along with right distal hydroureter, and the report suggested features of a malignant lesion in the right VUJ and the distal ureter. It also showed right moderate hydronephrosis with pelvic ureteric junction narrowing and multiple nonenhancing hypodensities in the inter and lower pole cortex of the right kidney with perinephric fat strandings suggestive of chronic pyelonephritis (Figure 1). Suspecting malignancy, cystoscopy was carried out which showed necrotic mass peeping from the right ureteric orifice. The histopathological examination of the sample showed fungus with broad-based, aseptate hyphae suggestive of mucormycosis. He was then started on amphotericin B deoxycholate (1 mg/kg/day). His serum creatinine rose to a maximum of 330 micromol/L during his stay. Amphotericin B deoxycholate was changed to liposomal amphotericin B. His serum creatinine subsequently decreased to 160 micromol/L before his surgery. He underwent right radical nephroureterectomy (Figure 2). The histopathological examination confirmed mucormycosis (Figures 3(a) and 3(b)). He was continued on oral posaconazole. His serum creatinine at discharge was 113 micromol/L. In follow-up of 1 month in OPD, he was doing fine with stable renal function.

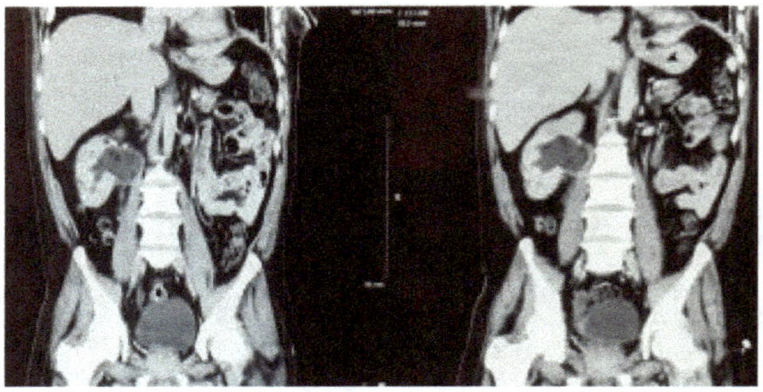

FIGURE 1: CT abdomen showed right-sided hydronephrosis.

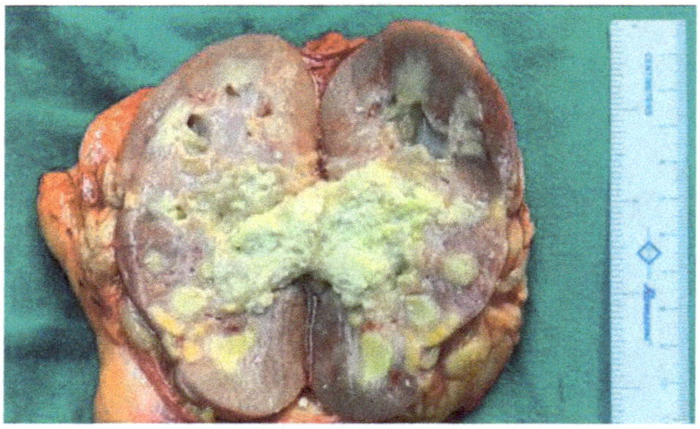

FIGURE 2: The cut section of the right kidney shows cheesy material infiltrating the renal pelvis and calyces.

3. Discussion

Mucormycosis is a rare infection characterized by invasion of vasculature resulting in infarction and necrosis of affected tissues [5]. Infection is almost exclusively found in immunocompromised hosts with the most common conditions being poorly controlled diabetes mellitus, previous solid organ or bone marrow transplant, high-dose steroids, and hematologic malignancy [6].

Renal mucormycosis in apparently healthy individuals is a very rare occurrence [7], and it typically develops from hematogenous spread in disseminated cases [8]. Isolated renal involvement is even more uncommon and speculated to be caused by ascending infection of the urinary tract [9]. Isolated renal mucormycosis usually presents with fever (88%), flank pain (70%), and hematuria or pyuria (70%) [6] with concomitant bacterial urosepsis in 53% [10]. Our case of renal mucormycosis had a rare presentation of unilateral hydronephrosis and pyelonephritis. Without early diagnosis and immediate aggressive treatment, renal mucormycosis is almost universally fatal [11].

In this era of COVID-19 infection, there has been a significant rise in invasive mucormycosis predominantly reported from Southeast Asia, especially India [12]. COVID-19 infection causes innate immune dysregulation which along with increased use of corticosteroids [13] and other immunosuppressants can lead to secondary bacterial and fungal infections. Along with these factors, the patient being in mechanical ventilation, administration of industrial-grade oxygen, use of multiple broad-spectrum antibiotics, prolonged hospital stay, exposure to invasive procedures, and generally poor hygiene of the patients also provide the perfect setting for secondary fungal infections [14]. Hyperglycemia also seems to be one of the predisposing factors which along with low pH leads to dysfunction of the polymorphonuclear cells and defective intracellular killing by both oxidative and nonoxidative mechanisms [15].

Definitive diagnosis is performed by positive cultures and histopathological demonstration of thick, nonseptate hyphae branching at the right angle [16]. Treatment of renal mucormycosis includes antifungals; amphotericin B, posaconazole, and isavuconazole are the only systemic antifungal drugs with activity against Mucorales, surgical debridement of the infected tissue (nephrectomy), and treatment of any predisposing condition [17, 18].

Given the high morbidity and mortality of these patients, a high degree of suspicion in appropriate clinical settings is of utmost importance in these cases for early diagnosis and treatment even if it is in an unusual location like in our case. The number of hospitals, multiple broad-spectrum antibiotics, high blood sugar levels, steroid administration, post-COVID-19 status, and lack of expertise in previous hospitals all played a significant role in delayed diagnosis of mucormycosis that could have been fatal. Computed tomography of the abdomen, cystoscopy, and histopathological examination

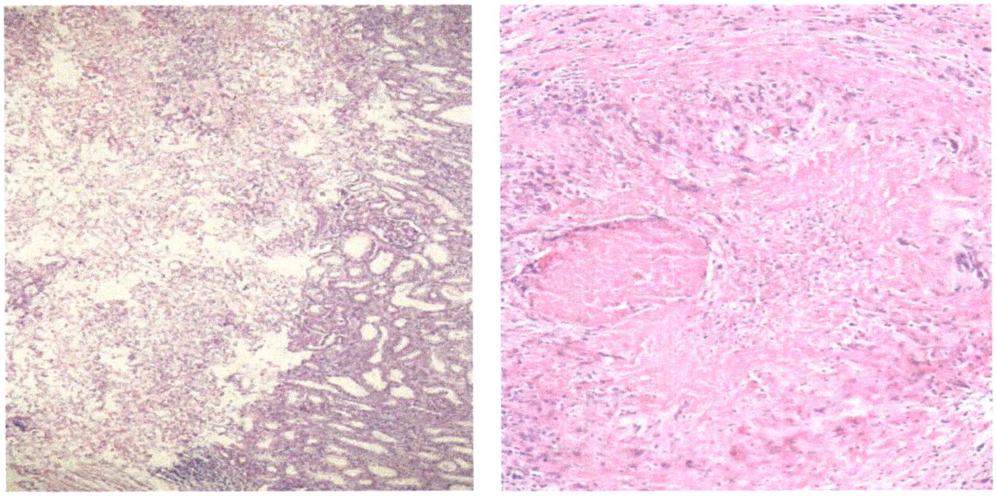

(a) (b)

Figure 3: (a) Renal parenchyma with abrupt necrosis and presence of broad-based, aseptate fungal hyphae showing 90° branching (HE × 100). (b) Invasion of the blood vessel by similar fungal profiles (PAS × 200).

should be performed urgently to reach a proper diagnosis. Forming multidisciplinary teams including nephrologists, urologists, pathologists, infectivologists, and microbiologists is essential for prompt management. Despite the high fatality in these cases, if proper treatment with antifungal agents and removal of the source by appropriate operation can be performed, a good outcome can be assured.

4. Conclusion

Timely identifying at-risk populations and having a high degree of suspicion with involvement of multidisciplinary teams are of utmost importance to diagnose and treat a rare and fatal infection like isolated renal mucormycosis presenting as unilateral hydronephrosis. The use of antifungal drugs and removal of the source can result in a good outcome.

Abbreviations

HIV:	Human immunodeficiency virus
Urine RE/ME:	Urine routine and microscopic examination
CT:	Computed tomography
VUJ:	Vesicoureteral junction
PUJ:	Pelvic ureteric junction.

Consent

Written informed consent for publication of clinical details and images was obtained from the patient.

Acknowledgments

The authors are grateful to the patient and family for allowing them to share the story of the patient. The authors would like to acknowledge Dr. Nishan Bhurtyal for helping in management of the patient.

References

[1] K. J. Kwon-Chung, "Taxonomy of fungi causing mucormycosis and entomophthoramycosis (zygomycosis) and nomenclature of the disease: molecular mycologic perspectives," *Clinical Infectious Diseases*, vol. 54, pp. S8–S15, 2012.

[2] B. Spellberg, J. Edwards, and A. Ibrahim, "Novel perspectives on mucormycosis: pathophysiology, presentation, and management," *Clinical Microbiology Reviews*, vol. 18, no. 3, pp. 556–569, 2005.

[3] S. K. Devana, V. G. Gupta, R. S. Mavuduru et al., "Isolated renal mucormycosis in immunocompetent hosts: clinical spectrum and management approach," *The American Journal of Tropical Medicine and Hygiene*, vol. 100, no. 4, pp. 791–797, 2019.

[4] L. Lansbury, B. Lim, V. Baskaran, and W. S. Lim, "Co-infections in people with COVID-19: a systematic review and meta-analysis," *Journal of Infection*, vol. 81, no. 2, pp. 266–275, 2020.

[5] H. S. Dhaliwal, A. Singh, S. K. Sinha et al., "Diagnosed only if considered: isolated renal mucormycosis," *The Lancet*, vol. 385, no. 9934, 2015.

[6] B. M. Marsh, R. Rajasingham, S. H. Tawfic, and M. S. Borofsky, "Successful conservative management of bilateral renal mucormycosis," *Urology*, vol. 120, pp. 2–5, 2018.

[7] A. Chakrabarti, A. Das, A. Sharma et al., "Ten years' experience in zygomycosis at a tertiary care centre in India," *Journal of Infection*, vol. 42, no. 4, pp. 261–266, 2001.

[8] D. Zygomycosis, "Report of four cases and review," https://academic.oup.com/cid/article-abstract/11/5/741/314198?redirectedFrom=fulltext.

[9] K. Gupta, R. Nada, K. Joshi, M. Rohilla, and R. Walia, "Can ascending infection from bladder serve as the portal of entry for primary renal zygomycosis?" *Mycopathologia*, vol. 170, no. 5, pp. 357–360, 2010.

[10] K. L. Gupta, K. Joshi, K. Sud et al., "Renal zygomycosis: an under-diagnosed cause of acute renal failure," *Nephrology Dialysis Transplantation*, vol. 14, no. 11, pp. 2720–2725, 1999.

[11] K. L. Gupta and A. Gupta, "Mucormycosis and acute kidney injury," *Journal of Nephropathology*, vol. 1, no. 3, pp. 155–159, 2012.

[12] A. Chakrabarti, H. Kaur, J. Savio et al., "Epidemiology and clinical outcomes of invasive mould infections in Indian intensive care units (FISF study)," *Journal of Critical Care*, vol. 51, pp. 64–70, 2019.

[13] The RECOVERY Collaborative Group, "Dexamethasone in hospitalized patients with COVID-19," *New England Journal of Medicine*, vol. 384, no. 8, pp. 693–704, 2021.

[14] V. Jain, G. Choudhary, A. Aggarwal, and R. Jena, "COVID-19 and fatal renal mucormycosis: contributory or coincidental?" *Indian Journal of Urology*, vol. 37, no. 3, 2021.

[15] A. S. Ibrahim, B. Spellberg, T. J. Walsh, and D. P. Kontoyiannis, "Pathogenesis of mucormycosis," *Clinical Infectious Diseases*, vol. 54, pp. S16–S22, 2012.

[16] E. Kursun, T. Turunc, Y. Z. Demiroglu, H. E. Alışkan, and A. H. Arslan, "Evaluation of 28 cases of mucormycosis," *Mycoses*, vol. 58, no. 2, pp. 82–87, 2015.

[17] B. Spellberg, T. J. Walsh, D. P. Kontoyiannis, J. Edwards Jr., and A. S. Ibrahim, "Recent advances in the management of mucormycosis: from bench to bedside," *Clinical Infectious Diseases*, vol. 48, no. 12, pp. 1743–1751, 2009.

[18] K. M. Parmar, S. Akif, S. Kumar, and P. Kaundal, "Isolated unilateral renal mucormycosis in a young immunocompetent male," *BMJ Case Reports*, vol. 14, no. 10, Article ID e245309, 2021.

24

"Recurrent Papillary Necrosis and Nephrocalcinosis Induced by Nonsteroidal Anti-Inflammatory Drugs for Gouty Arthritis Associated with Congenital Chloride-Losing Diarrhea: A Major Risk for Kidney Loss"

Kamel El-Reshaid,[1] **Shaikha Al-Bader**,[2] **and Hossameldin Sallam**[2]

[1]*Department of Medicine, Faculty of Medicine, Kuwait University, Kuwait City, Kuwait*
[2]*Department of Medicine, Nephrology Unit, Al-Amiri Hospital, Ministry of Health, Kuwait City, Kuwait*

Correspondence should be addressed to Kamel El-Reshaid; kamel_elreshaid@yahoo.com

Academic Editor: Yoshihide Fujigaki

Congenital chloride-losing diarrhea (CCLD) is a rare genetic disorder due to autosomal recessive mutation in the SLC26A3 gene on chromosome 7. It is characterized with chronic watery diarrhea with high fecal chloride (Cl: >90 mmol/L), low potassium (K), and metabolic alkalosis with low urinary Cl and K. The overall long-term prognosis is favorable with optimal life-long salt and K supplementation. In this case report, we describe a man with progressive renal failure and small kidneys that showed nephrocalcinosis and papillary necrosis. His disease was diagnosed since birth and was confirmed by our tests. He was incompliant with therapy and had developed gout. The latter complication of his disease has led to excessive NSAID use over the past years. Reinstitution of diet, drug therapy, and allopurinol had stabilized his renal disease for 1 year of follow-up. In conclusion, excessive analgesic use is a risk factor for renal failure in CCLD.

1. Introduction

Congenital chloride-losing diarrhea (CCLD) is a rare genetic disorder due to autosomal recessive mutation in the SLC26A3 gene on chromosome 7. The latter leads to defective intestinal chloride-bicarbonate exchanges, in epithelial sodium (Na)/hydrogen (H) transport through the Na/H exchangers (NHE2 and/or NHE3), with the resultant intestinal loss of chloride and retention of bicarbonate [1]. Consequently, the renin-angiotensin-aldosterone system is activated with Na reabsorption, potassium (K) excretion, and hypokalemia [2]. The first description of the disease was in 1945 by Gamble and Darrow, and nearly 250 cases have been reported to date [3]. Most of the cases have been reported from Finland, and their calculated prevalence was 1 in 43,000 newborns [4]. In Arab, only few cases have been reported in Saudi Arabia and Kuwait [5, 6]. The overall long-term prognosis is favorable with optimal life-long salt and K substitution though complications such as renal disease, hyperuricemia, inguinal hernias, spermatoceles, and decreased fertility reported in incompliant patients [7]. In this case report; we describe an adult patient, with this rare disease, who lost his kidneys due to chronic analgesic abuse for maltreated gouty arthritis.

2. The Case

A 30-year-old man presented with progressive nausea and vomiting over a few weeks. His past medical history revealed watery diarrhea since the age of 6 months. His investigations at that time have shown high stool chloride (Cl) >90 mmol/L with low serum and urinary Cl, potassium (K) and high uric acid (UA). Moreover, he had metabolic alkalosis. He had received high-salt diet in addition to slow K and calcium tablet. Twelve years ago, he had developed recurrent attacks of joint pains with high uric acid which was treated with

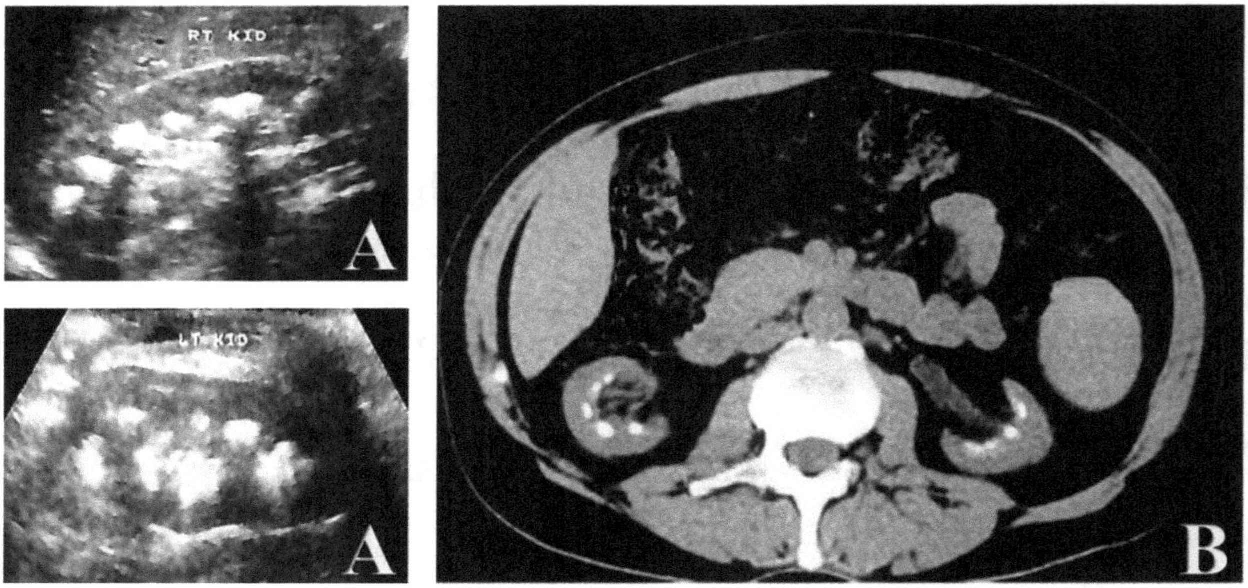

Figure 1: Ultrasound showing a small right kidney with nephrocalcinosis and calcified papilla (a) that was confirmed by CT scan (b).

multiple NSAIDs. On his initial presentation, the patient was conscious, oriented X3, and without distress of shortness of breath or pain. Blood pressure was 180/110 mmHg. He was afebrile with a body weight of 104 kg. He did not have jugular venous distension and oedema. Systemic examination did not show abnormality including lung auscultation. Laboratory investigations showed normal peripheral leucocytic and platelets counts. Hemoglobin was 104 g/L with normal MCV, transferrin saturation%, and vitamin B12. Serum urea and creatinine were elevated at 40 umol/L and 650 umol/L, respectively. Serum electrolytes revealed low sodium, Cl, calcium, and K at 129, 93, 1.8, and 2.9 mmol/L, respectively. Serum UA was elevated at 700 umol/L. Liver tests were normal with serum albumin at 41 g/L. Serum cholesterol and TSH were normal. Serum pH was 7.5, and bicarbonate was at 32 mmol/L. Urine routine and microscopy showed 1(+) proteinuria without hematuria and pyuria. Serum complements (C3 and C4), IgA level, and protein electrophoresis were normal. Anti-CCP, ANA, anti-ds DNA, ANCA, anti-GBM-antibodies, hepatitis B surface antigen, and anti-HCV antibodies were negative. Stool tests were negative for ova, parasites, and occult blood. Stool Cl was 120 mmol/L with zero urine Cl and K. Chest X-ray and ECG were normal. Abdominal and pelvic ultrasound did not show abnormality except for bilateral small kidneys at 8 cm with thin and echogenic cortex and few foci of papillary calcifications which were confirmed by CT scan examination (Figure 1). He was treated initially with intravenous KCl till K was >4 then with normal saline till establishing the euvolumic state. Subsequently, he required high salt and water with oral K supplementation (600 mg X2). Omeperazole 20 mg was added to protect KCl gastritis. His high uric acid was controlled with allopurinol 300 mg daily. With such measures, his electrolytes were corrected and serum creatinine decreased to 420 umol/L. On follow-up, he remained asymptomatic and his serum creatinine remained <500 umol/L for 1 year.

3. Discussion

Patients with CCLD have chronic watery diarrhea with high fecal Cl (>90 mmol/L), low K, and metabolic alkalosis with low urinary Cl and K [4]. Diagnosis is usually suspected with fetal abdominal distension and ultrasound features of polyhydramnios, hyperechoic bowel loops, honey comb appearance of the bowel, and dilated bowel loops with normal peristalsis [8]. Its differential diagnosis include Hirschsprung's disease, meconium ileus, anal atresia, and volvulus [9]. However, the characteristic laboratory findings assist in diagnosis and avoidance of unnecessary surgical interventions. Interestingly, it is the only diarrhea that produces metabolic alkalosis rather than metabolic acidosis. It can be differentiated from Barter's disease by having severe watery diarrhea, dehydration, failure to thrive, abdominal distention, and its electrolyte abnormalities. Contrary to Barter's, urine K is low with high Cl and its ease of correction of hypo K. Early diagnosis and treatment, with adequate salt and K, are essential for normal growth and development and prevention of other severe complications. The optimal dosage of electrolytes are Na 6 mmol/kg/day, K 6.5 mmol/kg/day, and Cl ranging from 12.5 mmol/kg/day, mmol/kg/day in infants, and less in older patients [5, 7]. The long-term disease complications have been attributed to chronic hypovolemia-induced nephrocalcinosis [10]. Virtually the majority of filtered Ca is absorbed passively in the paracellular route in the proximal convoluted tubules and ascending limb of Henle parallel to sodium. Only 10% is absorbed inversely to Na in the distal nephron [11]. Hence, with severe volume depletion, reabsorption of Ca is impaired leading to urine supersaturation and crystal precipitation with papillary calcification and nephrocalcinosis as in our patients. Moreover, maltreated gout, with NSAIDs, was a contributing factor in his papillary renal disease [12]. In conclusion; patients with CCLD should be adequately treated with salt and K supplementation and avoid NSAIDS for their associated gout.

References

[1] M. R. Dorwart, N. Shcheynikov, D. Yang, and S. Muallem, "The solute carrier 26 family of proteins in epithelial ion transport," *Physiology*, vol. 23, no. 2, pp. 104–114, 2008.
[2] M. W. Musch, D. L. Arvans, G. D. Wu, and E. B. Chang, "Functional coupling of the downregulated in adenoma Cl^-/base exchanger DRA and the apical Na^+/H^+ exchangers NHE2 and NHE3," *American Journal of Physiology—Gastrointestinal and Liver Physiology*, vol. 296, no. 2, pp. G202–G210, 2009.
[3] N. M. Kamal, H. Y. Khan, M. H. F. El-Shabrawi, and L. M. Sherief, "Congenital chloride losing diarrhea," *Medicine*, vol. 98, no. 22, Article ID e15928, 2019.
[4] C. Holmberg, "Congenital chloride diarrhoea," *Clinics in Gastroenterology*, vol. 15, no. 3, pp. 583–602, 1986.
[5] A. M. A. Abdullah, S. M. Katugampola, M. A. Abdullah, K. A. R. Adam, and N. Al-Jishi, "Congenital chloride-losing diarrhea in Saudi children," *Annals of Saudi Medicine*, vol. 10, no. 4, pp. 389–393, 1990.
[6] M. M. Lubani, K. I. Doudin, D. C. Sharda et al., "Congenital chloride diarrhoea in Kuwaiti children," *European Journal of Pediatrics*, vol. 148, no. 4, pp. 333–336, 1989.
[7] S. Hihnala, P. Höglund, L. Lammi, J. Kokkonen, T. Örmälä, and C. Holmberg, "Long-term clinical outcome in patients with congenital chloride diarrhea," *Journal of Pediatric Gastroenterology & Nutrition*, vol. 42, no. 4, pp. 369–375, 2006.
[8] N. Rose, P. Kaplan, S. Scott, A. Kousoulis, and R. Librizzi, "Prenatal presentation of congenital chloride diarrhea: clinical report and review of the literature," *American Journal of Perinatology*, vol. 9, no. 5-6, pp. 398–400, 1992.
[9] E. R. Peters and O. F. Redwin, "Ultrasound in the intrauterine diagnosis and treatment of fetal abnormalities," *Clinical Obstetrics and Gynecology*, vol. 25, no. 4, pp. 753–771, 1982.
[10] S. Wedenoja, T. Örmälä, U. B. Berg et al., "The impact of sodium chloride and volume depletion in the chronic kidney disease of congenital chloride diarrhea," *Kidney International*, vol. 74, no. 8, pp. 1085–1093, 2008.
[11] P. A. Friedman, "Codependence of renal calcium and sodium transport," *Annual Review of Physiology*, vol. 60, no. 1, pp. 179–197, 1998.
[12] R. S. Nanra, J. Stuart-Taylor, A. H. de Leon, and K. H. White, "Analgesic nephropathy: etiology, clinical syndrome, and clinicopathologic correlations in Australia," *Kidney International*, vol. 13, no. 1, pp. 79–92, 1978.

A Rare Case of Xanthogranulomatous Pyelonephritis with Spontaneous Renocolic Fistula and IVC Thrombosis

Daniele Sforza,[1] Leandro Siragusa,[2] Matteo Ciancio Manuelli,[1] Linda De Luca,[1] Bruno Sensi,[2] Simona Grande,[1] Renato Argirò,[3] Marco Nezzo,[3] Massimo Villa,[1] and Michele Grande[2]

[1]*Department of Emergency, Policlinico Tor Vergata Hospital, Rome, Italy*
[2]*Department of Surgery, Tor Vergata University of Rome, Rome, Italy*
[3]*Department of Diagnostic Imaging and Interventional Radiology, Tor Vergata University of Rome, Rome, Italy*

Correspondence should be addressed to Leandro Siragusa; leandros93@hotmail.it

Academic Editor: Rumeyza Kazancioglu

Xanthogranulomatous pyelonephritis (XGPN) is a rare disorder affecting the kidney which can fistulise to the colon in exceptional cases. We herein report a case of XGPN with renocolic fistula and large vessel thrombosis presenting with sepsis and pulmonary embolism. Preoperative diagnosis and strategic planning resulted in successful management. A 64-year-old woman presented to the emergency department with abdominal pain and a septic condition, corroborated by venous thromboembolism. Workup diagnosed a left renal abscess with calicocolic fistula. Scintigraphy confirmed a nonfunctioning left kidney. The patient underwent inferior vena cava filter placement and staged surgery. The first, damage control procedure was a loop ileostomy. Ten days later, when the patient's conditions improved, she underwent left nephrectomy and left colectomy with primary anastomosis. Finally, a year later, the ileostomy was closed. At follow-up, the patient was well, with unremarkable renal function. Scrupulous diagnostics, multidisciplinary decision making, and staged intervention have been key to optimal outcome.

1. Introduction

Xanthogranulamatous pyelonephritis (XGPN) is a rare cause of chronic renal disease, characterized by suppuration and accumulation of lipid-laden macrophages in the renal parenchyma [1]. A really uncommon sequela is the renocolic fistula, which is usually a consequence of primary bowel pathologies [2, 3].

We present a rare case of XGPN complicated by spontaneous renocolic fistula. Our patient presented with flank pain and clinical signs of deep vein thrombosis (DVT) and sepsis.

2. Case Report

A 64-year-old female was admitted to our emergency department for abdominal pain, fever, and signs of left lower limb DVT. She had no past medical or family history of thrombophilic disorders.

On physical examination, there were tenderness in the left lumbar region with mass and pain, edema, and swelling of superficial veins as well as increased skin temperature of the left lower limb. Her body temperature was 38.2°C, heart rate 105 beats/min, and blood pressure 100/60 mm Hg. Blood tests revealed anemia, leukocytosis, and increased C-reactive protein and D-dimer.

Ultrasonography confirmed the diagnosis of DVT; a CT scan revealed pleural effusion, massive pulmonary embolism, inferior vena cava thrombosis, voluminous retroperitoneal abscess of the left psoas muscle and left kidney with irregular borders, hypodense areas, and a staghorn calculus suspicious for XGPN (Figures 1(a) and 1(b)).

The patient received two units of packed red blood cells and fluid resuscitation therapy; she was also started on

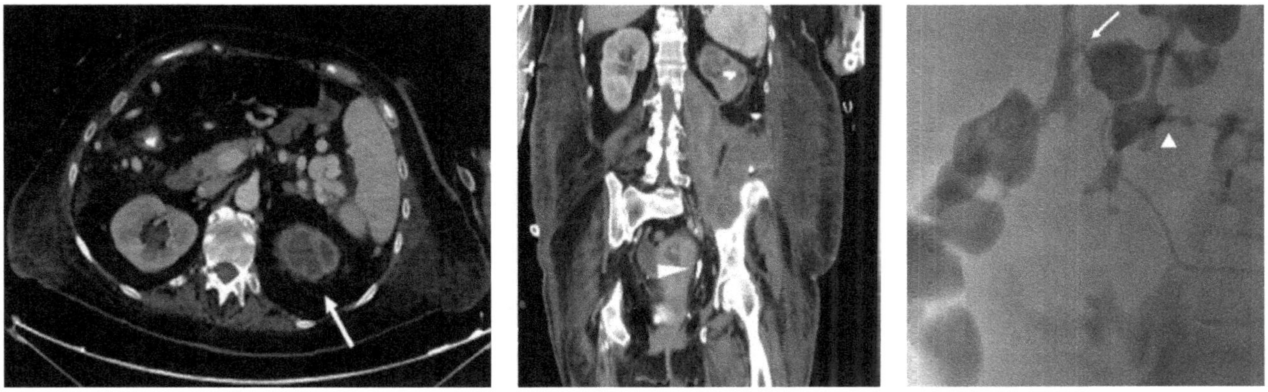

(a) (b) (c)

Figure 1: (a) Postcontrast CT images showed hypoperfusion of the left kidney with thinning of the cortex; dilatation of the left kidney excretory system with a "bear's paw sign" is also depicted suggesting diagnosis of xanthogranulomatous pyelonephritis (arrow); (b) postcontrast coronal reconstruction demonstrated ureteral stone (arrowhead) in the distal tract of the left ureter without significant dilatation of the proximal tract; (c) oblique projection pyelography after puncture of the inferior calix of the left kidney demonstrated leakage of contrast media with a double fistulous path form the pelvis directed anteriorly to the left colon (arrow) and posteriorly to the collection in the retroperitoneal collection (arrowhead).

empiric piperacillin/tazobactam antimicrobial therapy and enoxaparin sodium. After a multidisciplinary team meeting in the emergency area, the patient underwent an interventional radiologic procedure consisting of caval filter placement, left nephrostomy, and percutaneous drainage of the perinephric abscess; during the radiological procedure, contrast injected via the percutaneous drainage revealed a communication between the abscess, the lower pole calyx, and the descending colon (Figure 1(c)).

Therefore, the clinical and radiological features were suggestive of chronic pyelonephritis with spontaneous renocolic fistula, voluminous perinephric abscess, and reactive large vein thrombosis. We decided to treat the patient with a temporary ileostomy procedure, delaying definitive major surgical treatment, in order to ameliorate the clinical conditions. The postoperative course was uneventful, with a progressive improvement of general status. The early broad-spectrum antibiotic therapy was successful, with progressive decrease of inflammatory markers. Renal scintigraphy demonstrated a nonfunctioning left kidney, and a CT scan revealed resolution of pulmonary embolism. After 10 days from the first procedure, left nephrectomy and segmental left colectomy with terminoterminal anastomosis were performed. The patient had a good postoperative recovery and was discharged on day 38 from admission to the emergency department. On follow-up, the patient was asymptomatic and urinalysis, renal function tests, and colonoscopy were normal. After 12 months, the patient underwent ileostomy closure without complications.

Histopathological examination of the kidney showed an intense and widespread acute pyelonephritis, with abscessualization of the calices and pelvis and xanthogranulomatous chronic inflammation, with multinucleated giant cells, lipid-laden macrophages, and acute inflammatory cells, as well as loose "xanthoma" cells (Figure 2). Yellow tissue was present around many calices. There was evidence of papillary microadenoma but not carcinoma. These features were diagnostic of XGPN. The resected colon was the site of acute focally abscessed, diffuse serositis.

3. Discussion

XGPN was first described by Schlagenhaufer in 1916 [4]. This process is histopathologically characterized by suppuration, renal parenchyma destruction, and the presence of lipid-laden foamy macrophages [5]. Macroscopically, the affected kidney appears as a mass of yellow tissue with focal necrosis and hemorrhage. Histiocytes destroy the tissues, which leads to chronic pyelonephritis [6]. XGPN is more common in females and can occur at any age, although it is more usual during the fifth and sixth decades [7]. It affects both the kidneys with equal frequency, and the incidence is estimated to be approximately 8% in all kidneys removed or biopsied for inflammatory diseases (excluding glomerulonephritis) [8].

Precise etiology is unclear; however, it is thought to occur in association with infection and/or chronic urinary tract obstruction such as staghorn calculi [8]. Urinary tract calculi are present in 70–79% of patients with XGPN [9]. Other contributory factors include diabetes mellitus, immunocompromised states, and abnormal lipid metabolism. The disease can behave and appear somewhat like a renal cell carcinoma.

In this condition, inflammation of the renal parenchyma, with increased pressure inside the kidney, results in necrosis of the cortex. The consequent abscess formation is the cause of damage to neighboring organs; local invasion of adjacent structures has also been described, with cases of spleen, pancreas, or duodenum involvement or development of renocolic, renocutaneous, and renobronchial fistulas [10].

Classification of XPGN recognizes three stages based on disease extension:

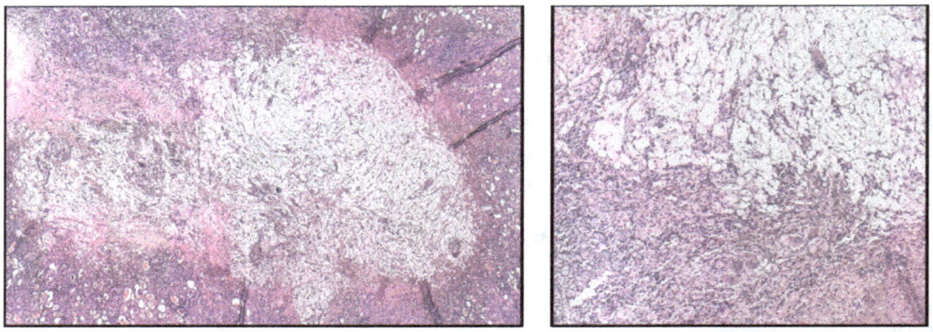

(a) (b)

Figure 2: (a) H & E 4x: acute pyelonephritis, with abscessualization of the calices and pelvis and xanthogranulomatous chronic inflammation; (b) H & E 10x: detailed image of the typical multinucleated giant cells in the context of XGPN.

(i) Stage I: nephric, disease is confined to the renal parenchyma only
(ii) Stage II: nephric and perinephric, the disease process involves the renal parenchyma along with perinephric fat
(iii) Stage III: nephric and perinephric, disease extending into the adjacent structure or diffused in the retroperitoneum

Classical features are those of an acute suppurative disease, frequently associated with a perinephric abscess. Clinical presentation is typically similar to pyelonephritis with dull, persistent flank pain, and associated fever, dysuria, malaise, and weight loss. Pneumaturia can be a presenting symptom. Evolution may be insidious with progressive weight loss, malaise, persistent renal sepsis, dehydration, anemia, and uremia. Rarely, there is cutaneous fistulation. Laboratory tests are nonspecific, with anemia and increased inflammatory markers being a common finding. Urine cultures are often positive for *Escherichia coli* and *Proteus* species.

Although renocolic fistulas were described by Hippocrates in 460 B.C., with a renal abscess invading the intestinal tract, the first modern report of renocolic fistula was in 1841 by Rayer. Since then, the advent of antimicrobial drugs and CT scan has made the pathology infrequent [11]. Etiology can be spontaneous, iatrogenic, or, rarely, traumatic, such as following severe abdominal trauma. Spontaneous renocolic fistulae are a consequence of primary chronic kidney disease, such as tuberculosis or hydatid cyst or malignancy [12, 13].

Renocolic fistulae are an uncommon complication of XGPN with no large case series in the literature to the best of our knowledge [13–15]. Anatomically, the left colon's posterior wall, devoid of serosa, is directly opposite the anterior surface of the left kidney. The inflammatory process can cause perforation of a thinned cortex and subsequent drainage of infected urine and necrotic material from perinephric abscess into the colon, resulting in a renocolic fistula [13, 14]. In XGPN, the kidney can be strongly adherent to adjacent structures, such as the psoas muscle and adrenal gland, with numerous new blood vessels extending from the inflamed kidney. Suspicion of a sinus or fistula should be assumed for purposes of surgical treatment when the renal parenchyma is adherent to structures such as the large or small bowel or the diaphragm [8, 13].

Radiological diagnosis of renocolic fistula in the setting of XGPN is often difficult in the absence of clinical suspicion, but some radiological signs are suggestive; frequently, the CT scan demonstrates the presence of a pelvic staghorn calculus and round areas of low density surrounded by a rim of contrast medium in the renal parenchyma (bear paw sign) [16, 17]. Radiological investigations allow diagnosis through CT scan, antegrade pyelography, barium enema, or, if there is cutaneous extension, fistulogram [1].

Parson et al. reported the first series of patients with fistulation in XGPN; since then, there have been few reports of this rare complication [8]. One case of preoperative diagnosis with retrograde pyelography was described. In another series, Majeed et al. similarly describe patients with renocolic fistulae as a complication of XGPN [18]. In this report, the renocolic fistulas were identified incidentally during surgery while the preoperative imaging did not detect radiological signs of fistulation.

In the majority of cases, the renal parenchyma is completely destroyed and nephrectomy is the definitive treatment. The affected colon is resected, and when conditions permit, a primary anastomosis is performed [6]. However, if the involved bowel was macroscopically normal and the fistulous opening was very small, primary suture closure is also possible. Usually, this is a unilateral process; however, in the rare case of bilateral XGPN, successful bilateral partial nephrectomy has been performed [19]. In our case, the extensive renal damage encouraged us to proceed with nephrectomy. Our choice to perform a defunctioning temporary ileostomy to exclude and protect the renocolic fistula and delay nephrectomy and colonic resection was conditioned by the patient's very poor general status; the patient was admitted with sepsis, severe anemia, and pulmonary embolism and also needed placement of an inferior vena cava filter because of extensive thrombosis.

The designation of XGPN as a separate entity is important because it is not only often recognizable as a clinicopathological syndrome but also unique among the inflammatory conditions of the kidney in closely mimicking the clinical, radiological, and even histological features of renal cell carcinoma [13].

Prognosis largely depends on the underlying etiology, renal failure stage, and the patient's general status.

XGPN is an unusual type of chronic pyelonephritis, resulting from chronic obstruction of the urinary tract by an infected stone. Spontaneous renocolic fistulas are extremely rare in this setting, especially after the progress of antimicrobial therapy and renal stone treatment. Scrupolous imaging is necessary for accurate diagnosis. The singularity of our case lies in the contemporaneity of pyelonephritis, renocolic fistula, pulmonary embolis and large vein thrombosis in the context of sepsis. The complexity of the clinical condition has imposed a successful two-stage management of the surgical complications of XGPN. [20]

Consent

Written informed consent was obtained from the patient for publication of this case report and any accompanying images.

Authors' Contributions

D.S. and L.S. wrote the manuscript and made substantial direct equal intellectual contribution. M.C.M., L.D.L., B.S., R.A., S.G., M.N, and M.V. contributed to the conception, design, and analysis and/or interpretation of data, and they made substantial intellectual contribution. M.G. critically revised the manuscript. All authors read and agreed to the published version of the manuscript.

References

[1] M. C. Karamchandani, R. Riether, J. Sheets, J. Stasik, L. Rosen, and I. Khubchandani, "Nephrocolic fistula," *Diseases of the Colon & Rectum*, vol. 29, no. 11, pp. 747–749, 1986.

[2] L. Numan, H. Zamir, N. M. Husainat, and M. Tahboub, "Xanthogranulomatous pyelonephritis causing renocolic fistula presenting as symptomatic anemia," *Cureus*, vol. 11, no. 6, p. e4947, 2019.

[3] Y. Matsuoka, G. Arai, H. Ishimaru, K. Takagi, J. Aida, and Y. Okada, "Xanthogranulomatous pyelonephritis with a renocolic fistula caused by a parapelvic cyst," *International Journal of Urology*, vol. 13, no. 4, pp. 433–435, 2006.

[4] F. Schlagenhaufer, "Ueber eigentumliche staphylomykosen der nieren und des pararenalen bindegewebes," *Frankfurter Zeitschrift für Pathologie*, vol. 19, pp. 139–148, 1916.

[5] M. A. Parsons, S. C. Harris, A. J. Longstaff, and R. G. Grainger, "Xanthogranulomatous pyelonephritis: a pathological, clinical and aetiological analysis of 87 cases," *Diagnostic Histopathology*, vol. 6, pp. 203–19, 1983.

[6] C.-K. Chuang, M.-K. Lai, P.-L. Chang et al., "Xanthogranulomatous pyelonephritis: experience in 36 cases," *The Journal of Urology*, vol. 147, no. 2, pp. 333–336, 1992.

[7] T. Yazaki, S. Ishikawa, Y. Ogawa et al., "Xanthogranulomatous pyelonephritis in childhood: case report and review of English and Japanese literature," *The Journal of Urology*, vol. 127, no. 1, pp. 80–83, 1982.

[8] M. A. Parsons, S. C. Harris, R. G. Grainger, B. Ross, J. A. R. Smith, and J. L. Williams, "Fistula and sinus formation in xanthogranulomatous pyelonephritis; a clinicopathological review and report of four cases," *British Journal of Urology*, vol. 58, no. 5, pp. 488–493, 1986.

[9] R. B. Rafal, P. A. Koscvsky, and J. A. Markisz, "Xanthogranulomatous pyelonephritis in an infant," *Urology*, vol. 37, no. 6, pp. 553–556, 1991.

[10] H. D. Flood, B. Jones, and R. Grainger, "Ureterocolic fistula: a unique complication of extracorporeal shock wave lithotripsy," *The Journal of Urology*, vol. 147, no. 1, pp. 122–124, 1992.

[11] R. P. Gibbons and J. D. Schmidt, "Reno-colic and reno-colic-cutaneous fistula: report of 3 cases," *The Journal of Urology*, vol. 94, no. 5, pp. 520–527, 1965.

[12] J. S. Pandya and N. Desai, "Reno-colo-cutaneous fistula," *Indian Journal of Urology*, vol. 17, pp. 62–64, 2000.

[13] S. Bhimreddeppa Patil, V. Shivanna Kundaragi, A. Nanagouda Biradar, and G. Siddanagouda Patil, "A case of xanthogranulomatous pyelonephritis with spontaneous renocolic fistula," *Türk Üroloji Dergisi/Turkish Journal of Urology*, vol. 39, no. 2, pp. 122–125, 2013.

[14] R. L. McDermott, C. M. Dowling, M. Alsinnawi, and R. Grainger, "Incidental renocolic fistula with xanthogranulomatous pyelonephritis," *International Journal of Surgery Case Reports*, vol. 4, no. 2, pp. 222–224, 2013.

[15] R. Parasher and K. Sasidharan, "Spontaneous reno-colic fistula," *Indian Journal of Urology*, vol. 17, pp. 64-65, 2000.

[16] P. Garrido Abad, M. A. Rodríguez-Cabello, R. Vera-Berón, and A. Platas-Sancho, "Bear paw sign: xanthogranulomatous pyelonephritis," *Journal of Radiology Case Reports*, vol. 12, no. 11, pp. 18–24, 2018.

[17] S. Goldman, D. Hartman, E. Fishman, J. Finizio, O. Gatewood, and S. Siegelman, "CT of xanthogranulomatous pyelonephritis: radiologic-pathologic correlation," *American Journal of Roentgenology*, vol. 142, no. 5, pp. 963–969, 1984.

[18] H. A. Majeed, K. A. Mohammed, and H. A. Salman, "Renocolic fistula as a complication to xanthogranulomatous pyelonephritis," *Singapore Medical Journal*, vol. 38, no. 3, pp. 116–119, 1997.

[19] L. M. Peréz, J. B. Thrasher, and E. E. Anderson, "Successful management of bilateral xanthogranulomatous pyelonephritis by bilateral partial nephrectomy," *The Journal of Urology*, vol. 149, no. 1, pp. 100–102, 1993.

26

Osmotic Demyelination Syndrome in a Patient with Hypokalemia but No Hyponatremia

Carolina Ormonde,[1] Raquel Cabral,[1] and Sara Serpa[2]

[1]*Nephrology Department, Hospital do Divino Espírito Santo, Ponta Delgada, Portugal*
[2]*Radiology Department, Hospital do Divino Espírito Santo, Ponta Delgada, Portugal*

Correspondence should be addressed to Carolina Ormonde; carolina.ormonde@hotmail.com

Academic Editor: Mahzuz Karim

Osmotic demyelination syndrome (ODS) is characterized by loss of myelin in various parts of the central nervous system. It is mainly caused by a rapid correction of hyponatremia, although other factors that may cause rapid rise in serum osmolality can also be associated with its development. Its prognosis is poor and the recovery rate is unknown. The authors report a rare case of a patient with multiple risk factors for ODS, without hyponatremia, who developed ODS and surprisingly recovered. This case report highlights the importance of recognizing risk factors for the development of ODS, even if the main one is not present.

1. Introduction

Osmotic demyelination syndrome (ODS) is a rare condition [1] characterized by loss of myelin in various parts of the central nervous system. It is subdivided into central pontine myelinolysis (CPM) and extrapontine myelinolysis (EPM), depending on what level the demyelination occurs [2]. The main risk factor consists in a rapid correction of chronic hyponatremia [3], but rare cases of ODS without the latter have been reported. Other known risk factors for ODS are malnutrition, alcoholism, hypokalemia, use of diuretics, and fluid resuscitation [2]. Symptoms may range from confusion to coma and can frequently be delayed some days after the trigger event [4]. Magnetic resonance imaging (MRI) is the key method for diagnosis, and its treatment is mainly supportive [5]. The overall prognosis seems to be poor, and the recovery rate is unknown [6]. We report a case of a patient who, unexpectedly, developed ODS without evidence of hyponatremia but also had multiple risk factors for its development.

2. Case Presentation

A 55-year-old male with a history of insulin dependent type 2 diabetes mellitus was admitted to the nephrology department with anasarca. He had a nephrotic syndrome for at least 2 years caused by diabetic nephropathy and had history of nonadherence to medication. Despite the generalized edema, he was noticeably malnourished. The patient was treated with high doses of furosemide and was also given ceftriaxone for a urinary tract infection. After eight days of hospital admission, he developed hypovolemic shock caused by a pseudomembranous colitis due to *Clostridium difficile*, for which aggressive fluid resuscitation was needed. He was given antibiotics for the pseudomembranous colitis—4 days of vancomycin to which he did not respond, and he was then switched to fidaxomicin. He also developed hypokalemia which was corrected with intravenous potassium chloride (60 meq a day for 5 days). Additionally, he had poor glycemic control for which insulin was instituted. Six days after this complication, he developed a slurred speech and a progressive decline in his level of consciousness throughout the course of the next two days. Neurologic examination revealed quadriplegia and, few days later, he developed a "locked-in syndrome."

There were no electrolyte disturbances in blood analysis by the time the patient developed these symptoms (Figure 1). The only relevant alterations were his usual severe hypoalbuminemia and hyperglycemia. Brain computed

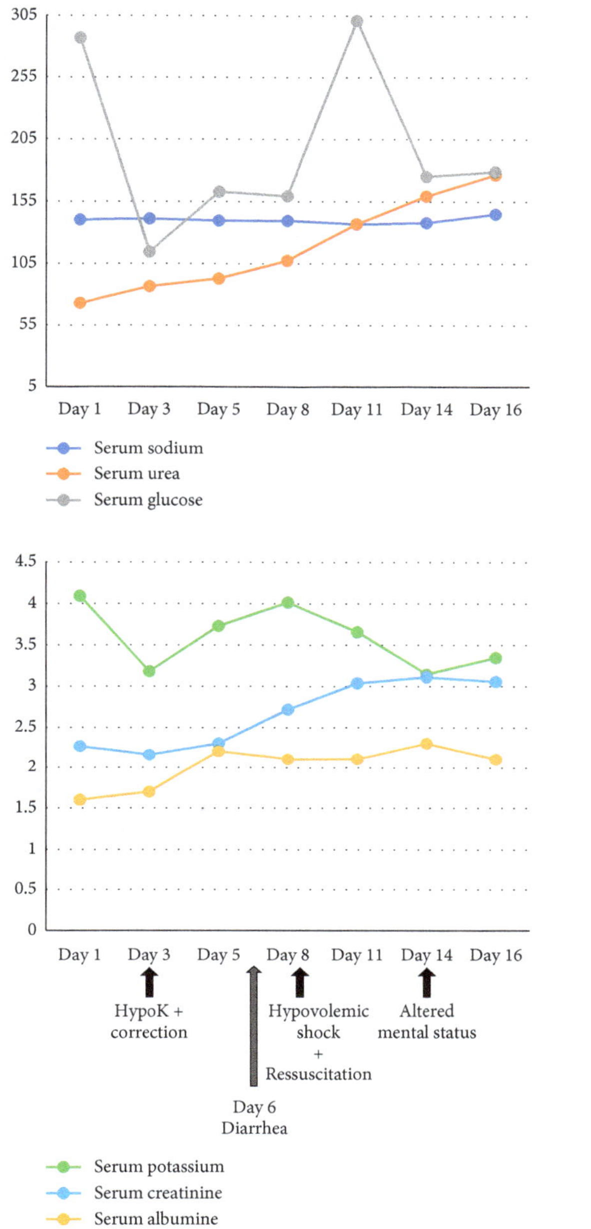

FIGURE 1: Correlation between sequence of events and serial laboratory results. Day 1 corresponds to the day of admission. Value units are the following: mg/dL for serum urea, creatinine, and glucose; mmol/L for serum sodium and potassium; g/dL for serum albumin.

tomography (CT) did not show acute lesions. Cerebrospinal fluid analysis showed 1 red blood cell/mm^3, normal glucose and protein levels, negative Gram stain, Ziehl–Neelsen stain and bacterial culture, and negative PCR for Herpes simplex virus. Electroencephalogram revealed diffuse and symmetric slow wave activity. An MRI was then performed revealing heterogeneous T1-hypointense, T2-hyperintense, and FLAIR-hyperintense areas located in the pons, cerebellar peduncles (mainly in the middle cerebellar peduncles), which were compatible with ODS (Figure 2). MRI also showed millimetric lacunae infarcts in corona radiata bilaterally and left cerebellum.

Supportive treatment was given to the patient, and, unexpectedly, he started recovering from coma over the following week. During this first week, he progressively recovered his level of consciousness with an intelligible speech. He also developed, during the recovery course, a bacteremia by *Acinetobacter baumannii* which was resolved with meropenem. Throughout the first month of recovery, he had a continuous and persistent program of physiotherapy and partially regained his legs and arms movements. When he was discharged, he was able to stand on orthostatic position and walk with bilateral support. He continued the rehabilitation program to regain complete autonomy.

3. Discussion

Adams et al. were the first to describe pontine myelinolysis in 1959 [7]. Today, it is known as ODS, and it is subdivided into CPM (the most frequent form) and EPM. [2] Although ODS is a rare condition, its true incidence is unknown and often underdiagnosed [1].

The main risk factor for ODS is rapid correction of chronic hyponatremia, particularly when it is lower than 120 meq/L [3]. Cerebral cells defend themselves from edema caused by chronic hyponatremia by altering their osmolality with gain in electrolytes and organic osmolytes. When hyponatremia is corrected too quickly, cells cannot readapt fast enough to the higher osmolality and are at risk of lysis. Oligodendrocytes are the most affected cells [1]. Other risk factors that may contribute to osmotic demyelination are as follows: malnutrition, chronic alcoholism, primary adrenal insufficiency, prolonged use of diuretics, hypokalemia, hyperglycemia, fluid resuscitation, hemodialysis, and liver transplant [2]. There are rare reports of ODS cases with mild or no hyponatremia, which demonstrates that a combination of other risk factors besides hyponatremia may also lead to ODS [3].

Frequently, symptoms are delayed for two to six days after rapid correction of osmolality and it can present in various ways [4]. Asymptomatic cases have also been described [3]. Clinical presentation of ODS is typically sequential [8], and the most common symptoms are confusion, muscle weakness, quadriplegia, oculomotor abnormalities, dysphagia, dysarthria, locked-in syndrome, and progressive deterioration of consciousness [9].

CT assessment of the skull base can be difficult due to beam hardening artifact. The preferable diagnostic method is MRI. Findings might be delayed up to four weeks after the initial symptoms [2]. It reveals T1-hypointense, T2-hyperintense, and FLAIR-hyperintense signals mainly in the pons. Moreover, there can be a typical sign of osmotic demyelination syndrome—"the trident sign"—where the symmetrical high T2/FLAIR signal abnormality appears located in central pons. This reflects the prevalent involvement of the transverse pontine fibers and relative sparing of the descending corticospinal tract. It may also be seen T1-hypointense, T2-hyperintense, and FLAIR-hyperintense signal changes in the basal ganglia, thalamus, cerebellum,

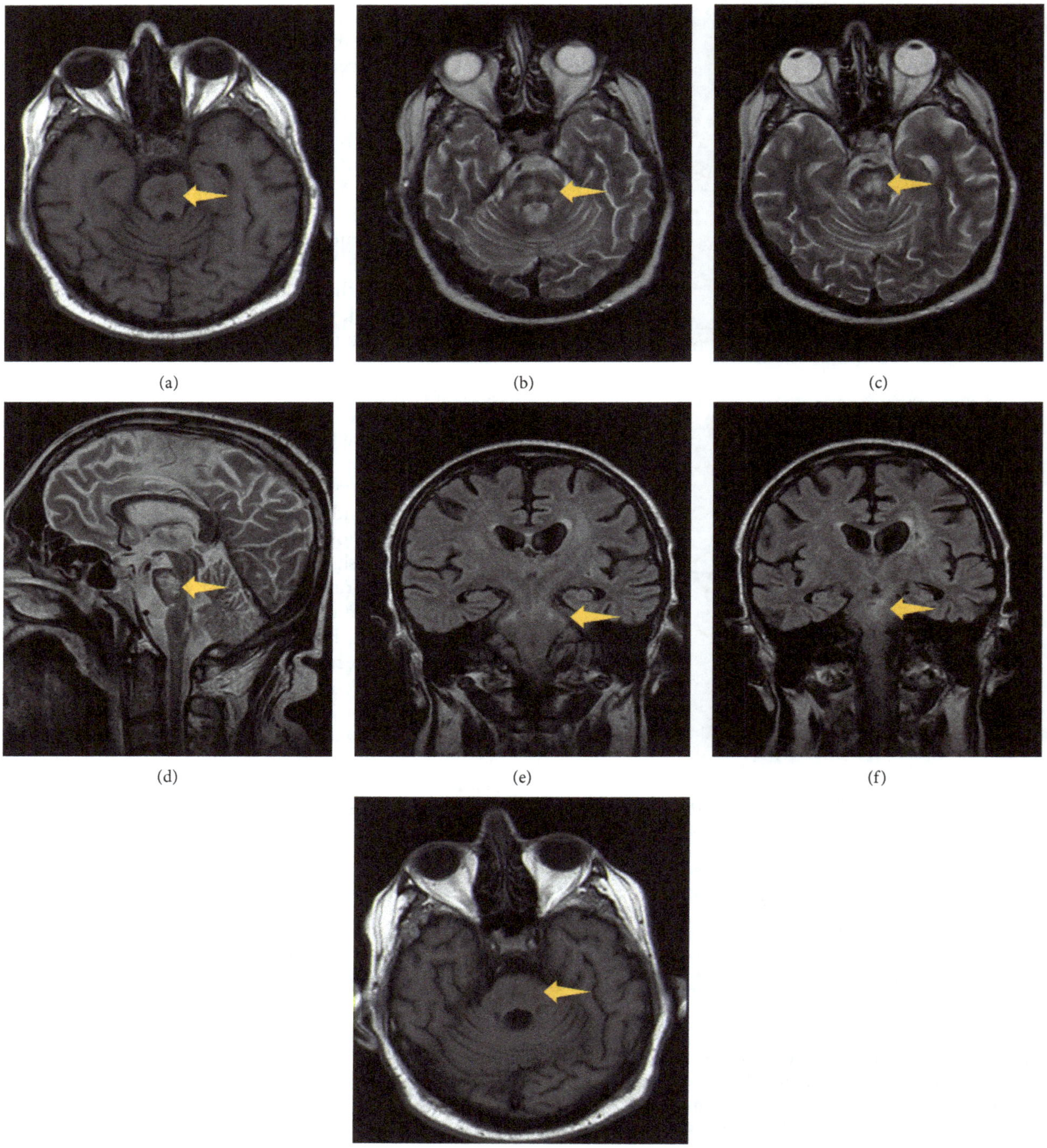

(a) (b) (c) (d) (e) (f) (g)

Figure 2: MRI images show central pontine T1 moderately hypointense areas (a), T2 and FLAIR areas of hyperintensity at the level of the pons (b, c, d, f), including an area trident-shaped of hyperintensity at the level of the pons on axial T2 (b) (typical appearances of the pons in osmotic demyelination syndrome), that extends to cerebellar peduncles (b, e); after gadolinium, there was no enhancement (g).

hippocampus, and cerebral cortex [5]. The earliest change is perceived on diffusion (diffusion-weighted (DWI) MRI) with restriction in the lower pons. This is apparent within 24 hours of the beginning of quadriplegia. On apparent diffusion coefficient (ADC) map, there is signal loss. Our exam was performed on 1 Tesla MRI without DWI capacity nor ADC map obtainable.

The most important therapy is prevention of rapid correction of hyponatremia, or in susceptible patients, prevention of rapid changes in plasma osmolality. Treatment is mainly supportive, but some case reports have shown that the use of intravenous immunoglobulin or plasmapheresis may be useful as they may remove myelotoxic substances from plasma [5].

Overall, ODS has a poor prognosis with a high mortality rate. Patients who survive may not recover if in a coma and irreversible sequelae may persist [6]. No clinical or radiological features predict the outcome [5]. A high level of suspicion for ODS is the most important factor for early diagnosis and better outcome. The level and time of recovery varies and are uncertain [4].

We reported an unusual case of CPM with no hyponatremia. After the unexpected diagnosis by MRI, we concluded that, even in the absence of the latter in our patient, the combination of multiple risk factors contributed to the development of ODS. First, he had a prolonged history of diabetes mellitus with nephrotic syndrome and poor glycemic control, which contributed to severe proteinuria and malnutrition. During the first days after admission, he was also given a high and prolonged course of diuretics to treat the anasarca. After the abrupt diarrhea that caused the hypovolemic shock and hypokalemia, he was given a large amount of fluids. From our point of view, this was the main trigger event that caused the rapid change in osmotic balance. After this event, the chronological presentation of neurologic manifestations is consistent with ODS.

There are rare, but similar, cases reported of ODS without hyponatremia. Jacob et al. described a similar case in a patient with no risk factors besides aggressive fluid resuscitation after acute bleeding [2]. Benders et al. also reported a case of CPM in a patient with multiple risk factors after the correction of electrolyte disturbances [3].

This case report also emphasizes the need to always be mindfulness with the therapeutic measures we take, even when we think they are innocuous.

References

[1] G. Dagur and S. A. Khan, "Current concepts in pontine myelinolysis: review of literature," *Translational Biomedicine*, vol. 6, no. 4, pp. 1–7, 2015.

[2] S. Jacob, H. Gupta, D. Nikolic, B. Gundogdu, and S. Ong, "Central pontine and extrapontine myelinolysis: the great masquerader-an autopsy case report," *Case Reports in Neurological Medicine*, vol. 2014, Article ID 745347, 5 pages, 2014.

[3] P. Benders, A. C. Heijckmann, and B. Van De Langerijt, "Central pontine myelinolysis: case report and short overview," *The Netherlands Journal of Critical Care*, vol. 25, no. 4, pp. 129–132, 2017.

[4] M. K. Sohn and J. H. Nam, "Locked-in syndrome due to central pontine myelinolysis: case report," *Annals of Rehabilitation Medicine*, vol. 38, no. 5, p. 702, 2014.

[5] D. L. Rebedew, "Is central pontine myelinolysis reversible?" *Wisconsin Medical Journal*, vol. 115, no. 6, pp. 326–328, 2016.

[6] C.-C. Lai, C.-K. Tan, S.-H. Lin, and H.-W. Chen, "Central pontine myelinolysis," *Canadian Medical Association Journal*, vol. 183, no. 9, p. E605, 2011.

[7] L. Jasmin, "Central pontine myelinolysis," *Journal of Neurology, Neurosurgery, and Psychiatry*, vol. 27, pp. 317–325, 1964.

[8] M. Saini, M. Mamauag, and R. Singh, "Central pontine myelinolysis: a rare presentation secondary to hyperglycaemia," *Singapore Medical Journal*, vol. 56, no. 4, pp. e71–e73, 2015.

[9] A. N. Tavare and D. Murray, "Central pontine myelinolysis," *New England Journal of Medicine*, vol. 374, no. 7, p. e8, 2016.

27

COVID-19 and APOL-1 High-Risk Genotype-Associated Collapsing Glomerulonephritis

Sasmit Roy,[1] Srikanth Kunaparaju,[2] Narayana Murty Koduri,[3] Vikram Sangani,[4] Mytri Pokal,[4] Venu Madhav Konala,[5] Mamtha Balla,[6] and Sreedhar Adapa[7]

[1]*Lynchburg Nephrology Physicians, 2091 Langhorne Road, Lynchburg, VA 24501, USA*
[2]*Richmond Nephrology Associates, 671 Hioaks Road, Suite B, Richmond, VA 23225, USA*
[3]*Great Plains Health, 601 W Leota St, North Platte, NE 69101, USA*
[4]*Quantum HC, Department of Internal Medicine, Navicent Health, 777 Hemlock Street, Macon, GA 31201, USA*
[5]*Precision Cancer Center, 122 St Christopher Dr, Ashland, KY 41101, USA*
[6]*Promedica Toledo Hospital, 2142 N Cove Blvd, Toledo, OH 43606, USA*
[7]*Adventist Medical Center, 115 Mall Drive, Hanford, CA 93230, USA*

Correspondence should be addressed to Sasmit Roy; docsasmit@gmail.com

Academic Editor: Hern n Trimarchi

Coronavirus Disease 2019 (COVID-19) caused by severe acute respiratory syndrome coronavirus 2 (SARS-CoV-2) primarily affects the lungs and can lead to acute respiratory distress syndrome (ARDS). The ongoing global pandemic has created healthcare and economic crisis for almost every nation of the world. Though primarily affecting the lungs, it has also affected the kidney in various ways including acute kidney injury (AKI), proteinuria, and hematuria. It has been increasingly shown that African American (AA) individuals affected with COVID-19 and presenting with AKI and nephrotic-range proteinuria are very susceptible to focal segmental glomerulosclerosis (FSGS). The APOL-1 gene, associated with the African American population, has been increasingly recognized as a risk factor for FSGS affected with COVID-19. Our case highlights a similar case of COVID-19 in a 65-year-old AA descendant with biopsy-proven FSGS and genetically confirmed APOL-1 alleles.

1. Introduction

Coronavirus Disease 2019 (COVID-19) caused by severe acute respiratory syndrome coronavirus 2 (SARS-CoV-2) primarily affects the lungs and can lead to acute respiratory distress syndrome (ARDS). The kidney is another major organ affected by the virus, which can cause acute kidney injury (AKI), proteinuria, and hematuria which are the independent predictive factors for mortality [1, 2]. COVID-19 infects disproportionately minorities and people with low socioeconomic status resulting in an increased risk of hospitalization and higher mortality [3].

We describe a case report of an African American male admitted with fever and shortness of breath and was diagnosed with COVID-19, who developed worsening renal function and proteinuria. The patient was subsequently started on hemodialysis and underwent kidney biopsy.

The kidney biopsy revealed collapsing glomerulonephritis, a rare entity that has reemerged in African American patients (who have a high-risk APOL1 gene), who were infected with COVID-19.

2. Case Presentation

A 65-year-old African American male was admitted to the hospital with chief complaints of fever and shortness of breath. The patient was exposed to a family member who has tested positive for COVID-19 and was subsequently confirmed with SARS-CoV-2 infection by reverse transcriptase polymerase chain reaction (RT-PCR) analysis. The patient's past medical history was significant for hypertension, diabetes mellitus type 2, hyperlipidemia, and chronic kidney disease stage 3A with the baseline glomerular filtration rate (GFR) of 50 mL/min. Home medications included amlodipine 10 milligrams (mg) daily, furosemide 40 mg daily, metformin 500 mg daily, and atorvastatin 40 mg daily. Physical examination was remarkable for a temperature of 101 degrees Fahrenheit, pulse rate of 89 beats/min, blood pressure of 108/75 mm Hg, and a respiratory rate of 22 breaths/min. The patient was in moderate respiratory distress using accessory muscles, and the auscultation of the lungs was significant for bilateral (b/l) wheezing and diffuse crackles. The rest of the physical examination was insignificant. The laboratory data are detailed in Table 1 (all admission) and Table 2 (progress in hospital up to 6 weeks after discharge, renal parameters).

The renal function was worse from baseline with the serum creatinine of 6.5 mg/dl, blood urea nitrogen (BUN) of 86 mg/dl, and spot urine protein-creatinine (UPC) ratio of 15.8 gm/gm (baseline values: creatinine 1.2 mg/dl, BUN 32 mg/dl, and UPC 2gm/gm 6 months ago). Renal ultrasound revealed b/l enlarged kidneys, with no hydronephrosis. Although he had nephrotic-range proteinuria, he did not present with other classic features of nephrotic syndrome such as severe albuminemia (i.e., serum albumin <2.5 mg/dl) or peripheral edema. Ocular examination for common diabetic retinopathy features such as glaucoma, macular edema, or microaneurysm were absent. The chest X-ray revealed diffuse infiltrates in b/l lung fields consistent with COVID-19. Other serologies including antinuclear antibody (ANA), complements (C3 and C4), antineutrophil cytoplasmic antibodies (ANCAs), antiglomerular basement membrane antibody, and antiphospholipase A2 receptor (anti-PLA2R) antibodies were normal. Serologies for hepatitis B and C virus, Human Immunodeficiency Virus (HIV), Epstein–Barr Virus (EBV), Cytomegalovirus (CMV), and Parvovirus B19 were all negative.

Serum immunofixation did not reveal any monoclonal protein. The patient was initially started on high-flow oxygen through a nasal cannula and was subsequently started on hemodialysis for worsening renal functions with oliguria on day five of admission.

The patient underwent renal biopsy for proteinuria and AKI to determine the etiology. Kidney biopsy revealed changes consistent with collapsing glomerulopathy, and light microscopy revealed intact glomeruli showing focal segmental sclerosis, associated with loop wrinkling, periglomerular fibrosis, and focal segmental podocyte hyperplasia with tuft collapse. No foci of endocapillary hypercellularity, crescent formation, or necrosis were identified. Out of the five glomeruli in light microscopy, one had global glomerulosclerosis, thereby suggesting roughly 20% renal tissue had global sclerosis. Around 50% globally showed collapsing lesions. The tubular epithelial cytoplasm demonstrated extensive protein resorption droplets, with the presence of focal microcystic dilatation. Interstitium revealed mild mixed inflammatory infiltrates with severe interstitial fibrosis, along with severe arterial intimal fibrosis and mild significant hyaline arteriosclerosis. Immunofluorescence did not show any significant immune deposits, while electron microscopy showed severe effacement of the podocyte foot process. No immune-type electron-dense deposits were identified on electron microscopy. Light and electron microscopy images are provided in Figures 1–5. In situ hybridization for SARS-CoV-2 was negative. Features of diabetic nephropathy such as increase in the mesangial matrix and cell content or decrease in the capillary lumen space were lacking though mild thickening of the glomerular capillary basement membrane was present.

The patient had two APOL1 risk variants detected through genetic testing which revealed compound heterozygosity for APOL1 G1 and G2 risk alleles.

The patient was subsequently treated with hydroxychloroquine, remdesivir, corticosteroids, and intravenous antibiotics during the hospital stay. The patient never needed invasive ventilation support nor intensive care unit (ICU) stay. He was discharged to the outpatient dialysis clinic on day 17 as he continued to require dialysis support. The renal function improved after six weeks, and he was taken off dialysis as his serum creatinine improved to 2.4 mg/dl with no further oliguria.

The patient continues to remain dialysis free till date, and his GFR has improved back to his baseline (pre-COVID-19 state), with the resolution of hematuria and proteinuria (Table 2). For immunosuppression, he completed a three-month course of oral prednisone with gradual tapering.

3. Discussion

The involvement of the kidney by COVID-19 is frequent and manifests as acute kidney injury, proteinuria, and hematuria often progressing to End-Stage Renal Disease (ESRD) requiring dialysis. Incidents of AKI, proteinuria, and hematuria in COVID-19 patients are 10%, 40%, and 26%, respectively [1, 2].

Patients with glomerulonephritis usually have hematuria, sustained proteinuria composed largely of albumin. There has been emerging evidence of collapsing glomerulopathy on kidney biopsy in genetically susceptible individuals with African ancestry, infected with COVID-19 [4, 5].

Collapsing glomerulopathy presents as segmental or global glomerular collapse with a rapid deterioration in renal function. Focal segmental glomerulosclerosis (FSGS) refers to a pattern of renal injury characterized by segmental glomerular scars that involves some, but not all, glomeruli, clinically largely manifested as proteinuria. FSGS is classified based on a variety of morphologies on the biopsy finding. Among them, collapsing glomerulopathy (CG) represents an aggressive variant that is characterized by a collapse of the glomerular tuft along with hyperplasia and hypertrophy of the podocytes [6]. Acute tubular injury, inflammation of the interstitium, and tubular dilatation with accompanying microcysts are the commonly associated findings of CG [6].

FSGS is more commonly seen in African Americans. Infections such as HIV, CMV, EBV, and Parvovirus B19 are commonly associated with CG. Malignancies, thrombotic microangiopathy, sickle cell disease, cholesterol embolization, genetic mutations, and certain drugs such as heroin,

TABLE 1: Admission labs with normal reference value.

	Value	Reference range
White blood cell count (10^9/L)	12.6	4.5 to 11.0
Hemoglobin (g/dL)	9.2	13.5–14.5
Platelets (10^9/L)	356	150–400
Sodium (mmol/L)	135	135–145
Potassium (mmol/L)	4.0	3.5–5.1
Carbon dioxide (mmol/L)	20	24
BUN (mg/dL)	52	7–20
Creatinine (mg/dL)	3.37	0.9–1.3
eGFR (mL/min)	23	>60
Albumin (g/dL)	3.5	4
Total protein (g/dL)	8.1	6–8.3
Creatinine kinase (U/L)	996	39–308
C-reactive protein (mg/dl)	12.5	0.0–0.60
Ferritin (ng/ml)	3624	26–388
Interleukin-6 (pg/ml)	104.5	0.0–15.5
UPCR (g/g)	15.8	0.0–.02
RBC on microscopy	>100/hpf	<3/hpf

TABLE 2: Renal parameters from admission to 6-week follow-up.

Laboratory value	Admission	Peak	Discharge	6 weeks after discharge
Creatinine	3.37	6.16	6.46	2.4
BUN	52	72	60	34
Urine protein/creatinine ratio	15.8	—	—	—
Hematuria	>100/hpf	—	—	—

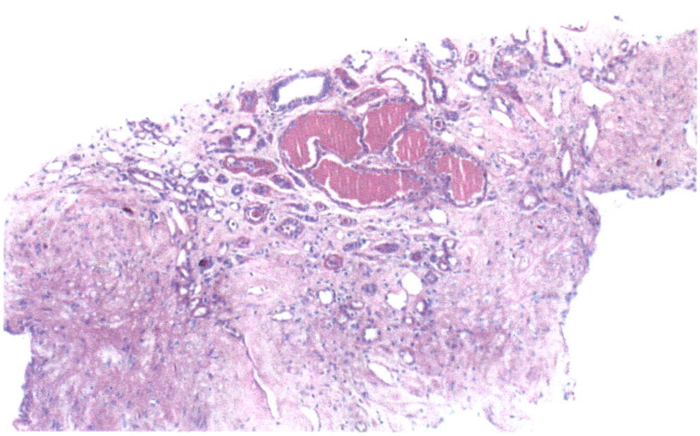

FIGURE 1: Focal microcystic tubular dilatation.

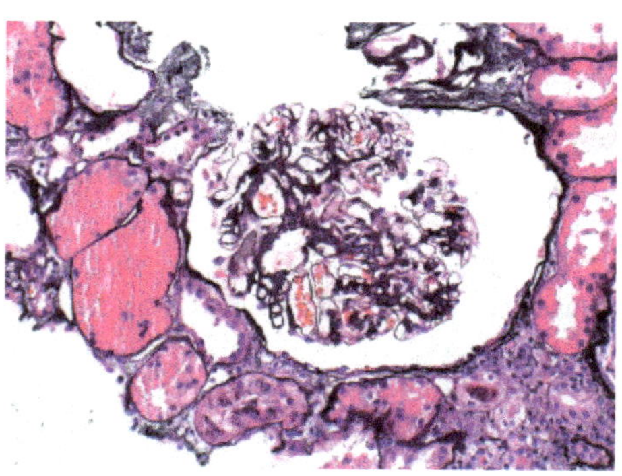

FIGURE 2: No proliferative glomerular changes.

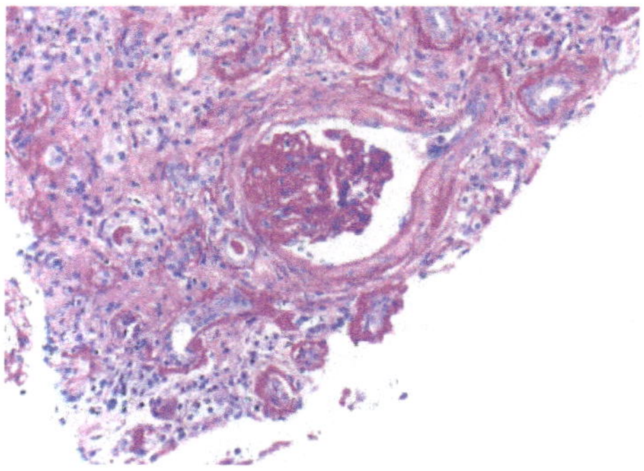

FIGURE 3: Segmental sclerosis and periglomerular fibrosis with tuft collapse.

calcineurin inhibitors, pamidronate, and interferon can also cause CG. It is also found in inflammatory and autoimmune conditions such as hemophagocytic syndrome and systemic lupus erythematous [6].

Polymorphism in the gene-encoding Apolipoprotein L1 (APOL1) is a major risk factor for nearly 10% of African Americans with nondiabetic ESRD, particularly FSGS. APOL1 alleles G1 and G2 inherited from each parent are required to increase the risk of kidney disease when compared to G0 which is considered as a low-risk allele [7]. Although, the exact mechanism on how these high-risk alleles transform the podocytes remains elusive [6]: mitochondrial dysfunction, endosome alteration, activation of protein kinases, cell membrane cation channel dysregulation, and interference with actinomycin in podocytes are the

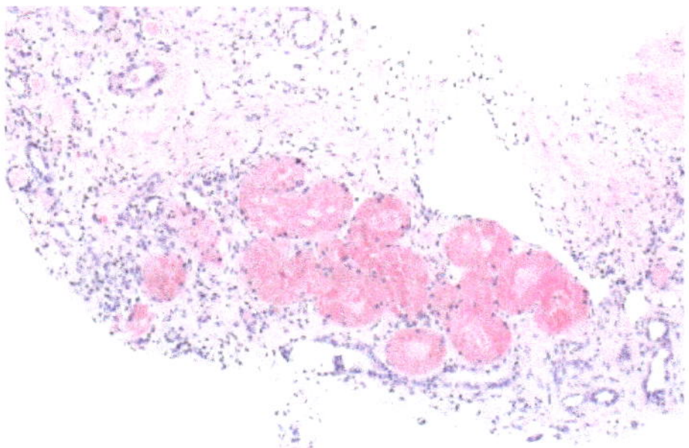

Figure 4: Tubules with protein resorption droplets.

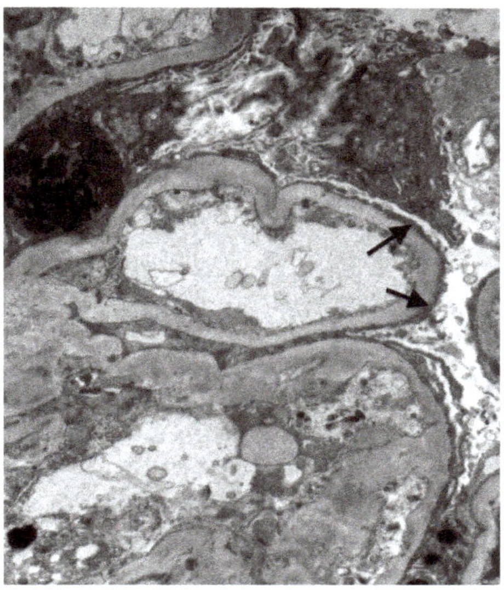

Figure 5: Electron microscopy showing diffuse foot process effacement (arrow).

multitude of cellular mechanisms put forth based on the cell culture and transgenic mice studies [6].

COVID-19 has been found to infect a disproportionate ratio of minorities and people of low socioeconomic background leading to increased hospitalization burden and higher mortality rate in these individuals [3]. Based on their study that included combined statistical areas (poverty prone/low – income areas as per the US office of Management and Budget) in 10 major US cities such as New York City, New Orleans, Atlanta, and Chicago, they found 63.5% of the confirmed COVID-19 cases (834126 of 1312679) in the United States as of May 10, 2020, were from those areas itself. In counties with high poverty (median income range, $36,850–$88,960), those with substantially nonwhite populations had an infection rate nearly eight times that of counties with substantially white populations (RR, 7.8; 95% CI, 5.1 to 12) and a death rate more than nine times greater (RR, 9.3; 95% CI, 4.7–18.4) [3].

Surprisingly, it has been found that, patients who had moderate pulmonary symptoms or who recovered from COVID-19, developed AKI and proteinuria and the AKI did not recover despite improvement in respiratory symptoms. This suggests that the effect on the lungs and kidneys are discrete [6]. Despite the initially proposed mechanism of direct renal cell infection [8–10], viral cytotoxic effect on podocyte contributing to AKI based on postmortem studies [6], and electron microscopy demonstrating possible viral particles in patients with CG [11], the follow-up case reports failed to demonstrate virus in a patient with CG by in situ hybridization studies or electron microscopy [6] or RT-PCR essay on renal tissue [12], suggesting an indirect effect of the virus on the kidneys.

Kudose et al. studied 17 patients with COVID-19-related AKI and their kidney biopsies and concluded that AKI in COVID-19 patients could be secondary to cytokine-mediated effects and heightened adaptive immune response but not related to direct viral injury [13]. Another multicentric study showed Acute Tubular Necrosis (ATN) and endothelial injury/thrombotic microangiopathy as a pathological process apart from collapsing GN [14].

SARS-CoV-2 enters ACE2 receptors located in proximal tubules and podocytes in kidneys per postmortem histology [7, 15]. In addition to the above mentioned mechanisms, imbalanced RAS activation, hypovolemia, high PEEP, and hemodynamic changes are suggested by Ahmadian et al. [16] Also, IgA nephropathy was seen as a causative agent for AKI in COVID-19 in one case [17].

3.1. Treatment. Treatment of COVID-19 is still an evolving process with various guidelines and studies conducted worldwide [18]. Treatment of secondary FSGS involves management of the etiology and reduction of proteinuria. The benefit of remdesivir is not observed in patients with eGFR <30, though our patient did receive it [19]. Anecdotal evidences of steroid use in collapsing GN is there without any definitive guidelines [20].

4. Conclusions

Kidney biopsy needs to be strongly considered, when there is clinical evidence of glomerulus involvement. Gene testing for APOL-1 should be performed if the patients are of African descent and are having nephrotic-range proteinuria with rapidly progressive renal failure. More evidence is needed through larger studies in terms of establishing prognostic markers, treatments, long-term effects of COVID-19 on the kidneys, and early interventions to improve outcomes.

Consent

The patient consented for publication of this study, and the written consent form is available to authors for submission if requested.

References

[1] Y. Cheng, R. Luo, K. Wang et al., "Kidney disease is associated with in-hospital death of patients with COVID-19," *Kidney International*, vol 97, no. 5, pp. 829–838, 2020.

[2] Z. Li, M. Wu, J. Yao et al., "Caution on kidney dysfunctions of COVID-19 patients," *medRxiv*, 2020, https://www.medrxiv.org/content/10.1101/2020.02.08.20021212v2.

[3] S. Adhikari, N. P. Pantaleo, J. M. Feldman, O. Ogedegbe, L. Thorpe, and A. B. Troxel, "Assessment of community-level disparities in coronavirus disease 2019 (COVID-19) infections and deaths in large US metropolitan areas," *JAMA Network Open*, vol. 3, no. 7, Article ID e2016938, 2020.

[4] A. A. Shetty, I. Tawhari, L. Safar-Boueri et al., "COVID-19-associated glomerular disease," *Journal of the American Society of Nephrology*, vol. 32, no. 1, pp. 33–40, 2021.

[5] H. Wu, C. P. Larsen, C. F. Hernandez-Arroyo et al., "AKI and collapsing glomerulopathy associated with COVID-19 and APOL1 high-risk genotype," *Journal of the American Society of Nephrology*, vol. 31, no. 8, pp. 1688–1695, 2020.

[6] S. H. Nasr and J. B. Kopp, "COVID-19-associated collapsing glomerulopathy: an emerging entity," *Kidney International Reports*, vol. 5, no. 6, pp. 759–761, 2020.

[7] D. J. Friedman, "COVID-19 and APOL1: understanding disease mechanisms through clinical observation," *Journal of the American Society of Nephrology*, vol. 32, no. 1, pp. 1-2, 2021.

[8] H. Su, M. Yang, C. Wan et al., "Renal histopathological analysis of 26 postmortem findings of patients with COVID-19 in China," *Kidney International*, vol. 98, no. 1, pp. 219–227, 2020.

[9] E. A. Farkash, A. M. Wilson, and J. M. Jentzen, "Ultrastructural evidence for direct renal infection with SARS-CoV-2," *Journal of the American Society of Nephrology*, vol. 31, no. 8, pp. 1683–1687, 2020.

[10] B. Diao, C. Wang, R. Wang et al., "Human kidney is a target for novel severe acute respiratory syndrome coronavirus 2 infection," *Nature Communications*, vol. 21, Article ID 2506, 2021.

[11] S. Kissling, S. Rotman, C. Gerber et al., "Collapsing glomerulopathy in a COVID-19 patient," *Kidney International*, vol. 98, no. 1, pp. 228–231, 2020.

[12] A. Couturier, S. Ferlicot, K. Chevalier et al., "Indirect effects of severe acute respiratory syndrome coronavirus 2 on the kidney in coronavirus disease patients," *Clinical Kidney Journal*, vol. 13, no. 3, pp. 347–353, 2020.

[13] S. Kudose, I. Batal, D. Santoriello et al., "Kidney biopsy findings in patients with COVID-19," *Journal of the American Society of Nephrology*, vol. 31, no. 9, pp. 1959–1968, 2020.

[14] S. Akilesh, C. C. Nast, M. Yamashita et al., "Multicenter clinicopathologic correlation of kidney biopsies performed in COVID-19 patients presenting with acute kidney injury or proteinuria," *American Journal of Kidney Diseases*, vol. 77, no. 1, pp. 82–93, 2021.

[15] A. Chenna, V. Madhav Konala, S. Bose et al., "Acute kidney injury in a case series of patients with confirmed COVID-19 (coronavirus disease 2019): role of angiotensin-converting enzyme 2 and renin-angiotensin system blockade," *Case Reports in Nephrology*, vol. 2020, Article ID 8811931, 8 pages, 2020.

[16] E. Ahmadian, S. M. Hosseiniyan Khatibi, S. Razi Soofiyani et al., "Covid-19 and kidney injury: pathophysiology and molecular mechanisms," *Reviews in Medical Virology*, vol. 31, no. 3, p. e2176, 2020.

[17] Y. Huang, X.-J. Li, Y.-Q. Li et al., "Clinical and pathological findings of SARS-CoV-2 infection and concurrent IgA nephropathy: a case report," *BMC Nephrology*, vol. 21, no. 1, p. 504, 2020.

[18] S. Bose, S. Adapa, N. R. Aeddula et al., "Medical management of COVID-19: evidence and experience," *Journal of Clinical Medicine Research*, vol. 12, no. 6, pp. 329–343, 2020.

[19] J. H. Beigel, K. M. Tomashek, L. E. Dodd et al., "Remdesivir for the treatment of covid-19-final report," *New England Journal of Medicine*, vol. 383, no. 19, pp. 1813–1826, 2020.

[20] L.-P. Laurin, A. M. Gasim, V. K. Derebail et al., "Renal survival in patients with collapsing compared with not otherwise specified FSGS," *Clinical Journal of the American Society of Nephrology*, vol. 11, no. 10, pp. 1752–1759, 2016.

28

Disseminated Mycobacterium Tuberculosis and IgA Nephropathy

Gordon Audley,[1] Bianca Davidson,[2] Erika Jones,[2] Brendon Price,[3] Brian Rayner,[2] Nicola Wearne,[2] and Zibya Barday[2]

[1]*Division of General Medicine, Department of Medicine, Faculty of Health Sciences, University of Cape Town and Groote Schuur Hospital, Cape Town, South Africa*
[2]*Division of Nephrology and Hypertension, Department of Medicine, Faculty of Health Sciences, University of Cape Town and Groote Schuur Hospital, Cape Town, South Africa*
[3]*Division of Anatomical Pathology, Department of Pathology, Faculty of Health Sciences, University of Cape Town/National Health Laboratory Services, Groote Schuur Hospital, Cape Town, South Africa*

Correspondence should be addressed to Gordon Audley; ggaudley@gmail.com

Academic Editor: David Mudge

Mycobacterium tuberculosis (MTB) is an under-recognised cause of genitourinary disease. IgA nephropathy (IgAN), a leading cause of glomerulonephritis worldwide, has been described as a rare consequence of disseminated MTB infection. In this case report, we present the first case of MTB associated IgAN in Africa. Finding IgAN on kidney biopsy in an MTB endemic area should prompt a thorough investigation for MTB to increase the chance of remission of IgAN and prevent inappropriate use of immunosuppression.

1. Introduction

After COVID -19, *Mycobacterium tuberculosis* (MTB) is the second leading infectious cause of mortality globally [1]. South Africa is one of eight countries that account for two-thirds of the MTB global burden [1]. Despite this high prevalence of MTB, genitourinary TB is an often under-recognised extrapulmonary site of infection [2].

IgA nephropathy (IgAN) is the leading cause of glomerulonephritis [GN] worldwide [3]. In most cases, the cause remains unclear, leading to the diagnosis of primary IgAN [4]. Secondary IgAN is most often associated with infections, immune disorders, and malignancy [5]. Finding and treating an identified cause remains central to the otherwise largely supportive management approach to the disorder [6]. In a small series of case reports, IgAN has been linked to MTB [4]. In this case report, we present a rare case of IgAN in the setting of disseminated MTB.

2. Case Presentation and Results

A 41-year-old male, previously well, presented with a 2-year history of progressively worsening constitutional symptoms (fever, weight loss, and night sweats) and a dry cough. Additionally, he noted progressively worsening chronic lower back pain without sensory or motor fallout and a painful nonhealing ulcer on his right hallux. During this period, he presented several times to his local primary health care clinic where he was tested twice for MTB with a sputum Gene Xpert (GXP) test, which were both negative. He received symptomatic treatment for his back pain with paracetamol, nonsteroidal anti-inflammatory drugs (NSAIDs), and antibacterial cream for the ulcer on his toe.

His first contact with our institute was via the vascular surgery outpatient clinic, where he was referred for the nonhealing ulcer on his right hallux (Figure 1(a)). Table 1 reveals the blood investigations. The inflammatory markers

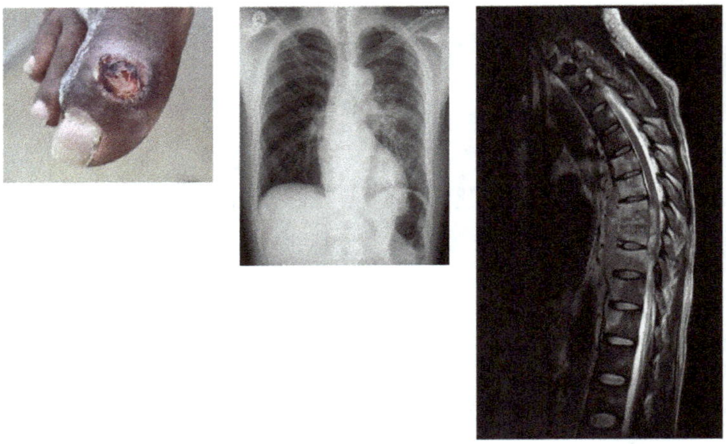

(a) (b) (c)

FIGURE 1: (a) Right hallux non-healing ulcer, (b) chest radiograph, and (c) magnetic resonance imaging (MRI) of the thoracic spine.

were markedly elevated (erythrocyte sediment rate >130 mm/hr (normal range: less than 20 mm/hr) and C-reactive protein 113 mg/ml (normal range: less than 10 mg/ml)). Immunoglobulin A (IgA) levels were raised at 6.2 g/L (normal range: 0.7–4 g/L), measurement of circulating IgA-MTB antigen complexes was not available at our laboratory. There was a mildly raised anti-DNase B of 259 IU/ml (normal range: less than 200 IU/ml), with a negative autoimmune antibody panel (antinuclear antibodies, antidouble-stranded DNA antibody, and antineutrophil cytoplasmic antibodies). Testing for human immune virus (HIV), hepatitis B and C virus and syphilis were all negative. A nephrology consult was requested for a raised urine protein-creatinine ratio (uPCR) of 0.242 g/mmol creatinine.

A clinical examination found him to be normotensive, apyretic, and cachectic with no peripheral lymphadenopathy nor oedema. Tenderness upon palpation of his thoracic spine was noted with no associated neurological fallout. On dipsticks, he had 3+ leucocytes and 3+ red blood cells, while urine microscopy revealed granular casts with no bacterial culture growth. Figure 1(b) shows a chest radiograph demonstrating bilateral reticular-nodular opacities.

An intensive MTB work up was performed. This included an induced sputum which tested trace positive for MTB on GXP and subsequently cultured MTB, sensitive to rifampicin and isoniazid. A biopsy of the right hallux ulcer (Figure 1(a)) revealed necrotising granulomatous inflammation with a solitary acid-fast bacillus seen on microscopy. Magnetic resonance imaging (MRI) of his spine (Figure 1(c)) revealed multi-level contiguous spondylitis at levels T6 to T10 with discitis and an epidural and paraspinal collection complicated by spinal cord compression but no oedema, in keeping with spinal MTB. No urine GXP nor urine TB cultures were sent.

The ultrasound showed bilateral normal-sized kidneys with increased echogenicity. A kidney biopsy was performed. The differential prior to kidney biopsy was acute interstitial nephritis (AIN) secondary to NSAIDs, direct infection of the kidney by MTB, or postinfectious glomerulonephritis.

Kidney biopsy demonstrated a total of 59 glomeruli, four of which were globally sclerosed, three were segmentally sclerosed, and one showed a cellular crescent to be present. Haematoxylin and eosin (H&E) showed glomeruli with diffuse mesangial hypercellularity with no evidence of endocapillary hypercellularity (Figure 2(a) and 2(b)). The Jones methenamine silver stain revealed no double contours or spikes present, and the Congo Red did not show any evidence of amyloidosis. Immunohistochemical stains revealed diffuse strong IgA (3+) staining within the mesangium with lesser amounts noted within the paramesangium region (Figure 2(c) and 2(d)). Weak staining for IgM and C3 were noted (1+ intensity). IgG and C1q stains were negative. The background kidney showed mild tubular atrophy and interstitial fibrosis with a chronicity score of 2/10 (mild) as per Sethi et al. criteria [7,8]. No granulomata nor acid-fast bacilli were seen and no MTB were cultured. The diagnosis of IgAN ($M_0E_0S_0T_0$-C_1) was assessed in the setting of disseminated MTB (pulmonary, spinal and skin) [9]. Early secreted antigenic target-6 staining was not available at our laboratory.

A multidisciplinary consultation (nephrology, orthopaedics, infectious diseases, and dermatology) advised first line MTB treatment with an extended course of 12 months (2 months intensive phase – (rifampicin/isoniazid, pyrazinamide/ethambutol), followed by 10 months of continuation phase (rifampicin/isoniazid)). An angiotensin-converting-enzyme inhibitor (enalapril) was prescribed for the proteinuria. At four months follow-up, the patient reported marked improvement in constitutional symptoms and back pain, while estimated GFR increased and uPCR also improved (Table 1).

3. Discussion

This report describes a rare case of secondary IgAN in the setting of MTB. To our knowledge, MTB-associated IgAN is limited to case reports and small case studies, with no cases described from Africa, despite the high prevalence and incidence of MTB throughout the continent. Kidney

TABLE 1: Blood and urine investigation results.

	8 weeks prior to admission	7 weeks prior to admission	Admission	1st week of admission	1 month follow-up	4 month follow-up
Sodium (136–145 mmol/l)	133	137	131	133	139	
Potassium (3.5–5.1 mmol/l)	5, 4	5, 4	5, 1	4, 6	4, 6	4.6
Urea (2.1–7.1 mmol/l)	6, 4	6, 2	4, 6	4, 3	2, 8	
Creatinine (64–104 umol/l)	90	102	94	87	67	70
Estimated GFR (ml/min/1.73 m^2)	91	78	86	85	113	111
Calcium (2.20–2.55 mmol/l)	2, 15			2, 14	2, 32	
Magnesium (0.63–1.05 mmol/l)	0, 85			0, 71	0, 75	
Phosphate (0.78–1.42 mmol/l)	1, 12			1, 3	1, 21	
Total Protein (60–78 g/l)		76		71		
Albumin (35–52 g/l)	30	32		25	34	
White cell Count (3.90–12.60 × 10^9/l)	7, 38	8, 34	9, 29	9, 76	5, 88	
Lymphocytes (1.40–4.50 (3.90–12.60 × 10^9/l)		1, 29		1, 55		
Haemoglobin (13–17 g/dl)	12, 2	12, 1	11	9, 6	13, 1	
Platelets (186–454 × 10^9/l)	587	646	710	603	529	
Total cholesterol (<5 mmol/l)	3, 33			3, 04		
Urine protein creatinine ratio (g/mmol creatinine)	0, 242		0, 137		0, 149	0.055

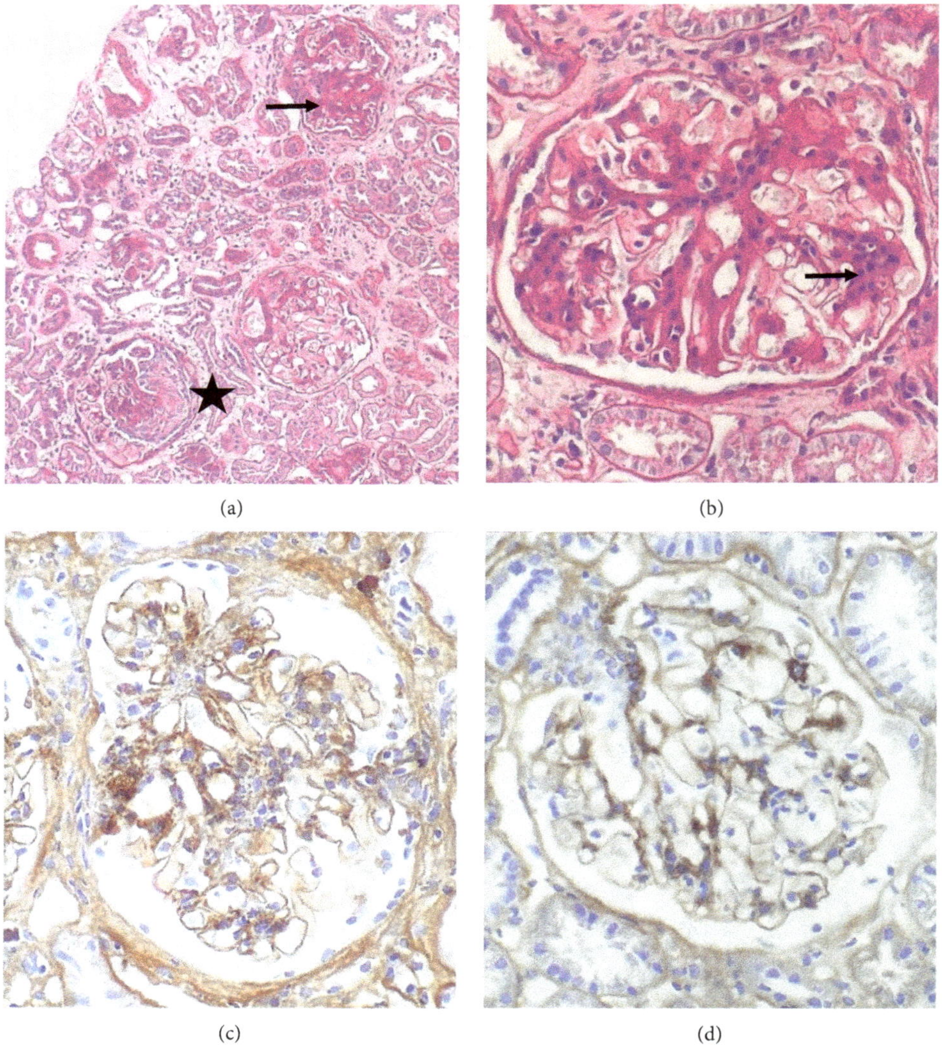

Figure 2: (a) Periodic acid-Schiff stained paraffin sections showing mesangial hypercellularity (arrow) and a focal cellular crescent (star) (x 100). (b) Higher magnification of glomerulus exhibiting mesangial hypercellularity (arrow) (x 400). (C) and (D) Immunohistochemical staining for IgA–strong mesangial and focal paramesangial staining, early subendothelial deposits are also appreciated (C). Strong mesangial staining was noted in occasional glomeruli which did not exhibit mesangial hypercellularity (D).

manifestations of MTB are diverse and heterogeneous, ranging from genitourinary TB, granulomatous interstitial nephritis, amyloidosis, treatment-related drug reactions, but rarely glomerulonephritis (GN). [2,10,11].

IgAN is the most prevalent primary cause of GN worldwide. The global prevalence rates vary according to ethnicity and geographical regions. It accounts for 40% of kidney biopsies in China and Japan, 30% in Europe, and 20% in the United States. [5] In Africa, IgAN appears to be comparatively less common and rare in the African black population [12]. In a 10-year retrospective analysis of native kidney biopsy reports in a tertiary centre in South Africa, IgAN was an infrequent cause of primary GN (5.8% of all identified cases) [13,14]. Furthermore, a meta-analysis of kidney biopsy findings across Africa between 1980 and 2004 found the prevalence of IgAN to be 2.8% [12]. The reasons for this are multifactorial and poorly understood.

The exact pathogenesis of MTB-IgAN is not well defined and an appropriate disease model is unavailable [4]. IgA, specifically against mycobacterial antigens, has been demonstrated in the sera of patients with active MTB, as have immune complexes of IgA antibodies and mycobacterial antigens [15]. The pathogenesis of IgAN is hypothesised to result from abnormally glycosylated IgA antibodies, which are mainly produced by mucosa-localized plasma cells in response to mucosal inflammation [4]. MTB antigens can stimulate $\gamma\delta$T cell activation and proliferation on the human mucosal surface to secrete a large amount of T cell-secreted transforming growth factor β1 (TGFβ1) [4]. High TGFβ1 levels stimulate B cells to differentiate into plasma cells [4]. These plasma cells subsequently produce defective IgA1 and promote IgA1 deposition in the mesangial areas of the kidney [4]. Deposition of these immune complexes, with subsequent activation of the alternative complement and the lectin pathway, with resultant local injury, leads to IgAN [15]. Identification in serum and demonstration on kidney biopsy of specific IgA-MTB antigen complexes and high TGFβ1 levels, although not available in our laboratory, would strengthen the causal link between MTB and IgAN. Furthermore, why certain individuals develop this pathological IgA response to MTB is still unclear and requires further investigation.

When MTB infection affects the kidney or genitourinary tract, the diagnosis may be difficult. The conventional methods of diagnosis include: urine MTB culture, urine GXP, and urine lipoarabinomannan (LAM). Urine microscopy and mycobacterial culture remain the gold standards for diagnosis of genitourinary MTB; however, sensitivity is low, with a culture yield reported as around 46% in HIV-negative persons, and results take up to six weeks to become available [16]. Although data is limited, urine and renal tissue GXP have shown diagnostic promise in MTB-associated granulomatous interstitial nephritis (direct renal granulomatous infection) [17]. The utility of GXP on urine has been reported to have a sensitivity of 87% and specificity of 91% in a meta-analysis by Hillemann et al. in this setting [18]. Urine LAM is a valuable diagnostic tool in diagnosing renal involvement in disseminated MTB; however, its utility has only been demonstrated in human immune deficiency (HIV) positive patients with advanced immunosuppression and is thus not applicable in our case [19]. The role of urine MTB culture, GXP, and LAM in the setting of MTB associated IgAN (indirect immune mediated disease) has to our knowledge not been explored. Early secreted antigenic target-6 (ESAT-6), an antigen secreted by MTB, is implicated in the virulence and pathogenicity of MTB. Two case studies from China have demonstrated that ESAT-6 staining of the kidney tissue can assist in the diagnosis of MTB in the kidney [5,15]. Li et al. showed that when the culture is negative and ESAT-6 is positive, the chance of progressing to overt clinical MTB with immune suppression is high if no MTB prophylaxis is provided [15]. MTB treatment on the other hand, in the setting of IgAN and MTB, is associated with resolution of the proteinuria and haematuria [15].

In our resource-limited setting, without the advanced diagnostic techniques discussed above, we are unable to conclusively prove that our patient's disseminated MTB infection was indeed the cause of the IgAN; however, the rapid improvement in proteinuria as well as the clearance of haematuria with TB treatment strengthens our case of cause and effect.

4. Conclusion

In conclusion, in the setting where IgAN is a rare disease and MTB is common, the histological diagnosis of IgAN should prompt an extensive MTB workup. This will expedite the diagnosis and allow timely initiation of MTB treatment to increase the chance of remission of IgAN and prevent inappropriate use of immunosuppression with the increased risk of MTB dissemination [15].

Additional Points

1. MTB is an important, albeit rare, secondary cause of IgAN. 2. Despite a high MTB prevalence in Africa–no cases of MTB associated IgAN have previously been described. 3. Finding IgAN in a MTB endemic area should prompt extensive work-up for MTB.

Acknowledgments

The authors would like to thank all staff in the E13 renal unit at Groote Schuur Hospital for their tireless dedication to their patients.

References

[1] World Health Orginization, "Tuberculosis," 2021, https://www.who.int/news-room/fact-sheets/detail/tuberculosis.

[2] J. B. Eastwood, C. M. Corbishley, and J. M. Grange, "Tuberculosis and the kidney," *Journal of the American Society of Nephrology*, vol. 12, no. 6, pp. 1307–1314, 2001.

[3] L. De Siati, M. Paroli, C. Ferri, A. O. Muda, G. Bruno, and V. Barnaba, "Immunoglobulin A nephropathy complicating pulmonary tuberculosis," *Annals of Diagnostic Pathology*, vol. 3, no. 5, pp. 300–303, 1999.

[4] Y. Wang and Y. Tao, "Tuberculosis-associated IgA nephropathy," *Journal of International Medical Research*, vol. 46, no. 7, pp. 2549–2557, 2018.

[5] N. Zhao, J. Y. Sun, H. F. Xu, and F. Y. Sun, "Early diagnosis of tuberculosis-associated IgA nephropathy with ESAT-6," *Tohoku Journal of Experimental Medicine*, vol. 241, no. 4, pp. 271–279, 2017.

[6] B. H. Rovin, S. G. Adler, J. Barratt et al., "KDIGO 2021 clinical practice guideline for the management of glomerular diseases," *Kidney International*, vol. 100, no. 4, pp. S1–S276, 2021.

[7] S. Sethi and F. C Fervenza, "Standardized classification and reporting of glomerulonephritis," *Nephrology Dialysis Transplantation*, vol. 34, no. 2, pp. 193–199, 2019 Feb 1.

[8] S. Sethi, V. D. D'Agati, C. C Nast et al., "A proposal for standardized grading of chronic changes in native kidney biopsy specimens," *Kidney International*, vol. 91, no. 4, pp. 787–789, 2017.

[9] I. S. D. Roberts, H. T. Cook, S. Troyanov et al., "The Oxford classification of IgA nephropathy: pathology definitions, correlations, and reproducibility," *Kidney International*, vol. 76, no. 5, pp. 546–556, 2009.

[10] B. Davidson, D. Nel, E. S. W. Jones et al., "Granulomatous interstitial nephritis on renal biopsy in human immunodeficiency virus positive patients: prevalence and causes in Cape Town, South Africa," *Nephrology*, vol. 24, no. 7, pp. 681–688, 2019.

[11] Y. Solak, A. Gaipov, M. Anil et al., "Glomerulonephritis associated with tuberculosis: a case report and literature review," *The Kaohsiung Journal of Medical Sciences*, vol. 29, no. 6, pp. 337–342, 2013.

[12] I. G. Okpechi, O. I. Ameh, A. K. Bello, P. Ronco, C. R. Swanepoel, and A. P. Kengne, "Epidemiology of histologically proven Glomerulonephritis in Africa: a systematic review and meta-analysis," *PLoS One*, vol. 11, no. 3, Article ID e0152203, 2016.

[13] I. Okpechi, C. Swanepoel, M. Duffield et al., "Patterns of renal disease in Cape Town South Africa: a 10-year review of a single-centre renal biopsy database," *Nephrology Dialysis Transplantation*, vol. 26, no. 6, pp. 1853–1861, 2011 Jun.

[14] A. Vermeulen, C. N. Menezes, M. Mashabane et al., "Patterns of renal disease: a 30-year renal biopsy study at chris hani baragwanath academic hospital, soweto, johannesburg, South Africa," *South African Medical Journal*, vol. 109, no. 7, pp. 486–492, 2019.

[15] S. Li, T. Siyuan, F. Jiangmin et al., "Analysis of the association between *Mycobacterium tuberculosis* infection and Immunoglobulin A nephropathy by early secreted antigenic target 6 detection in renal biopsies: a prospective study," *Postgraduate Medicine*, vol. 129, no. 3, pp. 307–311, 2017.

[16] Y. Pang, Y. Shang, J. Lu et al., "GeneXpert MTB/RIF assay in the diagnosis of urinary tuberculosis from urine specimens," *Scientific Reports*, vol. 7, no. 1, p. 6181, 2017.

[17] A. K. Hemal, N. P. Gupta, T. P. Rajeev, R. Kumar, L. Dar, and P. Seth, "Polymerase chain reaction in clinically suspected genitourinary tuberculosis: comparison with intravenous urography, bladder biopsy, and urine acid fast bacilli culture," *Urology*, vol. 56, no. 4, pp. 570–574, 2000 Oct 1.

[18] D. Hillemann, S. Rüsch-Gerdes, C. Boehme, and E. Richter, "Rapid molecular detection of extrapulmonary tuberculosis by the automated GeneXpert MTB/RIF system," *Journal of Clinical Microbiology*, vol. 49, no. 4, pp. 1202–1205, 2011.

[19] A. Gupta-Wright, K. L. Fielding, J. J. van Oosterhout et al., "Rapid urine-based screening for tuberculosis to reduce AIDS-related mortality in hospitalized patients in Africa (the STAMP trial): study protocol for a randomised controlled trial," *BMC Infectious Diseases*, vol. 16, no. 1, p. 501, 2016.

29

Calciphylaxis: A Long Road to Cure with a Multidisciplinary and Multimodal Approach

Vasiliki Zoi, Dimitra Bacharaki, Aggeliki Sardeli, Minas Karagiannis, and Sophia Lionaki

Department of Nephrology, National and Kapodistrian University of Athens, Attikon Hospital, Athens, Greece

Correspondence should be addressed to Sophia Lionaki; sofia.lionaki@gmail.com

Academic Editor: Yoshihide Fujigaki

Calciphylaxis is a rare yet potentially fatal condition, resulting from ectopic calcification of the small arterioles of the dermis with resulting necrotic lesions infection, sepsis, and death. In hemodialysis patients, its prevalence ranges between 1 and 4%, while mortality amounts to 30–80%. We present in here a 45-year-old female on chronic dialysis with morbid obesity, who was admitted for painful nodules in the lower abdomen and necrotic lesions at the lower extremities. Severe uremia and uncontrolled secondary hyperparathyroidism were the main characteristics in this patient, and thus, a clinical diagnosis of calciphylaxis was made. Treatment modalities included wound care plus antibiotics and analgesics, daily hemodialysis, and strategies targeting calcification with sodium thiosulfate, cinacalcet, and non-calcium-containing binders. A crucial factor for overcoming the infection-lesion vicious circle is thorough and daily care of the lesions. Nursing attention was focused on the motivation of her self-care, for the prevention of institutionalization and the psychological support of the patient and her family. The most intriguing feature was the fact that she experienced several exacerbations during the follow-up time. During the final relapse, she was prescribed hyperbaric oxygen sessions that actually put the disease under control thereafter. The good outcome for this patient was probably related to the combination of close follow-up along with a multidisciplinary approach.

1. Introduction

Calciphylaxis or uremic arteriolopathy (CUA) is a rare necrotic lesion of dermal and subcutaneous tissue resulting from ectopic calcification of the medial layer of arterioles and small arteries. These changes cause tissue ischemia, necrosis, ulceration, and finally sepsis. It was first described in 1968 by Anderson et al. as a necrotic lesion of dermal and subcutaneous tissue in patients with hyperparathyroidism and hypercalcemia [1]. Calciphylaxis primarily affects patients on dialysis or after renal transplantation; however, exceptions have been reported. The average age of onset is between 50 and 60 years with a clear female predominance [2, 3]. Major risk factors include Caucasian ethnicity, female gender, diabetes mellitus, dialysis, obesity, hypoalbuminemia in the context of malnutrition and chronic inflammation, hyperphosphatemia, elevated calcium x phosphate product, and combined use of active vitamin D analogues with high doses of calcium-containing phosphate binders [4, 5] and the use of vitamin K antagonists. Among hemodialysis patients, the incidence rate has been estimated at 35 cases per 10,000 patients in the United States and 4 cases per 10,000 patients in Europe. The mortality rate however amounts to 30–80% and is more often related to infectious complications resulting in sepsis. Furthermore, the overall one-year survival does not exceed 40% [6]. Clinically, it frequently develops in the lower extremities but may also manifest around the abdomen and hips and may affect peripheral sites or even skeletal muscle. Management of CUA is primarily based on wound care with surgical debridement and systemic antibiotics, elimination of all possible precipitating factors of ectopic calcification, administering agents capable of inhibiting the progress of calcification, and controlling risk factors to avoid recurrences.

We describe in here a patient with calciphylaxis, who experienced multiple relapses for more than a year necessitating the application of all available treatments. In our experience, patient survival was probably related to close monitoring, personalized medicine, and exploitation of a multidisciplinary strategy [1, 7].

2. Case Description

A 45-year-old obese female on hemodialysis presented to the emergency department with extremely painful nodules of the lower abdomen area and necrotic lesions at the buttocks and inner surface of the thighs (Figures 1(a)–1(c)). She had been dialyzed for two months, through a temporary central venous catheter, that was malfunctioning. She had poorly controlled Hashimoto thyroiditis and suffered from morbid obesity (BMI: 53 Kg/m^2). Laboratory results at presentation were suggestive of uncontrolled uremia and severe hyperparathyroidism (Table 1). Notably, the product of phosphate x calcium (Ca) was 81.34 with high serum parathormone (PTH) of 1500 pg/μL, but ultrasonography of the parathyroid area was negative for adenomas.

A definitive diagnosis of calciphylaxis was made by a skin biopsy (Figure 2), which revealed medial calcification of dermal arterioles or small arteries and fibrointimal hyperplasia, microthrombi, and vascular narrowing or occlusion, often with evidence of necrosis. Calcification of small- to medium-sized blood vessels was also seen. The intimal layer of blood vessels was significant for fibrosis, and intravascular thrombi were seen. The main feature was the diffuse calcification of small capillaries in the adipose tissue.

A nuclear bone scan (Figure 3(a)) using scintigraphy with technetium 99 m revealed increased radiotracer uptake in the soft tissue of the thighs, homogenously and bilaterally, as well as in all areas of the skin lesions. Notably, a three-phase technetium 99 m methylene diphosphate bone scan is not required for the diagnosis of CUA but it may be a helpful adjunct, especially in early lesions, since it is highly sensitive and specific to identify the extent of cutaneous calcifications. In this case, bone scintigraphy was helpful in order to demonstrate the response to treatment (as decreased radiotracer uptake).

2.1. Management and Outcome. Treatment strategies aimed to maintain phosphorus levels at less than 5.5 mg/dL. Dialysis frequency was increased (six times per week for 3-4 hours daily) to optimize the clearance of uremic molecules and improve bone-mineral markers while the central venous catheter was replaced by a permanent one. Calcium supplements and calcium-based phosphate binders were discontinued and converted to non-calcium-containing binders (800 mg, 3 TID). High calcium dialysate baths (greater than 2.5 mEq/L) were avoided. In order to manage hyperparathyroidism, cinacalcet, a calcimimetic agent, was introduced. Sodium thiosulfate was given intravenously at the end of hemodialysis, in low doses at first to inhibit soft tissue calcification. Side effects of sodium thiosulfate included metabolic acidosis and gastrointestinal disturbances such as nausea and vomiting. However, the patient was thoroughly informed and supported, in order to accept the treatment in carefully incremented doses.

Skin lesions were challenging to treat, with wound care and pain management being extremely important. Debridement was utilized to remove devitalized and necrotic tissue, prevent infection, and promote healing. Appropriate antibiotics were given culture-guided, regularly, and by clinical indication. During the final relapse, she was offered hyperbaric oxygen therapy to facilitate wound healing. Specifically, she underwent 10 sessions of hyperbaric oxygen sequentially and then once monthly, leading to completely healed lesions. The patient was reluctant to follow the recommendation for a minimum of 20 treatments, i.e., 5–7 sessions per week. However, we believe that this treatment played a tremendous role in the final outcome. Eventually, all the ulcers were replaced by a new epithelium (Table 2).

Nursing care included precise administration of the medication and handling of the increased incidents during hemodialysis, including vomiting due to the thiosulfate treatment. The new permanent central venous catheter was cared for on a daily basis. The treatment included the patient's immense pain to be cured with narcotic analgesic medication, and the lesions required daily cleaning. To avoid institutionalization, efforts were made to promote her self-care, motivate her, and prevent hospitalization's depression. She was assisted to keep in touch with her work and friends through telephone and internet and restart one of her hobbies, which was knitting. Gradually, she was able to bathe herself, get off the bed on her one, and walk through the hospital. Great deal of time was given for psychological support of the patient and her family with the assistance of a psychologist, as this ensured their compliance to the treatment and their full support. Additional care was paid by the nursing staff and the dietician to not skip meals, since adequate nutrition is imperative for wound healing. Pain of the lesions which was accentuated during hemodialysis, a characteristic feature of calciphylaxis, already made her anorectic. She was finally discharged 70 days after admission, but she was closely followed up for a total of 13 months. At that point, she had also lost 30 kg and had regained ambulatory capacity with regular physical therapy. Nowadays, she receives hemodialysis treatment with no relapses in terms of calciphylaxis (Figures 1(d) and 3(b)).

3. Discussion

Calciphylaxis is a rare, potentially life-threatening syndrome characterized by progressive and painful skin ulcerations associated with medial calcification of medium-sized and small cutaneous arterial vessels. Superinfection of necrotic skin lesions with subsequent sepsis significantly contributes to this outcome and, most of the time, leads to death [4]. This case of calciphylaxis was dominated by multiple relapses for more than a year, which were successfully managed using a personalized approach with multiple therapeutical modalities including increased dialysis frequency, non-calcium-containing binders, cinacalcet, sodium thiosulfate, and hyperbaric oxygen therapy. We considered organizing a clinical trial, but we did not pull through, due to low enrollment.

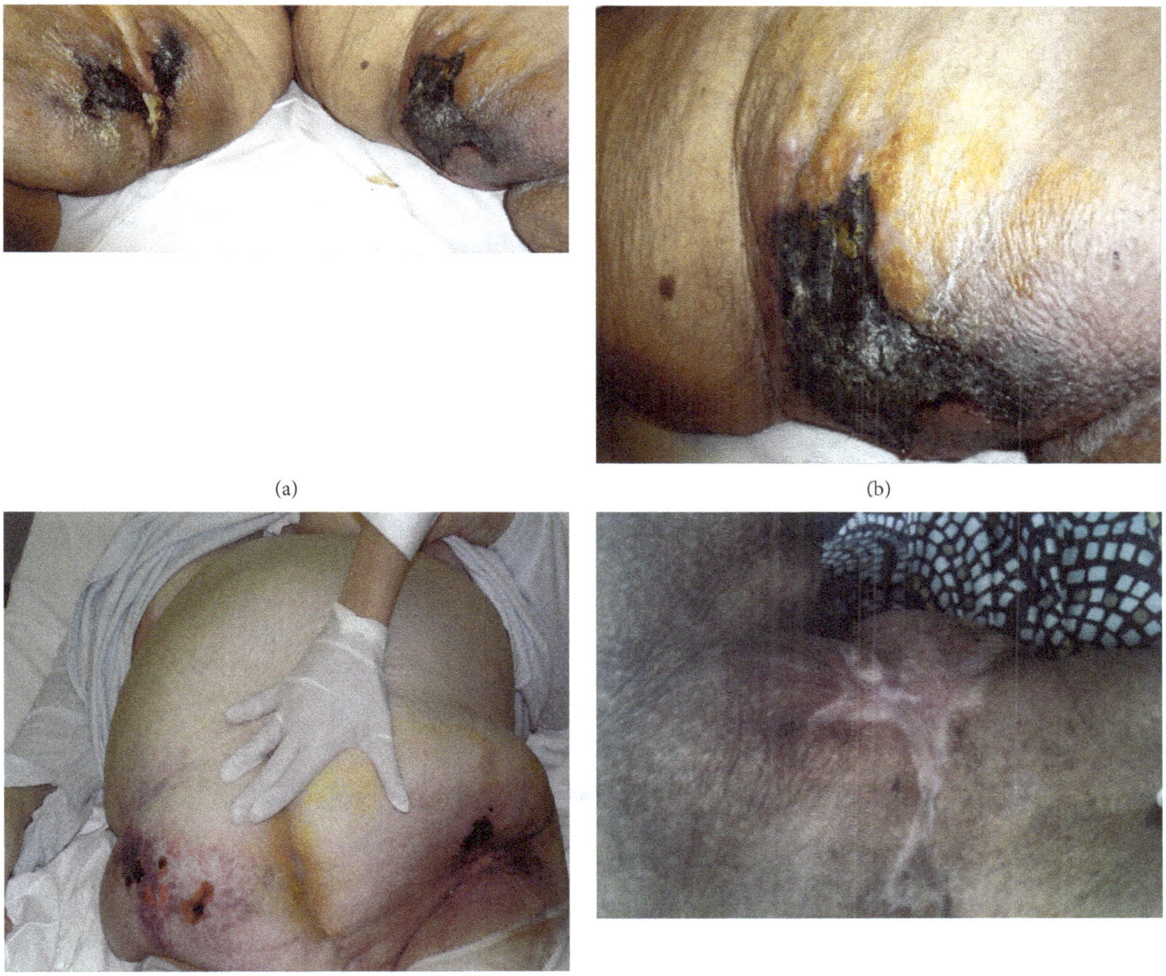

(a) (b) (c) (d)

FIGURE 1: (a) Necrotic tissues of the thighs; (b) necrotic tissues; (c) abdomen ulcers; (d) healed necrotic lesions with scars.

TABLE 1: Laboratory measurements at different points during the follow-up time.

Laboratory outcomes (serum)	On admission	1st month	6th month	End of follow-up
WBC (K/μl)	14.41 K/μl	7.33	12.81	8.05
NEUT. (K/μl)	11.71	4.76	8.96	4.52
Hct (%)	22.3	28.7	29.9	27.5
Hb (g/dl)	6.6	8.6	8.7	9.1
Ca (mg/dl)	8.3	9.3	8.9	8.5
Urea (mg/dl)	227	92	34	32
Creatinine (mg/dl)	11.3	3.5	3	3.4
P (mg/dl)	9.8	3.6	2.4	2.7
PTH (pg/ml)	1500	48.6	45	42
CRP (mg/dl)	288	34.7	59.6	15

In most occasions, calciphylaxis is a clinical diagnosis. The biological content includes secondary hyperparathyroidism and obvious phosphorus and calcium metabolism disorders. Although pathogenesis remains incompletely understood, elevated calcium x phosphate product, increased serum PTH, warfarin, iron therapy, corticosteroids, and administration of activated vitamin D have been associated with the development of calciphylaxis. Yet, abnormalities of bone-mineral parameters are not sufficient to cause calciphylaxis on their own in most patients [9, 15]. Deficiency of vascular calcification inhibitors such as fetuin-A, osteoprotegerin, and matrix Gla protein may play a role in the development of calciphylaxis. Fetuin-A is a glycoprotein that binds calcium and phosphorus, and it is

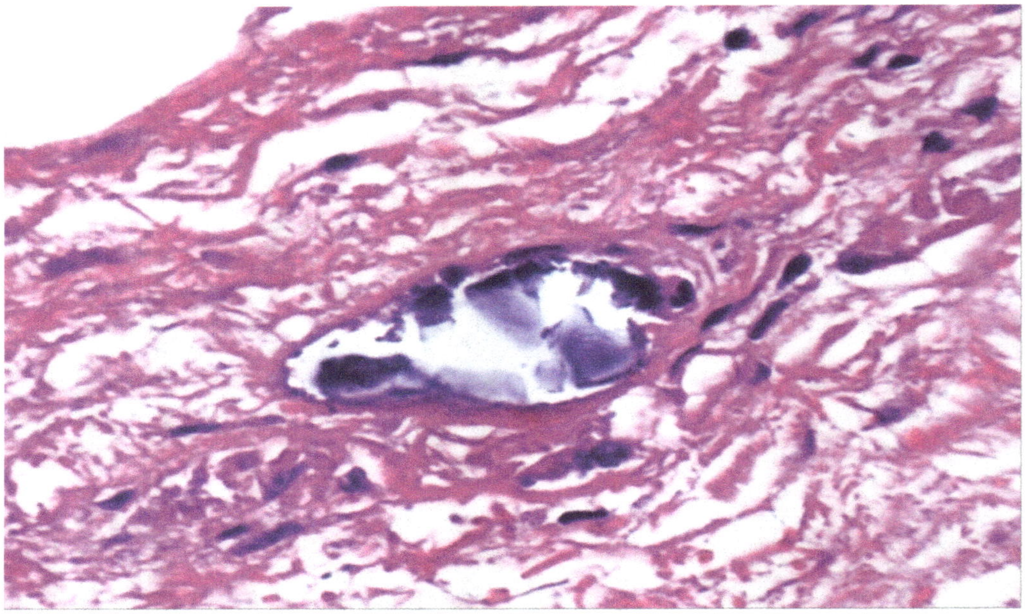

FIGURE 2: Skin biopsy.

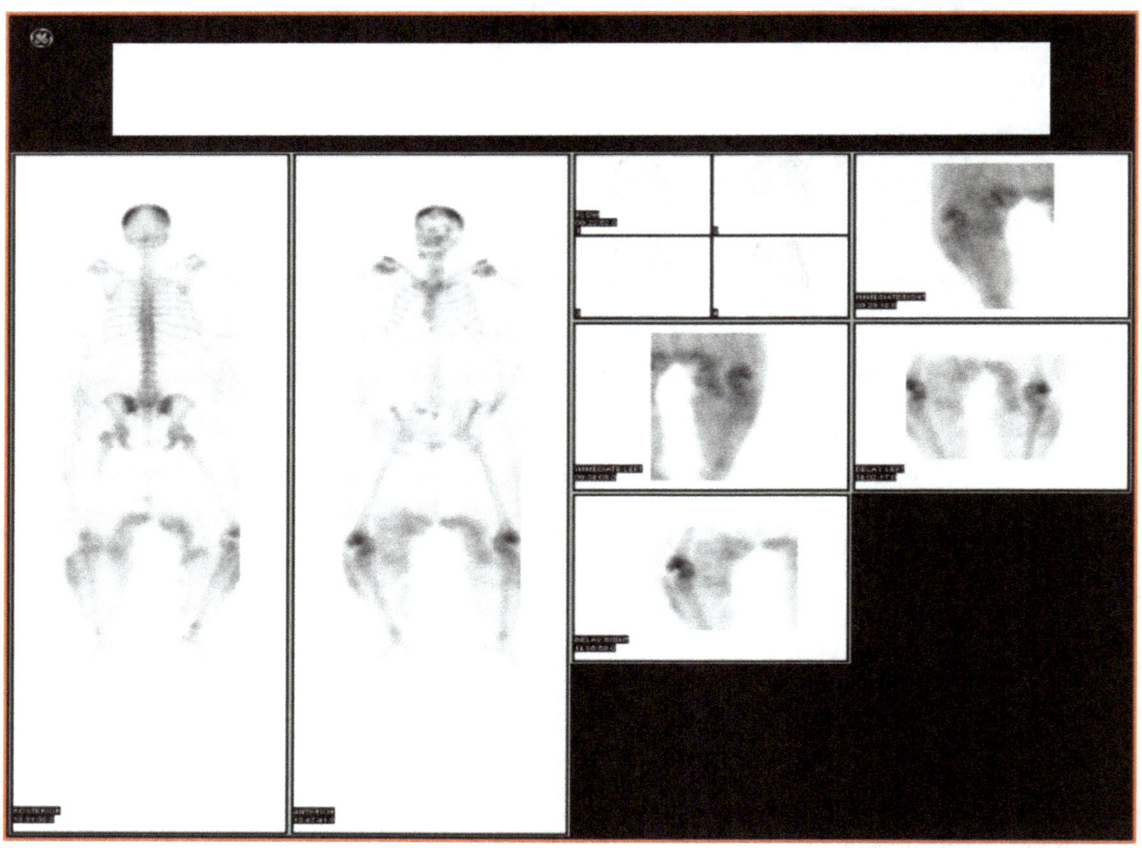

(a)

FIGURE 3: Continued.

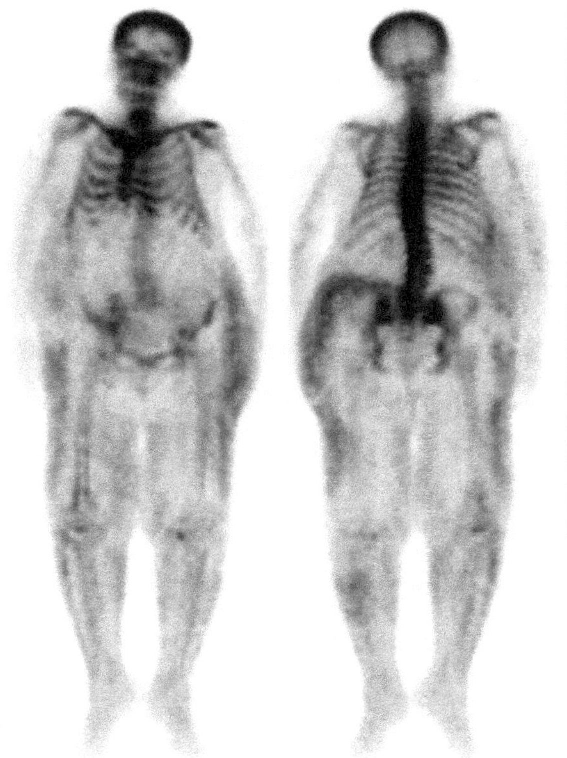

(b)

FIGURE 3: (a) Bone scintigraphy with technetium 99 m before therapy; (b) bone scintigraphy with technetium 99 m after therapy.

TABLE 2: Therapies used for the management of patients with calciphylaxis and mechanisms of action.

Therapies	Mechanism of action
Increased dialysis frequency	Clearance of uremic molecules [3, 4, 8]
Dialyzate calcium 1,25 mmol/L	Slowing down calcification [3, 4, 6]
Non-calcium-containing binders	Avoiding hypercalcemia—high phosphorus [3, 4, 9]
Cinacalcet	Controlling parathyroid hormones [10, 11]
Sodium thiosulfate	Inhibiting calcification [12, 13]
Debridement	Ulceration treatment [6]
Hyperbaric oxygen therapy	Tissue oxygenation—wound healing [8, 14]

downregulated in dialysis patients. Osteoprotegerin plays an important role in bone metabolism. Matrix G1a protein may also prevent vascular calcification and is dependent on vitamin K-dependent carboxylation for its activity [10, 16].

Thiosulfate is a chelating agent, with high affinity to calcium ions, which may interfere with calcium and phosphate precipitation producing soluble calcium thiosulfate which can potentially be removed by dialysis [12, 13]. It may also interfere with the local inflammation process by antioxidant properties [17]. Treatment with sodium thiosulfate is off-label but has been routinely used in calciphylaxis and is considered the cornerstone of its treatment [12, 13]. The mechanism by which sodium thiosulfate treats calcific uremic arteriolopathy remains unknown. Previously, it was believed to work only through calcium chelation; however, recent studies suggest that sodium thiosulfate may also inhibit soft tissue calcification through mechanisms independent of calcium binding.

Moreover, Basile et al. [18] reported successful hyperbaric oxygen therapy in a small number of calciphylaxis patients. This approach is based on the attempt to improve wound healing in ischemic tissues. In that study, the patients were exposed to 100% oxygen under 2.5-fold elevated atmospheric pressure in a closed chamber for 90 minutes per session in order to significantly increase local oxygen pressure in the ulcerated and necrotic areas (the number of sessions per patient ranged between 20 and 108) while 8 of 11 patients showed effective healing of ulcerations [8, 17]. Finally, management of calciphylaxis aims at the restoration of phosphocalcic balance, effective detoxification of affected areas, and the elimination of as many risk factors as possible. Cinacalcet was introduced to lower PTH in place of activated vitamin D in order to control serum calcium and phosphorus levels [11].

In conclusion, the majority of cases with calciphylaxis is seen in the setting of end-stage kidney disease, as a result of secondary hyperparathyroidism and elevation of the serum calcium-phosphate product. A multifactorial etiology is likely. In this case, factors such as morbid obesity, inadequate dialysis, uncontrolled hyperparathyroidism, and history of vitamin D deficiency were possibly involved. Various treatment options were employed. Supportive management methods like pain control and wound care with sodium thiosulfate, hyperbaric oxygen therapy, tissue plasminogen activator, vitamin D and vitamin K supplementation, parathyroidectomy, and daily hemodialysis have been described. Sodium thiosulfate is thought to work by enhancing the solubility of calcium phosphate and removing calcifications. Importantly, a multidisciplinary approach is often needed to fight calciphylaxis including input from a nephrologist, dermatologist, dietician, wound surgeon, wound nurse, dialysis nurse, pain management specialist, palliative care team, and hyperbaric oxygen provider combined with close follow-up and escalation of treatment choices in autoimmune diseases.

Consent

Written informed consent for publication of clinical details and clinical images were obtained from the patient.

References

[1] D. C. Anderson, W. K. Stewart, and D. M. Piercy, "Calcifying panniculitis with fat and SKIN necrosis in a case of uraemia with autonomous hyperparathyroidism," *Lancet*, vol. 292, no. 7563, pp. 323–325, 1968.

[2] A. Jovanovich and M. Chonchol, "Calcific uremic arteriolopathy revisited," *Journal of the American Society of Nephrology*, vol. 27, no. 11, pp. 3233–3235, 2016.

[3] S. U. Nigwekar, C. A. Solid, E. Ankers et al., "Quantifying a rare disease in administrative data: the example of calciphylaxis," *Journal of General Internal Medicine*, vol. 29, pp. S724–S731, 2014.

[4] S. U. Nigwekar, D. Kroshinsky, R. M. Nazarian et al., "Calciphylaxis: risk factors, diagnosis, and treatment," *American Journal of Kidney Diseases*, vol. 66, no. 1, pp. 133–146, 2015.

[5] S. U. Nigwekar, S. Zhao, J. Wenger et al., "A nationally representative study of calcific uremic arteriolopathy risk factors," *Journal of the American Society of Nephrology*, vol. 27, no. 11, pp. 3421–3429, 2016.

[6] S. Udomkarnjananun, K. Kongnatthasate, K. Praditpornsilpa, S. Eiam-Ong, B. L. Jaber, and P. Susantitaphong, "Treatment of calciphylaxis in CKD: a systematic review and meta-analysis," *Kidney International Reports*, vol. 4, no. 2, pp. 231–244, 2019.

[7] V. M. Brandenburg, R. Kramann, H. Rothe et al., "Calcific uremic arteriolopathy (calciphylaxis): data from a large nationwide registry," *Nephrology Dialysis Transplantation*, vol. 32, no. 1, pp. 126–132, 2017.

[8] C. Basil, A. Montanaro, M. Masi, G. Pati, P. De Maio, and A. Gismondi, "Hyperbaric oxygen therapy for calcific uremic arteriolpathy: a case series," *Journal of Nephrology*, vol. 15, 2002.

[9] M. Ketteler, P. H. Biggar, V. M. Brandenburg, G. Schlieper, R. Westenfeld, and J. Floege, "Epidemiology, pathophysiology and therapy of calciphylaxis," *Deutsches Arzteblatt*, vol. 104, no. 50, pp. 3481–3485, 2007.

[10] P. A. Price, M. K. Williamson, T. M. T. Nguyen, and T. N. Than, "Serum levels of the fetuin—mineral complex correlate with artery calcification in the rat," *Journal of Biological Chemistry*, vol. 279, no. 3, pp. 1594–1600, 2004.

[11] J. Floege, Y. Kubo, A. Floege, G. M. Chertow, and P. S. Parfrey, "The effect of cinacalcet on calcific uremic arteriolopathy events in patients receiving hemodialysis: the EVOLVE trial," *Clinical Journal of the American Society of Nephrology*, vol. 10, no. 5, pp. 800–807, 2015.

[12] S. U. Nigwekar, S. M. Brunelli, D. Meade, W. Wang, J. Hymes, and E. Lacson, "Sodium thiosulfate therapy for calcific uremic arteriolopathy," *Clinical Journal of the American Society of Nephrology*, vol. 8, no. 7, pp. 1162–1170, 2013.

[13] G. F. Cohen, S. Nikki, and B. S. Vyas, "Sodium thiosulfate in the treatment of calciphylaxis," *Journal of Clinical and Aesthetic Dermatology*, vol. 6, no. 5, pp. 41–44, 2013.

[14] J. An, B. Devaney, K. Y. Ooi, S. Ford, G. Frawley, and S. Menahem, "Hyperbaric oxygen in the treatment of calciphylaxis: a case series and literature review," *Nephrology*, vol. 20, no. 7, pp. 444–450, 2015.

[15] T. Ghosh, D. S. Winchester, M. D. P. Davis, R. El-Azhary, and N. I. Comfere, "Early clinical presentations and progression of calciphylaxis," *International Journal of Dermatology*, vol. 56, no. 8, pp. 856–861, 2017.

[16] A. S. Dobry, L. N. Ko, J. St John, J. M. Sloan, S. Nigwekar, and D. Kroshinsky, "Association between hypercoagulable conditions and calciphylaxis in patients with renal disease: a case-control study," *JAMA Dermatol*, vol. 154, no. 2, p. 182, 2018.

[17] S. U. Nigwekar, "Multidisciplinary approach to calcific uremic arteriolopathy," *Current Opinion in Nephrology and Hypertension*, vol. 24, no. 6, pp. 531–537, 2015.

[18] C. Basile, "Hyperbaric oxygen therapy in the treatment of calciphylaxis? Yes, more than hope," *Kidney International*, vol. 62, no. 6, 2002.

30

An Unusual Case of Kidney Injury in a Young Woman with a Connective Tissue Disease

Roberto Rivera and Salvador Vila

Department of Medicine, University of Puerto Rico School of Medicine, Guillermo Arbona Building Room A824A, PO Box 365067, San Juan, PR 00936-5067, USA

Correspondence should be addressed to Salvador Vila; svilaperez@hotmail.com

Academic Editor: Yoshihide Fujigaki

A 32-year-old female was admitted to our institution with thrombocytopenia, fever, serositis, hepatosplenomegaly, diffuse lymphadenopathy, and renal insufficiency. A diagnosis of systemic lupus erythematosus was made. Due to recalcitrant thrombocytopenia, serositis, and renal insufficiency methylprednisolone was prescribed in high doses. In addition to proteinuria and hematuria, she was found to have uric acid crystals in her urinalysis. A serum uric acid was found elevated at 18 mg/dL. Rasburicase infusions were started. Within 5 days of commencing rasburicase and continuing high-dose methylprednisolone, her serum creatinine normalized and proteinuria resolved. The microhematuria disappeared within 2 weeks of beginning rasburicase. The rapid reversal of renal insufficiency and all urinary abnormalities after the start of rasburicase infusions suggests that the renal injury was most likely due to uric acid-mediated renal injury and not lupus nephritis. Our case illustrates the co-occurrence of 2 distinct clinical entities, one common for the patient's age, sex, and foremost clinical findings, while the other uncommon and unexpected, but both associated to kidney injury. Clinicians must be aware that careful evaluation of symptoms and laboratory tests is needed to make a thorough differential diagnosis and provide the right treatment at the most opportune moment.

1. Case Report

A 32-year-old female was transferred to our institution due to recalcitrant thrombocytopenia and suspicion of lymphoma. Three months prior to her referral, she started to experience fever, chills, and abdominal pain. She was found to have an enlarged liver and spleen as well as lymph node enlargement in multiple body sites. An oncologist evaluated the patient and ordered diagnostic laboratory tests. However, she was hospitalized 3 days prior to return appointment with the oncologist at a different hospital due to hemoptysis and easily bruised skin. Anemia, thrombocytopenia, and renal insufficiency were noted. Blood products transfusions were given without improvement in the thrombocytopenia. She was then referred to our institution with a presumptive diagnosis of lymphoma.

Upon admission, a history of bouts of inflammatory arthritis in the past was obtained. Episodes of Raynaud's phenomena were observed. The CBC showed a white blood cell count of 6 930/μL, hemoglobin of 7.1 gm/dL, platelet count of 3 000/μL, Westergren sedimentation rate (WSR) of 150 mm/hr, and C-reactive protein (CRP) of 188.2 mg/dL. Serum chemistries were abnormal for blood urea nitrogen of 50.2 mg/dL, serum creatinine (SCr) of 2.36 mg/dL, calcium of 7.4 mg/dL, phosphorus of 4.9 mg/dL, albumin of 1.6 gm/dL, alkaline phosphatase of 246 IU/L, and serum uric acid (SUA) of 18 mg/dL. Total bilirubin and direct/indirect bilirubin ratio were normal. The urinalysis was abnormal for 35–40 RBC/HPF, and the presence of many uric acid crystals. Spot urine for protein creatinine ratio (SUPCR) was 0.815 mg/mg. Computerized tomography of the chest and abdominopelvic areas revealed bilateral pleural effusions, lymphadenopathy, hepatosplenomegaly, and ascites (Figure 1).

Immediately upon arrival a clinical diagnosis of systemic lupus erythematosus with multiorgan involvement was

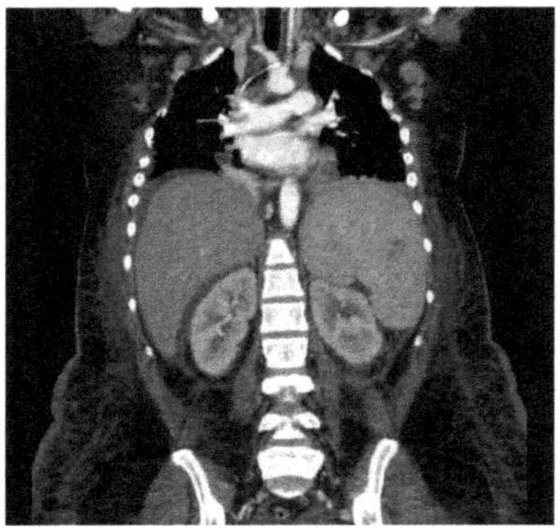

FIGURE 1: Abdominopelvic CT showing pleural effusions, lymphadenopathies, hepatosplenomegaly, and ascites.

made based on gender, age, serositis, prior history of inflammatory arthritis, renal insufficiency, and Raynaud's phenomena. Lupus nephritis was considered the cause of the kidney insufficiency and intravenous (IV) methylprednisolone, 1 gm daily for 3 days followed by 1 mg/kg/day, was started. However, the presence of uric acid crystals in the urinalysis and elevated SUA made us suspicious of urate nephropathy. Rasburicase infusions were started. Within 5 days of starting rasburicase infusions, the Scr normalized, and proteinuria resolved. Microhematuria resolved at the end of week 2 of rasburicase infusions. Urine output also increased from approximately 600 cc/day to around 1000 cc/day (Figure 2).

The platelet count failed to increase after 4 weeks of corticosteroids use and IV immune globulin (IVIG) at 0.4 gm daily for 5 days was started. One month after the IVIG infusions ended, she persisted with platelet counts below 10000/μL and rituximab 750 mg IV weekly infusions for four consecutive weeks was started. Nineteen days after the start of rituximab, the platelet count began to increase, and the pleural effusions and ascites improved.

Additional investigations include a positive FANA at a titer of 1 : 2560, speckled pattern, C_3 of 87.3 (normal range (NR) 88–201), C_4 of 8.8 (NR 12–45), anti-SSA Ab >240 EU/mL, anti-U1 RNP Ab >206 EU/mL, RF IgM of 34 IU/mL (NR < 20),and positive lupus anticoagulant. Anti-cardiolipin, anti-β2 glycoprotein-1, anti-ds-DNA, anti-Sm, and anti-CCP Ab were all negative. Serum cryoglobulins were not detected. Bone marrow biopsy showed a normocellular bone marrow with megakaryocytic hyperplasia. Core needle biopsy of axillary lymphadenopathy revealed polytypic plasmacytosis with normal kappa/lambda ratios and HHV-8 negative. Flow cytometry was unremarkable and chromosomal analysis failed to reveal karyotypic abnormalities.

One year later, the patient is on prednisone 15 mg daily and hydroxychloroquine at 5 mg/Kg/day. She is not taking allopurinol. The blood counts are normal, Scr is 0.78 mg/dL, microhematuria is not present, SUPCR is 0.144 mg/mg, SUA 7.6 mg/dL, fractional excretion of uric acid (FEUA) is 6.6%, with hourly uric acid (UA) urine excretion of 18.5 mg/1.73 M^2, WSR is 27 mm/hr, and serum complement levels are normal. During the year of follow-up, she has repeatedly tested positive for anti-ds-DNA Ab and lupus anticoagulant and has developed synovitis of hand joints. A positron emission tomography showed F-18 FDG avidity in lymph nodes of the cervical, axillary, retroperitoneal, and pelvic areas. Excisional cervical lymph node biopsy was conducted, and a polytypic lymphoplasmacytic infiltrate was seen. Neither storiform fibrosis nor obliterative phlebitis was observed. Markers for lymphoproliferative malignancies remained negative. She has not required further rituximab infusions.

2. Discussion

Autoimmune rheumatic diseases may start as illnesses that involve multiple body organs from its outset [1, 2]. In such cases, organ damage is usually considered to be due to the autoimmune disease. Our patient meets criteria for a definitive diagnosis of systemic lupus erythematosus (SLE) [3, 4]. The prevalence of SLE in the Hispanic population in the US has been reported around 84.6/100 000 [5]. The prevalence of SLE in Puerto Ricans has been reported to be higher with an overall prevalence of 159/100 000, and of 277/100 000 in females [6]. Kidney injury is a frequent manifestation of SLE with a prevalence of lupus nephritis (LN) upward of 50% [7]. LN has to be aggressively treated to prevent irreversible loss of renal function, chronic renal insufficiency, and the potential need for renal replacement therapy.

Other potential causes of kidney disease in a patient with a lymphoplasmacytic infiltrate in a lymph node biopsy and an inflammatory process include multicentric Castleman disease (CD) and IgG4-related disease. Since she is HHV-8- and HIV-Ab-negative, idiopathic Castleman disease (ICD) and its variant thrombocytopenia, anasarca, retroperitoneal fibrosis, renal dysfunction, and organomegaly (TAFRO) syndrome have to be considered. ICD and TAFRO have a strong inflammatory process with systemic symptoms such as fever, elevation of the CRP and WSR, organomegaly, lymphadenopathies in multiple body sites, and cytopenia. However, international diagnostic criteria state that in order to make a diagnosis of ICD/TAFRO, inflammatory diseases such as SLE must be ruled out [8]. More recently, case reports have been published where an initial diagnosis of definitive SLE has been made, only to be changed to ICD/TAFRO over time [9, 10]. The authors described SLE as a mimicker for ICD/TAFRO. In our patient, long-term observation validated the diagnosis of SLE since over time, she developed arthritis, documented by a rheumatologist, the anti-ds-DNA Ab became positive, and the ANA positivity persisted. IgG4-related disease (igg4-rd) is highly unlikely despite the presence of lymph node biopsy showing lymphoplasmacytic infiltrates. Absence of storiform fibrosis and obliterative phlebitis in the lymph node biopsy does not rule out igg4-rd as these pathological findings are not seen in lymph nodes. However, igg4-rd is usually a disease of males in their middle age, clinical presentation and inflammatory markers tend to be more indolent, and she lacks typical renal radiographic CT changes such as enlarged kidneys and multiple nodules. In addition, patients with igg4-rd and renal disease not infrequently have retroperitoneal, pancreas, thyroid, or other organ involvement all absent in this patient [11, 12].

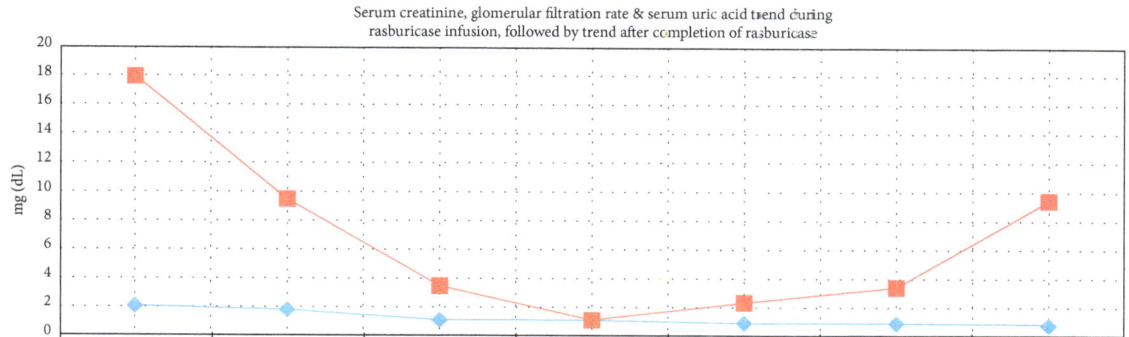

	Day 1 of rasburicase	Day 2 of rasburicase	Day 3 of rasburicase	Day 4 of rasburicase	Day 1 after rasburicase	Day 2 after rasburicase	Day 207 after rasburicase
creatinine	2.02	2.16	1.72	1.2	0.8	0.81	0.78
serum uric acid	18	9.5	3.4	0.8	2.3	3.4	9.5
GFR	33	30	40	62	100	99	103

FIGURE 2: Serum creatinine, estimated glomerular filtration rate (GFR), and serum uric acid during and after rasburicase infusions.

Uric acid nephropathy is suggested by SUA above 15 mg/dL, presence of uric acid crystals in the urine sediment, renal insufficiency, and ratio of urine uric acid to creatinine above 1.0 [12]. Hyperuricemia is believed to injure the kidney through several mechanisms including uric acid intrarenal stone formation and obstruction, tubular cell inflammation and apoptosis, decreased renal circulation, and increased oxidative stress [13]. In our patient, uric acid nephropathy is suggested by a SUA above 15 mg/dL, presence of uric acid crystals in the urine, renal insufficiency that reverted back to a normal SCr within 5 days of starting rasburicase together with an increase in urine output, and quick resolution of the microhematuria. A renal biopsy to document the presence of LN was initially not performed due to the protracted thrombocytopenia. Later, in the patient's clinical course, it was not considered due to normal SCr levels and urine sediment and the fact the authors have never seen a patient with LN with moderate renal insufficiency achieving a full renal remission within 14 days of starting corticosteroid therapy. A renal biopsy to make a tissue diagnosis of urate nephropathy was considered. However, we decided against recommending the biopsy taking in consideration the patient's risk vs benefit ratio. It was possible the kidney biopsy would not show urate acid crystals because by the time the platelet count stabilized and the biopsy could have been conducted in a safer manner, she had already finished all rasburicase infusions and was on allopurinol. In addition, even if the biopsy had shown urate deposits in the renal tubules, the probability of a change in therapy was considered remote.

The cause of the SUA elevation at admission is not clear. Conditions associated to an abrupt rise in SUA such as tumor lysis syndrome [14], rhabdomyolysis [15], and repeated epileptic seizures [16] were absent. Conditions associated to a gradual increase in the SUA were also not identified [16–19]. A genetic cause for serum uric acid elevation is highly unlikely as she has a large family with many first and second degree relatives and a negative family history of gout or uric acid stones. One year after her discharge she continues to have a slight elevation of the SUA off allopurinol. The FEUA is normal suggesting the SUA elevation is not caused by an overproduction of uric acid. It is possible she may have experienced an increase in the SUA level several weeks prior to her admission presumably due to active tissue necrosis resulting in increased uric acid renal clearance and uric acid nephropathy.

In summary, we report a case of a woman with kidney insufficiency in whom 2 different clinical entities that cause kidney injury co-occurred. SLE, a not uncommon disease in females in their 4th decade of life that causes kidney injury through autoimmune mechanisms, and urate nephropathy, an extremely rare cause of kidney injury, were seen in a young female in the absence of an identifiable cause for severe hyperuricemia, that causes kidney injury through uric acid deposition in renal tissues and immune-mediated mechanisms. Methylprednisolone infusions alone, prescribed specifically for LN, would have most likely controlled the urate nephropathy through its anti-inflammatory effects since there was no evidence of uric acid stones physically obstructing urinary flow. In this respect, steroids alone would have treated two different pathogenic causes of renal injury that share similar mechanisms of injury. However, the combination of methylprednisolone and rasburicase infusions most likely accelerated the control of urate nephropathy reducing the possibility of long-term renal damage [20, 21].

Clinicians must not forget that performing a differential diagnosis is necessary in arriving at a correct diagnosis and to provide opportune treatment, in order to prevent unnecessary morbidity, particularly, since it is not always the case that different clinical entities respond to the same treatment.

References

[1] T. Dörner and R. Furie, "Novel paradigms in systemic lupus erythematosus," *Lancet*, vol. 393, no. 10188, pp. 2344–2358, 2019.

[2] K. J. John, M. Sadiq, T. George et al., "Clinical and immunological profile of mixed connective tissue disease and a

comparison of four diagnostic criteria," *International Journal of Rheumatology*, vol. 2020, Article ID 9692030, 6 pages, 2020.

[3] M. Petri, A. M. Orbai, G. S. Alarcón et al., "Derivation and validation of the systemic lupus international collaborating clinics classification criteria for systemic lupus erythematosus," *Arthritis & Rheumatism*, vol. 64, no. 8, pp. 2677–2686, 2012.

[4] M. Aringer, K. Costenbader, D. Daikh et al., "2019 European league against rheumatism/american college of rheumatology classification criteria for systemic lupus erythematosus," *Annals of the Rheumatic Diseases*, vol. 78, no. 9, pp. 1151–1159, 2019.

[5] G. Stojan and M. Petri, "Epidemiology of systemic lupus erythematosus: an update," *Current Opinion in Rheumatology*, vol. 30, no. 2, pp. 144–150, 2018.

[6] M. J. Molina, A. M. Mayor, A. E. Franco, C. A. Morell, M. A. Lopez, and L. M. Vila, "Prevalence of systemic lupus erythematosus and associated comorbidities in Puerto Rico," *Journal of Clinical Rheumatology*, vol. 13, no. 4, pp. 202–204, 2007.

[7] S. Almaani, A. Meara, and B. H. Rovin, "Update on lupus nephritis," *Clinical Journal of the American Society of Nephrology*, vol. 12, no. 5, pp. 825–835, 2017.

[8] D. C. Fajgenbaum, T. S. Uldrick, A. Bagg et al., "International evidence-based consensus diagnostic criteria for HHV-8-negative/idiopathic multicentric castleman disease," *Blood*, vol. 129, no. 12, pp. 1646–1657, 2017.

[9] L. Wang, H. Chen, J. Shi et al., "Castleman disease mimicking systemic lupus erythematosus. A case report," *Medicine*, vol. 97, no. 38, Article ID e12291, 2018.

[10] G. Puerta, D. De Paz, D. Aguirre-Valencia et al., "TAFRO syndrome mimicking systemic lupus erythematosus: case report and literature review," *Revista Colombiana de Reumatología*, 2021.

[11] A. Martínez-de-Alegría, S. Baleato-González, R. García-Figueiras et al., "IgG4-related disease from head to toe," *RadioGraphics*, vol. 35, no. 7, pp. 2007–2025, 2015.

[12] B.-W. Yoo, J. J. Song, Y.-B. Park, and S.-W. Lee, "2019 American college of rheumatology/european league against rheumatism classification criteria for IgG4-related disease," *Annals of the Rheumatic Diseases*, 2020.

[13] S. A. Fathallah-Shaykh and M. T. Cramer, "Uric acid and the kidney," *Pediatric Nephrology*, vol. 29, no. 6, pp. 999–1008, 2014.

[14] A. A. Ejaz, R. J. Johnson, M. Shimada et al., "The role of uric acid in acute kidney injury," *Nephron*, vol. 142, no. 4, pp. 275–283, 2019.

[15] F. P. Wilson and J. S. Berns, "Tumor lysis syndrome: new challenges and recent advances," *Advances in Chronic Kidney Disease*, vol. 21, no. 1, pp. 18–26, 2014.

[16] G. Efstratiadis, A. Voulgaridou, D. Nikiforou, A. Kyventidis, E. Kourkouni, and G. Vergoulas, "Rhabdomyolysis updated," *Hippokratia*, vol. 11, no. 3, pp. 129–137, 2007.

[17] C. Patel, C. P. Wilson, N. Ahmed, and Y. Hattab, "Acute uric acid nephropathy following epileptic seizures: case report and review," *Case Reports in Nephrology*, vol. 2019, Article ID 4890287, 6 pages, 2019.

[18] M. A. McAdams-DeMarco, A. Law, J. W. Maynard, J. Coresh, and A. N. Baer, "Risk factors for incident hyperuricemia during mid-adulthood in african american and white men and women enrolled in the ARIC cohort study," *BMC Musculoskeletal Disorders*, vol. 14, p. 347, 2013.

[19] C. Ben Salem, R. Slim, N. Fathallah, and H. Hmouda, "Drug-induced hyperuricaemia and gout," *Rheumatology*, vol. 56, no. 5, Article ID kew293, 2016.

[20] P. Richette and F. Perez-Ruiz, "Serum uric acid and metabolic risk," *Current Medical Research and Opinion*, vol. 29, pp. 9–15, 2013.

[21] C. Réategui-Sokolova, M. F. Ugarte-Gil, R. V. Gamboa-Cárdenas et al., "Serum uric acid levels contribute to new renal damage in systemic lupus erythematosus patients," *Clinical Rheumatology*, vol. 36, no. 4, pp. 845–852, 2017.

31

Pontine Myelinolysis Caused by Hypovolemic Hypernatremia

D. O. Beraldo,[1,2] S. B. C. P. Duarte,[1,3] R. B. Santos,[1] C. G. Mendes,[1] M. P. Silveira,[1] A. S. Neto,[1] M. M. Silva,[1] L. G. Oliveira,[1] A. V. Bonfim,[1] A. A. Teixeira,[1,2] and R. A. Teixeira[1,3]

[1]*Hospital Renascentista, Pouso Alegre, MG, Brazil*
[2]*Escola Paulista de Medicina—UNIFESP, São Paulo, Brazil*
[3]*Instituto do Coração—FMUSP, São Paulo, Brazil*

Correspondence should be addressed to D. O. Beraldo; daniel_beraldo@hotmail.com

Academic Editor: Hern n Trimarchi

Introduction. Central pontine myelinolysis is characterized by the occurrence of acute demyelinating lesions of cells in the pons secondary to abrupt oscillations of serum osmolarity. Its exact incidence is not well defined, but studies show a prevalence of 0.25 to 0.5% in the general population, 2.5% in the intensive care unit, and up to 10% in patients with risk factors, such as chronic liver disease and hepatic transplantation, alcoholism, malnutrition, diuretic therapy, electrolyte imbalance, hypoglycemia, and hyperglycemia. *Case Report*. A 70-year-old white female with extranodal diffuse large B-cell non-Hodgkin's lymphoma (extensive mass on the left anterior chest wall), stage IVA, developed pontine myelinolysis secondary to hypovolemic acute hypernatremia, which occurred due to diarrhea caused by chemotherapy (rituximab, cyclophosphamide, doxorubicin, and vincristine). *Discussion*. Pontine myelinolysis occurs most often due to the rapid correction of chronic hyponatremia. But here, we describe a case of the disease secondary to the occurrence of hypovolemic acute hypernatremia in a patient with a hematological malignancy under treatment, who was on chronic treatment with thiazide diuretics and who presented with other electrolyte disturbances as risk factors for the development of pontine myelinolysis.

1. Introduction

Central pontine myelinolysis (CPM) was first described in 1959 by Adams et al. as a disease that affected alcoholic and malnourished patients and was characterized by acute demyelinating lesion of pontine cells secondary to abrupt oscillations of serum osmolarity [1]. The term myelinolysis was intentionally used to highlight the predominance of noninflammatory lesions to the myelin as opposed to other neuronal structures [1]. It is within the spectrum of the osmotic demyelination syndrome (ODS), which is divided into CPM and extrapontine myelinolysis, which in turn are distinguished by involvement of the central region of the pons or regions outside it, respectively [2, 3].

The exact incidence of the disease is not well defined, but studies show a prevalence of 0.25 to 0.5% in the general population, 2.5% in the intensive care unit, and up to 10% in patients undergoing liver transplantation [4–7]. Some groups are more predisposed to the development of ODS, such as alcoholics; malnourished individuals; those with liver disease; chronic users of diuretics; patients with other electrolyte disturbances (hypokalemia, hypophosphatemia, and hypernatremia); individuals with hypoglycemia and hyperglycemia, central and nephrogenic diabetes insipidus, and adrenal insufficiency; those with Wilson's disease, celiac disease, and psychiatric conditions such as psychogenic polydipsia, and women during pregnancy and puerperium [8–15].

The main etiopathogenic mechanism of ODS is the rapid correction of hyponatremia, especially in the scenario of hyponatremia with chronic evolution. A low serum sodium concentration leads to serum hyposmolarity and the consequent passage of free water into the intracellular environment of the cells of the central nervous system, which promotes cellular edema. In cases of chronic evolution, cells adapt and lose osmoles (electrolytes and organic osmoles, such as myoinositol, taurine, glutamine, glutamate, creatinine, and glycerophosphorylcholine) and free water as a compensatory mechanism. In the scenario of rapid correction of hyponatremia, there is an acute increase in serum osmolarity and consequent dehydration of cells of the central nervous system, leading to noninflammatory demyelinating lesions and apoptosis [9, 16–20].

This case report describes the occurrence of CPM related to hypovolemic acute hypernatremia secondary to diarrhea. It is a rare cause of ODS, which is often related to the correction of hyponatremia.

2. Case Report

A 70-year-old white female was diagnosed in June 2017 with extranodal diffuse large B-cell non-Hodgkin's lymphoma (extensive mass on the left anterior chest wall), stage IVA. Chemotherapy was initiated with the R-CHOP regimen (rituximab, cyclophosphamide, doxorubicin, and vincristine) in the same month, performing the first two cycles using a Port-a-Cath catheter, without complications and with a substantial reduction of the left anterior thoracic mass. Comorbidities included hypertension for 3 years, hemorrhoidal disease (conservative treatment), bilateral knee arthrosis with total left knee arthroplasty 3 years earlier, and esophageal hiatus hernia (conservative treatment). Associated with this was a history of an imagining finding of an asymptomatic pulmonary thromboembolism during the staging of the hematological malignancy and history of poliomyelitis at 8 years of age with motor sequelae in the lower limbs (with unaided walking ability maintained). The patient had no history of smoking or drinking, and medications consisted in chronic use of chlortalidone 25 mg once daily, omeprazole 40 mg once daily, rivaroxaban 20 mg once daily, bromopride 10 mg once daily, and sulfamethoxazole/trimethoprim 800/160 mg 3x a week.

The patient underwent the third cycle of chemotherapy in September 2017, and 10 days later, she began to suffer from general malaise, hyporexia, prostration, lesions of the oral mucosa, acute voluminous diarrhea without pathological products, and fever (38.3°C). She was admitted to the intensive care unit of Hospital Renascentista with a diagnosis of high-risk febrile neutropenia with no defined infectious focus (MASCC score of 11 points), severe mucositis of the gastrointestinal tract with considerable oral lesions and diarrhea, prerenal acute renal failure, and severe pancytopenia after chemotherapy. Physical examination showed that the patient was dehydrated (3/4+), prostrate, less communicative and febrile (38.3°C), had poor peripheral perfusion with blood pressure 80/50 mmHg and heart rate 110 bpm, and had substantial oral mucositis, with no other changes in the general and neurological examination. Laboratory tests showed the following results: hemoglobin 6.7 g/dL, leukocytes 270 cells/mm^3 (20% neutrophils), platelets 8000 cells/mm^3, creatinine 2.6 mg/dL, urea 194 mg/dL, fasting glucose 82 mg/dL, sodium 164 mEq/L, magnesium 1.4 mEq/L, phosphorus 2.2 mg/dL, potassium 2.2 mEq/L, AST 23 IU/L, ALT 20 IU/L, albumin 2.1 g/dL, bilirubins normal, coagulation tests normal, arterial lactate 31 mg/L, pH 7.21, HCO3 16 mEq/L, chest X-ray normal, urinalysis normal, urine culture negative, and blood cultures negative.

Immediate empirical antibiotic treatment was initiated with piperacillin-tazobactam and vancomycin due to high-risk febrile neutropenia with multiple risk factors for Gram-positive infection (mucositis, long-term invasive device, acute neurological disorder, multiple organ dysfunction, and hypotension), in addition to hemodynamic support of sepsis, volume resuscitation, transfusion support, and correction of water-electrolyte imbalance. She evolved with hemodynamic improvement, resolution of fever, improvement of renal function, and improvement of hypomagnesemia, hypokalemia, and hypophosphatemia, with progressive and slow sodium correction (<0.5 mEq/L/hour) until normalization after several days. However, considerable diarrhea and pancytopenia followed, which began to improve after two weeks of hospitalization. From a neurological point of view, despite clinical and laboratory improvement, she maintained prostration and developed a fluctuating lowered level of consciousness, grade I paresis of upper limbs and grade III paresis of lower limbs, mild dysarthria, upper and lower limb hyporeflexia, no signs of pyramidal release, and normal brain stem reflexes and ocular motricity. A complementary investigation was performed with cranial computed tomography, which showed only a previous small left lacunar stroke (Figure 1); electroencephalogram, which showed changes suggestive of toxic-metabolic damage to the central nervous system; cerebrospinal fluid analysis, which was normal; and cranial magnetic resonance, which revealed changes suggestive of pontine myelinolysis (Figure 2).

The patient continued with clinical and laboratory improvement, with complete resolution of pancytopenia, water-electrolyte imbalance, renal dysfunction, and diarrhea. She had a slow neurological improvement and was discharged with normal level of consciousness and progressive recovery of motor deficits. After two years, her neurological status was the same as before the central pontine myelinolysis event, and her cranial computed tomography revealed a hypoattenuating focal area in the central region of the pons (Figure 3).

3. Discussion

The clinical picture of CPM includes a variety of neurological manifestations, which include flaccid quadriparesis with subsequent evolution to the spastic phase, dysarthria and dysphagia (pseudobulbar palsy), oculomotor and pupillary changes, and lowered level of consciousness. In some situations, locked-in syndrome may occur. These neurological changes are due to the involvement of the pontine structures to different degrees, particularly the base of the pons (corticobulbar and corticospinal tracts) and tegmentum of the pons [9]. The symptoms usually appear 2 to 7 days after the electrolyte changes [21], and there is no apparent relationship between the severity of the clinical condition and the initial sodium values, the rate of sodium correction, and the presence of associated comorbidities [8].

The diagnosis of CPM should be considered in cases of acute onset of neurological symptoms related to sodium imbalance, especially rapid correction of hyponatremia

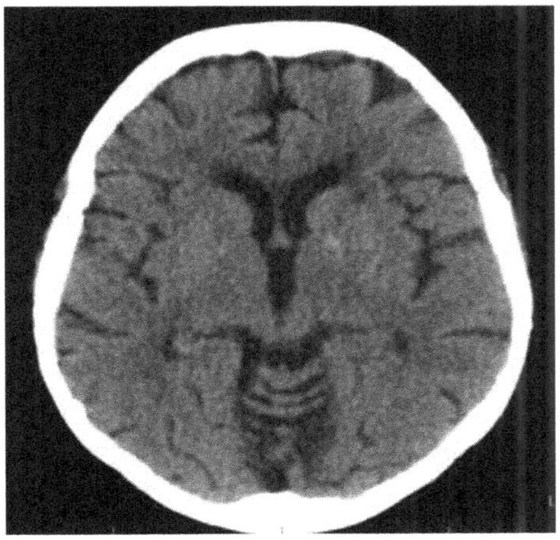

FIGURE 1: Cranial computed tomography showing previous left lacunar stroke.

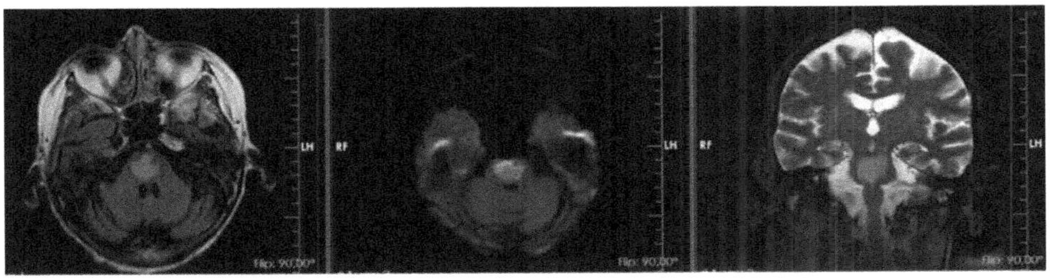

FIGURE 2: Cranial magnetic resonance showing findings in the pons suggestive of pontine myelinolysis (sequences: axial T2, diffusion, and coronal T2).

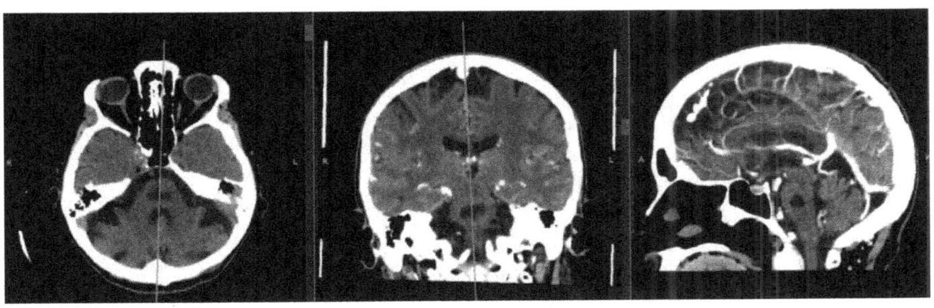

FIGURE 3: Cranial computed tomography showing a hypoattenuating focal area in the central region of the pons (sequences: axial, coronal, and sagittal).

(>0.5 mEq/L/hour), where it is confirmed by imaging of the central nervous system, with prominence for magnetic resonance, whose findings are bilateral hypersignal in the central region of the pons in the T2 and FLAIR sequences and hyposignal in the T1 sequence [22]. Radiological changes usually appear days after clinical manifestations, and the diffusion sequence in MRI has been shown to be effective for an earlier diagnosis [23, 24].

The approach in CPM consists mainly in preventive measures based on the correct handling of the correction of sodium imbalance since there are no well-established treatments. Some approaches have been studied in recent years, with emphasis on immunoglobulin therapy or plasmapheresis, which possibly promote remyelinization and reduction of myelotoxicity. Rodriguez et al. described 3 cases of pontine myelinolysis treated with immunoglobulin and observed clinical improvement after treatment [25]. Also, Saner et al. evaluated immunoglobulin and plasmapheresis therapy in a renal transplant patient and also found an improvement in neurological status [26].

Pontine myelinolysis occurs most often due to rapid correction of chronic hyponatremia [27]. However, there are rare reports in the literature of CPM secondary to other osmolal disorders (hyperglycemia and hypoglycemia) [28, 29], in addition to cases with normal serum sodium [30] or in the presence of rapid onset hypernatremia in patients with risk factors for OSD (34). Kilinç et al. described an episode of pontine myelinolysis with normal serum sodium in a 34-year-old male patient on chronic renal dialysis [30]. Additionally, Varanda et al. reported a case of pontine myelinolysis caused by multifactorial hypernatremia in a female patient with liver cirrhosis who was a regular alcohol drinker, which is in agreement with our findings [31].

4. Conclusion

We describe here a case of CPM related to the occurrence of hypovolemic acute hypernatremia secondary to diarrhea in a patient with a hematological malignancy under treatment, presenting with the risk factors such as chronic use of a thiazide diuretic and the presence of other electrolyte disturbances (hypophosphatemia, hypokalemia, and hypomagnesemia).

References

[1] R. D. Adams, M. Victor, and E. L. Mancall, "Central pontine myelinolysis," *A.M.A. Archives of Neurology & Psychiatry*, vol. 81, no. 2, pp. 154–172, 1959.

[2] R. Laureno, "Central pontine myelinolysis following rapid correction of hyponatremia," *Annals of Neurology*, vol. 13, no. 3, pp. 232–242, 1983.

[3] A. M. Alleman, "Osmotic demyelination syndrome: central pontine myelinolysis and extrapontine myelinolysis," *Seminars in Ultrasound, CT and MRI*, vol. 35, no. 2, pp. 153–159, 2014.

[4] B. K. Kleinschmidt-Demasters, A. M. Rojiani, and C. M. Filley, "Central and extrapontine myelinolysis: then and now," *Journal of Neuropathology and Experimental Neurology*, vol. 65, no. 1, pp. 1-11, 2006.

[5] C. Lampl and K. Yazdi, "Central pontine myelinolysis," *European Neurology*, vol. 47, no. 1, pp. 3-10, 2002.

[6] R. Abbott, E. Silber, J. Felber, and E. Ekpo, "Osmotic demyelination syndrome," *BMJ-British medical journal*, vol. 331, no. 7520, pp. 829-830, 2005.

[7] P. B. Rao, A. Azim, N. Singh et al., "Osmotic demyelination syndrome in intensive care unit," *Indian Journal of Critical Care Medicine*, vol. 19, pp. 166–169, 2015.

[8] F. Y. Ismail, A. Szóllics, M. Szólics, N. Nagelkerke, and M. Ljubisavljevic, "Clinical semiology and neuroradiologic correlates of acute hypernatremic osmotic challenge in adults: a literature review," *American Journal of Neuroradiology*, vol. 34, no. 12, pp. 2225-2232, 2013.

[9] R. J. Martin, "Central pontine and extrapontine myelinolysis: the osmotic demyelination syndromes," *Journal of Neurology, Neurosurgery, and Psychiatry*, vol. 75, no. 3, pp. 22–28, 2004.

[10] A. S. Patel, L. Matthews, and W. Bruce-Jones, "Central pontine myelinolysis as a complication of refeeding syndrome in a patient with anorexia nervosa," *The Journal of Neuropsychiatry and Clinical Neurosciences*, vol. 20, no. 3, pp. 371-373, 2008.

[11] J. Wadhwa, R. Ananthakrishnan, S. Sadashiv, and A. Hamide, "Extrapontine myelinolysis: rare manifestation of a well-known disorder," *BMJ Case Reports*, vol. 2013, no. 1, Article ID bcr2013200808, 2013.

[12] H. Uchida, S. Sakamoto, K. Sasaki et al., "Central pontine myelinolysis following pediatric living donor liver transplantation: a case report and review of literature," *Pediatric Transplantation*, vol. 18, pp. 120–123, 2014.

[13] J. W. Wu, P. N. Wang, and J. F. Lirng, "Extrapontine myelinolysis in a patient with primary adrenal insufficiency," *Acta Neurologica Taiwanica*, vol. 23, no. 4, pp. 146-152, 2014.

[14] R. Verma and D. Rai, "Central pontine myelinolysis associated with Wilson disease in a 7-year-old child," *BMJ Case Report*, vol. 2013, no. 1, Article ID bcr2012007408, 2013.

[15] P. Sharma, S. Sharma, N. Panwar et al., "Central pontine myelinolysis presenting with tremor in a child with celiac disease," *Journal of Child Neurology*, vol. 29, no. 3, pp. 381–384, 2014.

[16] M. D. Mahto, "Central pontine myelinolysis: historical and mechanistic considerations," *Metabolic Brain Disease*, vol. 25, no. 1, pp. 97–106, 2010.

[17] A. M. Rojiani, J. W. Prineas, E.-S. Cho et al., "Electrolyte-induced demyelination in rats," *Acta Neuropathologica*, vol. 88, no. 4, pp. 287–292, 1994.

[18] A. M. Rojiani, E.-S. Cho, L. Sharer, and J. W. Prineas, "Electrolyte-induced demyelination in rats," *Acta Neuropathologica*, vol. 88, no. 4, pp. 293–299, 1994.

[19] R. H. Sterns, D. J. Thomas, and R. M. Herndon, "Brain dehydration and neurologic deterioration after rapid correction of hyponatremia," *Kidney International*, vol. 35, no. 1, pp. 69–75, 1989.

[20] J. D. King and M. H. Rosner, "Osmotic demyelination syndrome," *The American Journal of the Medical Sciences*, vol. 339, no. 6, pp. 561-567, 2010.

[21] R. Laureno and B. I. Karp, "Myelinolysis after correction of hyponatremia," *Annals of Internal Medicine*, vol. 126, no. 1, pp. 57–62, 1997.

[22] G. M. Miller, H. L. Baker, H. Okazaki, and J. P. Whisnant, "Central pontine myelinolysis and its imitators: MR findings," *Radiology*, vol. 168, no. 3, pp. 795–802, 1988.

[23] D. Le Bihan, R. Turner, P. Douek, and N. Patronas, "Diffusion MR imaging: clinical applications," *American Journal of Roentgenology*, vol. 159, no. 3, pp. 591–599, 1992.

[24] P. W. Schaefer, P. E. Grant, and R. G. Gonzalez, "Diffusion-weighted MR imaging of the brain," *Radiology*, vol. 217, no. 2, pp. 331–345, 2000.

[25] M. Rodriguez, D. J. Miller, and V. A. Lennon, "Immunoglobulins reactive with myelin basic protein promote CNS remyelination," *Neurology*, vol. 46, no. 2, pp. 538–545, 1996.

[26] F. H. Saner, S. Koeppen, M. Meyer et al., "Treatment of central pontine myelinolysis with plasmapheresis and immunoglobulins in liver transplant patient," *Transplant International*, vol. 21, no. 4, pp. 390-391, 2008.

[27] T. D. Kohnle, J. E. Fugate, and A. A. Rabinstein, "Central pontine and extrapontine myelinolysis: a systematic review," *European Journal of Neurology*, vol. 21, no. 12, pp. 1443–1450, 2014.

[28] A. Akyol, "Association of central pontine myelinolysis and extra-pontine myelinolysis in diabetic patient," *Neuro Enocrinology Letters*, vol. 28, pp. 252–254, 2007.

[29] L. E. Morales-Buenrostro, J. F. Tellez-Zenteno, J. G. Posadas-Calleja et al., "Pontine myelinolysis after a hypoglycemic episode," *Revista de Investigacion Clinica*, vol. 54, pp. 181–184, 2002, in Spanish.

[30] M. Kilinç, U. S. Benli, and U. Can, "Osmotic myelinolysis in a normonatremic patient," *Acta Neurologica Belgica*, vol. 102, no. 2, pp. 87–89, 2002.

[31] S. Varanda, S. Costa, R. Carvalho, F. Sousa, and G. Carneiro, "Central pontine myelinolysis caused by hypernatremia," *Journal of the Neurological Sciences*, vol. 370, pp. 274–276, 2016.

32

Acute Oxalate Nephropathy Caused by Excessive Vegetable Juicing and Concomitant Volume Depletion

Harshad Chaudhari,[1] Jennine Michaud,[2] Nityasree Srialluri,[1] Smita Mahendrakar,[1] Christine Granz,[2] and Michael Yudd[2]

[1]*Rutgers University Department of Nephrology and Hypertension, Newark, NJ, USA*
[2]*Department of Veterans Affairs, Renal Section, East Orange, NJ, USA*

Correspondence should be addressed to Harshad Chaudhari; hc835@njms.rutgers.edu

Academic Editor: Sophia Lionaki

Acute oxalate nephropathy (AON) induced by high dietary intake of oxalate-rich food is a rare cause of acute kidney injury and end-stage renal disease (ESRD). We describe a 68-year-old man with adequate baseline renal function who developed severe AON and ESRD. Six months earlier, he started a daily oxalate-rich fruit and vegetable juice diet high in spinach, with a calculated daily oxalate dietary intake of 1500 mg, about 10 times a typical diet. Renal biopsy showed extensive tubular oxalate deposits and acute tubular damage; the renal tissue was relatively free of chronic changes such as glomerulosclerosis, tubular atrophy, and interstitial fibrosis. A year later, he remains dialysis dependent.

1. Introduction

Oxalate is an end-product of glyoxalate metabolism in the liver. Diets rich in leafy vegetables and nuts also contribute oxalate and precursors of oxalate. Oxalate is cleared solely by the kidneys. We describe a patient with relatively good baseline renal function and free of microalbuminuria who developed severe acute oxalate nephropathy and end-stage renal disease because of excessive dietary intake of oxalate and volume depletion.

2. Case History

A 68-year-old Caucasian man with a medical history of insulin-dependent diabetes for 18 years and poorly controlled hypertension presented with weakness and was found to have acute kidney injury.

Six months before admission, he started a vegetable juicing regimen, thinking this diet was best for his overall health and may help with diabetic control. Hemoglobin A1c was 8.1 two months before admission and averaged 8.3 during the three years before admission. He blended one-third of a pound of raw baby spinach leaves with Swiss chard and added broccoli, cauliflower, green beans, asparagus, kale, beets, cilantro, parsnips, mushrooms, onions, and blueberries or raspberries. He added 4 ounces of water to the mix and drank one quart daily. For breakfast, he consumed oatmeal and vegetables. Lunch and dinner included pureed yams, spinach, Swiss chard, tofu, and garbanzo beans. He snacked on pumpkin seeds and pine nuts. His daily intake of oxalate was approximately 1500 mg/day, about 10 times that of a typical diet. This dietary oxalate amount was based on estimates of intake by the nutritionist and calculations utilizing the Harvard database [1]. Some of these foods had a very high oxalate-producing content, particularly spinach. Others did not. Table 1 contains a list of the highest oxalate content foods consumed by the subject, along with the estimated oxalate content of his daily blended vegetable beverage.

He had had long-standing achalasia, which was treated with a myotomy and a Nissen fundoplication 16 years earlier. Associated with the achalasia, the patient had intermittent nausea, regurgitation, and vomiting for many years. However, 6 weeks before admission, these symptoms

Table 1: Subject's estimated daily oxalate intake (food item/serving size/amount of oxalate).

Food item	Estimated quantity (serving size)	Oxalate content
Ingredients with the highest oxalate content included in the daily vegetable juicing regimen		
Raw baby spinach leaves	2 cups	1312 mg
Swiss chard	1 cup	347 mg
Asparagus	4–8 spears	6–12 mg
Beets	1 cup	152 mg
Parsnips	½ cup	15 mg
Raspberries	½ cup	24 mg
		Estimated total = 1862 mg
Additional potential high-oxalate dietary sources (not consumed consistently by the patient)		
Yams (pureed)	1-2 cups	28–56 mg
Cooked spinach	½-1 cup	755–1510 mg
Tofu	3.5 oz	13 mg
Pumpkin seeds	½ cup	19.5 mg

worsened, and he regurgitated small volumes about 6–8 times a day. He described having a poor appetite and an unintentional weight loss of 10 pounds. There was no history of chronic diarrhea, steatorrhea, or malabsorption.

An initial physical exam revealed a blood pressure of 180/72 mm Hg and heart rate of 55 beats per minute. His skin appeared to be dry with decreased turgor. The lungs were clear, the heart rhythm was regular with normal S1 and S2, and the abdomen was nontender with no peripheral edema. Antihypertension medications were amlodipine, lisinopril, doxazosin, and clonidine patch.

The initial labs showed a blood urea nitrogen (BUN) of 92 mg/dL and serum creatinine level of 9.6 mg/dL. The urinalysis performed by the nephrologist showed 1+ protein, a few clumps of white cells, and a moderate number of muddy brown casts. There were no crystals or bacteria. Two months and eight months before admission, serum creatinine was 1.4 mg/dl and the estimated glomerular filtration rate was 50 ml/min. Two months before admission, urine microalbumin was 8 mg/L, normal. Multiple microalbumin values before this were also normal over the previous 2 years.

He was aggressively hydrated, but the renal function did not improve. Hemodialysis was started, and a renal biopsy was performed. A 24 h urine collected one month after the patient started dialysis while he was ingesting a dialysate diet (2 g sodium, 2.5 g potassium, and 100 g protein diet) revealed a low urine oxalate level of 10 mg in 1400 ml of urine. He was in severe renal failure during the collection, so interpretation of this low oxalate is difficult.

The renal biopsy had 40 glomeruli, 3 of which were globally sclerosed. The glomeruli appeared normal in size and cellularity. The mesangial matrix was not expanded. Glomerular basement membranes were normal in thickness and contour. There was minimal chronicity noted in the tubulointerstitial compartments. There was acute tubular injury with simplification of the lining epithelium and dilatation of the lumen. Numerous and diffuse intratubular calcium oxalate deposits were noted (Figures 1 and 2), which demonstrated birefringence when viewed under polarizing light. There was severe arteriosclerosis and multifocal severe arteriolar hyalinosis.

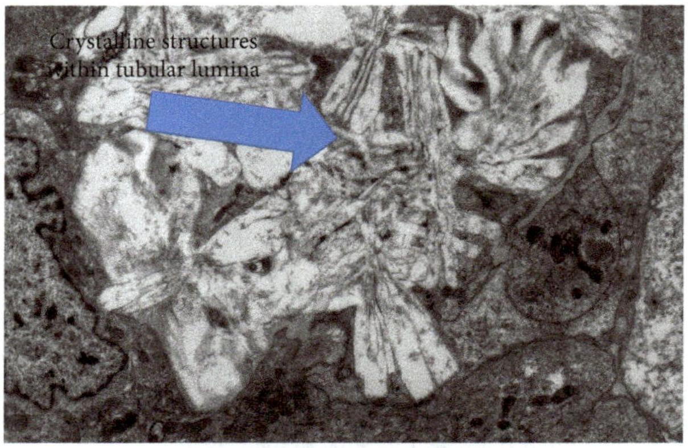

Figure 1: EM showing multiple oxalate crystals in the lumen of the kidney tubule.

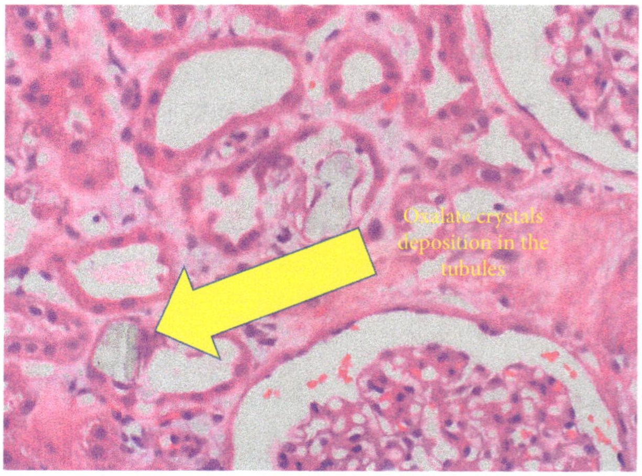

Figure 2: Oxalate crystals seen again in the kidney tubules.

The acute kidney injury was due to acute oxalate nephropathy. Upon further questioning, he denied ingestion of vitamin C or ethylene glycol, and he had no history of nephrolithiasis. Aside from the achalasia symptoms, he denied any other GI complaints or surgical procedures. There was no history of primary hyperoxaluria in his family.

One year after this admission, he remained dialysis dependent.

3. Discussion

Oxalate nephropathy is classified as primary (genetic) or secondary (see Table 2). Primary hyperoxaluria (PH) is a rare collection of genetic diseases due to inborn errors of glyoxalate metabolism and characterized by overproduction of oxalate [2]. The genetic abnormalities of 3 hepatic enzymes can give heterogeneous clinical presentations for PH types 1, 2, and 3. PH type 1, usually the most severe, is the predominant type, making up 80% of the cases. The clinical manifestations of PH usually present early in life; the median age of onset for PH type 1 is 5.5 years, for type 2 is 3.2 years, and for type 3 is 2 years. However, cases of PH, particularly types 2 and 3, can present later in life, even for patients in their 70s [3]. The most common clinical picture is recurrent calcium oxalate renal stones. This can progress to nephrocalcinosis and CKD from oxalate deposits and, in the most severe cases, to oxalalosis, a diffuse systemic deposition of oxalate leading to a myriad of symptoms. A definitive diagnosis for PH requires genetic testing. Although we did not rule out PH, the clinical picture, an elderly man with no history of renal stones suddenly developing acute kidney injury from acute oxalate nephropathy, makes this diagnosis unlikely.

Secondary oxalate nephropathy is most commonly found in inflammatory small bowel disease, malabsorption syndromes, and intestinal bypass resections, known collectively as enteric hyperoxaluria [4, 5]. In these states, excessive oxalate is absorbed in the gut by several mechanisms. Increased gut luminal free fatty acids in these states increase colonic permeability to oxalates. Also, intestinal calcium binds to free fatty acids and biliary acids. This leaves more luminal oxalate unbound, which can then be absorbed. The increased oxalate that is absorbed will eventually be filtered and cleared by the kidneys, resulting in hyperoxaluria. Typical settings for this are Crohn's disease, celiac sprue, and pancreatic insufficiency. Ileal resection and Roux-en-Y gastric bypass surgery and treatment with orlistat, a bowel and pancreatic lipase inhibitor, have been complicated by oxalate nephropathy [6–8]. Our patient had no symptoms of malabsorption or intestinal disease.

Secondary oxalate nephropathy has been described in ethylene glycol toxicity and excessive ingestion of vitamin C. Both substances are metabolized to oxalate. Less commonly, oxalate nephropathy has been described in patients with excessive intake of plant-based foods high in oxalate, including the juicing of certain vegetables and fruits [4, 9, 10].

Oxalate nephropathy is a rare finding on renal biopsy. In a recent report of more than 7,000 renal biopsies over 25 years at one institution, only 65 (less than 1%) had calcium oxalate deposits causing renal failure, and of these cases, only 3 were attributed to diets rich in oxalate [10]. All three of those cases were in patients who also had some degree of CKD. A recent systematic review of secondary oxalate nephropathy found 33 cases of biopsy-proven oxalate nephropathy, which were attributed to diets rich in oxalate [4]. The primary sources of oxalate in those cases were ascorbic acid and starfruit. Other dietary sources included spinach, rhubarb, Chaga mushrooms, black tea, and nuts (i.e., peanuts, cashews, and almonds) [10–12].

Table 2: Primary and secondary causes of hyperoxaluria.

Primary (inherited)
PH1: deficiency of alanine-glyoxylate aminotransferase
PH2: deficiency of glyoxylate reductase/hydroxypyruvate reductase
PH3: deficiency of 4-hydroxy-2-oxo-glutarate aldolase
Secondary (acquired)
Enteric hyperoxaluria: fat malabsorption states, pancreatic insufficiency, intestinal bypass surgeries, and orlistat
Ethylene glycol
Excessive vitamin C ingestion
Excessive ingestion of high-oxalate foods, in particular star fruit
Deficiency of oxalate-degrading bacteria from antibiotic use

Why only a small number of oxalate-rich consumers develop oxalate nephropathy is not known. The vegetarian diet is a popular diet, with millions of people worldwide safely consuming an oxalate-rich diet. Besides the high-oxalate dietary consumption, there must be other environmental or genetic factors working together to cause oxalate nephropathy. In our patient, intravascular volume depletion probably played a major role. We presume that, in the setting of volume depletion, the ensuing avid sodium and water reabsorption in the renal tubules led to higher concentrations of the excessive luminal oxalate and favored calcium oxalate precipitation in the distal tubules.

Dietary calcium influences the gut absorption of oxalate [13, 14]. Oxalate in the intestinal lumen binds with calcium; this bound oxalate is poorly absorbed, and it will be passed out with the stool. If dietary calcium is low, more luminal oxalate will be unbound, and therefore, oxalate absorption will be increased. In healthy adults eating a customary free-choice diet and then fed a controlled diet containing a 20-fold normal oxalate load (2200 mg) and an adequate calcium intake (1200 mg), daily urinary oxalate more than doubled, from 28 mg on the customary diet to 70 mg on the extremely-high-oxalate diet (normal daily urinary oxalate is up to 45 mg). When they were fed the same high-oxalate diet but now with a very-high-calcium diet (3800 mg), daily urinary oxalate was unchanged from the free-choice diet, 29 mg. [13]. Our patient's dietary calcium may have been very low; a low-calcium diet combined with a high-oxalate diet would lead to greater oxalate gut absorption and greater hyperoxaluria.

Increased gut absorption of oxalate may be present even in patients with apparently normal gastrointestinal systems. The increased oxalate absorption may result from hyperactivity of the main oxalate gut transporters, the anion exchangers belonging to the SLC-26 gene family [15].

Recent evidence has shed light on the role of gut bacteria in degrading intestinal oxalate, thereby decreasing intestinal absorption of oxalate and decreasing urinary oxalate. The human microbiota harbors bacteria known as the oxalobiome, which can encode an oxalate degradation pathway

[16, 17]. The oxalobiome members include *Oxalobacter formigenes*, *Escherichia coli*, Bifidobacterium spp., and *Lactobacillus* spp. Alterations and loss of the oxalabiome members can lead to hyperoxaluria and an increase in calcium oxalate stones. Settings for this are antibiotic therapy, malabsorption, and intestinal bypass surgeries.

In summary, we present a case of acute oxalate nephropathy leading to acute kidney injury and end-stage renal disease due to excessive intake of oxalate-rich foods and intravascular volume depletion. It might be prudent for people with a tendency for volume depletion to avoid this diet.

References

[1] Harvard, *Oxalate Content of Foods*, Department of Nutrition, Harvard T.H. Chan School of Public Health, Boston, MA, USA, 2008, https://regepi.bwh.harvard.edu/health/nutrition.html.

[2] P. Cochat, G. Rumsby, and P. Hyperoxaluria, "Primary hyperoxaluria," *New England Journal of Medicine*, vol. 369, no. 7, pp. 649–658, 2013.

[3] S. F. Garrelfs, G. Rumsby, and H. Peters-Sengers, "OxalEurope Consortium Patients with primary hyperoxaluria type 2 have significant morbidity and require careful follow-up," *Kidney International*, vol. 96, no. 6, p. 1389, 2019.

[4] N. Lumlertgul, M. Siribamrungwong, B. L. Jaber, and P. Susantitaphong, "Secondary oxalate nephropathy: a systematic review," *Kidney International Reports*, vol. 3, no. 6, pp. 1363–1372, 2018.

[5] L. Nazzal, S. Puri, and D. S. Goldfarb, "Enteric hyperoxaluria: an important cause of end-stage kidney disease," *Nephrology Dialysis Transplantation*, vol. 31, no. 3, pp. 375–382, 2016.

[6] N. Demoulin, Z. Issa, R. Crott et al., "Enteric hyperoxaluria in chronic pancreatitis," *Medicine*, vol. 96, no. 19, Article ID e6758, 2017.

[7] L. Karamadoukis, G. H. Shivashankar, L. Ludeman, and A. J. Williams, "An unusual complication of treatment with orlistat," *Clinical Nephrology*, vol. 71, no. 4, pp. 430–432, 2009.

[8] J. Forryan, V. Mishra, and E. Gibbons, "When the cause is not crystal clear," *Forryan New England journal of medicine*, vol. 382, no. 1, pp. 74–78, 2020.

[9] S. Makkapati, V. D. D'Agati, and L. Balsam, ""Green smoothie cleanse" causing acute oxalate nephropathy," *American Journal of Kidney Diseases*, vol. 71, no. 2, pp. 281–286, 2018.

[10] J. E. Getting, J. R. Gregoire, A. Phul, and M. J. Kasten, "Oxalate nephropathy due to "juicing": case report and review," *The American Journal of Medicine*, vol. 126, no. 9, pp. 768–772, 2013.

[11] A. K. Barman, R. Goel, M. Sharma, and P. J. Mahanta, "Acute kidney injury associated with ingestion of star fruit: acute oxalate nephropathy," *Indian Journal of Nephrology*, vol. 26, pp. 446–448, 2016.

[12] G. Bakul, V. N. Unni, N. V. Seethaleksmy, A. Mathew, R. Rajesh, and P. P. Jose, "Acute oxalate nephropathy due to "Averrhoa bilimbi" fruit juice ingestion," *Indian Journal of Nephrology*, vol. 23, no. 4, pp. 297–300, 2013.

[13] B. Hess, C. Jost, L. Zipperle, R. Takkinen, and P. Jaeger, "High-calcium Intake Abolishes Hyperoxaluria and reduces urinary crystallization during a 20-fold normal oxalate load in humans," *Nephrology Dialysis Transplantation*, vol. 13, no. 9, pp. 2241–2247, 1998.

[14] R. P. Holmes, H. O. Goodman, and D. G. Assimos, "Contribution of dietary oxalate to urinary oxalate excretion," *Kidney International*, vol. 59, no. 1, pp. 270–276, 2001.

[15] J. M. Whittamore and M. Hatch, "The role of intestinal oxalate transport in hyperoxaluria and the formation of kidney stones in animals and man," *Urolithiasis*, vol. 45, no. 1, pp. 89–108, 2017.

[16] M. Liu and L. Nazzal, "Enteric hyperoxaluria," *Current Opinion in Nephrology and Hypertension*, vol. 28, no. 4, pp. 352–359, 2019.

[17] M. Mehta, D. S. Goldfarb, and L. Nazzal, "The role of the microbiome in kidney stone formation," *International Journal of Surgery*, vol. 36, pp. 607–612, 2016.

33

Multiple Focal Brown Tumors (Osteitis Fibrosa Cystica) in a Renal Transplant Recipient

Thavathurai Priyanthan,[1] **Anne Pernille Hermann**,[2,3] **Jonas Asgaard Bojsen**,[3,4] **Anne Bruun Krøigaard**,[5] **Claus Bistrup**,[1,3] **and Erik Bo Pedersen**[1,3]

[1]*Department of Nephrology, Odense University Hospital, Odense, Denmark*
[2]*Department of Endocrinology, Odense University Hospital, Odense, Denmark*
[3]*Department of Clinical Research, University of Southern Denmark, Odense, Denmark*
[4]*Department of Radiology, Odense University Hospital, Odense, Denmark*
[5]*Department of Pathology, Odense University Hospital, Odense, Denmark*

Correspondence should be addressed to Thavathurai Priyanthan; tpriyanthan@hotmail.com

Academic Editor: Anja Haase-Fielitz

Brown tumors (BTs) are manifestations of osteitis fibrosa cystica that develops due to increased osteoclast activity secondary to hyperparathyroidism (HPTH). The name comes from its characteristic brown color due to high hemosiderin level and hemorrhage surrounded by osteoclastic giant cells, fibrous tissue, and bone fragments. Presentation can be either unifocal or rarely multifocal. Misdiagnosis of BT compared to malignant giant cell tumor is not uncommon. Early diagnosis and intervention may prevent destructive bone changes. Treatment of BTs due to chronic renal failure should be aimed primarily at its prevention with phosphate binders, vitamin D (analogues), calcimimetics, and prolonged dialysis sessions. Parathyroidectomy can be the option in nonresponsive cases. In this report, we present an unusual case of multiple brown tumors in a 54-year-old female renal transplant patient involving the spine, jaw, and scapula, initially misdiagnosed as giant cell tumor. Five years later, the patient was diagnosed with BT because of the medical history, morphology, and negative p63 staining in combination with secondary/tertiary hyperparathyroidism. The patient subsequently underwent subtotal parathyroidectomy.

1. Introduction

Brown tumors (BTs) were first described by Friedrich Daniel von Recklinghausen in 1891 [1]. They are seen in osteitis fibrosa cystica (OFC), where giant cell focal lesions consisting of osteoclasts and fibrous tissue give rise to lytic skeletal lesions. The name comes from its characteristic brown color due to the high hemosiderin level from the collection of osteoclastic giant cells, fibrous tissue, and blood in the surrounding stroma. They are well documented in both primary and secondary/tertiary hyperparathyroidism (HPTH) and occur due to increased osteoclast activity. Prevalence of these tumors is lower in secondary HPTH (1.5–1.7%), compared to primary HPTH (3%) [2–4]. Presentation can be either unifocal or rarely multifocal [3]. BTs have been reported in various locations such as jaw bones, ribs, and vertebrae [2, 4, 5]. BTs have no malignant potential; however, they can present as expansive lesions compressing surrounding structures or produce facial disfigurement [3, 4, 6].

The incidence of these tumors in dialysis patients is unknown but increasing due to longevity of these patients [2, 3, 7]. Solitary BTs have been reported previously in renal transplant patients [8]; in this report, we present an unusual case of multiple focal brown tumors in a renal allograft recipient at predialysis stadium involving the spine, initially misdiagnosed as giant cell tumor.

2. Case Report

A 54-year-old female with a 35-year history of type-1 diabetes mellitus, complicated by retinopathy (blindness), neuropathy (Charcot's foot, gastroparesis), and chronic kidney failure, received a deceased-donor renal allograft in 2002. She was on triple immunosuppressive therapy including cyclosporine A, mycophenolate mofetil, and prednisolone. Thirteen years posttransplant, she presented with abdominal pain; a positron emission tomography-computed tomography (PET-CT) revealed several fluorodeoxyglucose (FDG) absorbing bone lesions corresponding to the transverse process of the thoracic vertebra (T12), the body of T8, and the scapulae bilaterally. Subsequent magnetic resonance imaging (MRI) confirmed the tumors in T8 and T12, each measuring approximately 3 cm with a T2-weighted hypointense lesion with paravertebral expansion (Figure 1). Reevaluation of previous scans brought attention to changes in the jaw bones. Specifically, no pathological lymph nodes were seen. A biopsy from T12 suggested a giant cell tumor, although a final diagnosis was not established.

No progression was seen during the insuring three years on serial MRI of the spine. However, 44 months following the initial MRI, the patient developed irregular bone changes in her left shoulder and emergence of a new large mass in S3/S4 (7.5 × 22 mm). Subsequent scans revealed further growth of these tumors in both scapulae and T8. Due to the clinical picture with the absence of pathological lymph nodes, morphology, and the absence of the p63 tumor marker, the giant cell tumor diagnosis was excluded.

Two years later, an MRI revealed a lumbar spine (L1) tumor (Figure 2). A biopsy raised suspicion of a new giant cell tumor. The patient developed severe radicular pain accompanied by weakness of left lower extremity due to neural compression from this lesion. In addition, new spinal lesions developed in corpus of C6 and the right pedicle of L4. Due to the previously described medical history, morphology, negative p63 staining, and the presence of secondary/tertiary hyperparathyroidism (PTH 40–50 pmol/L (1.6–6.0 pmol/L)), a reevaluation of the biopsy material was performed. A giant cell reparative granuloma was described, as shown in Figure 3, and it was concluded that her tumors were indeed BTs. The patient subsequently underwent parathyroidectomy with removal of 3½ parathyroid glands. Postoperative PTH levels were in the normal range 1.0–1.5 pmol/L.

Her pain and symptoms in the lower extremities improved within the first postoperative week. She received short-term dialysis treatment but was discharged on the sixth postoperative day with plasma creatinine approximately 325 micromol/L without further dialysis requirement. There had been neither progression nor regression of the tumor on MRI scanning three months after parathyroidectomy, and her radicular pain and sensory disturbances in the extremities have reduced significantly, with reduced analgetic requirement.

3. Discussion

Chronic kidney disease–mineral and bone disorder (CKD-MBD) is a broader clinical syndrome that develops as a systemic disorder of the mineral and bone metabolism due to CKD. It comprises several components including bone pathology, laboratory abnormalities (calcium, phosphorus, FGF23, vitamin D, and PTH), and extra skeletal calcification. Renal osteodystrophy is part of the syndrome of CKD-MBD, being an exclusive term used to describe morphological bone changes associated with CKD. According to the TMV (bone turnover, mineralization, and volume) system of KDIGO guidelines, renal osteodystrophy comprises of OFC, adynamic bone disease, osteomalacia, and mixed uremic osteodystrophy [9, 10]. Brown tumor is a manifestation of OFC in which there is high bone turnover due to increased osteoclast activity caused by hyperparathyroidism. The histologic features include osteoclastic giant cells, which erodes blood vessels and therefore is located around areas of hemorrhage, admixed with the fibrous tissue and woven bone. A characteristic zonal pattern is seen, as the clusters of giant cells aggregate around red blood cells, surrounded by a zone of reactive fibrosis, which, in turn, is bounded by the reactive bone. The location of BT has most frequently been described in the long bones, facial bones, jaws, sternum, ribs, and the pelvic bones [2–4, 6].

As illustrated in our case, misdiagnosis of BT compared to (malignant) neoplastic giant cell tumor of the bone (GCTB) is not uncommon, as both have very similar imaging presentations and histologic findings. These histologic similarities are already described by Jaffe in 1940 [11]. In BT, these multinucleated giant cells are generally arranged in clusters, sometimes with focal hemorrhage and hemosiderin deposition, but cellular atypia and mitotic figures are absent. In comparison, in giant cell tumors, these giant cells tend to be distributed regularly and uniformly with the presence of atypia and mitotic figures. However, there is no accepted histologic criteria presently available to differentiate BT from giant cell tumors [3].

Unfortunately, characterization of the tumors as BTs in our patient was delayed despite morphological changes that did not include neither atypical cells nor regularly distributed multinucleated giant cells in combination with presence of hemorrhage (hemosiderin) and absence of p63 staining. In addition, lack of pathological lymph nodes ruled out the metastatic malignant process. Above all, the clinical presentation (including hyperparathyroidism) in combination with multiple radiologic findings was not consistent with a giant cell tumor of the bone. Our patient had symptoms that may suggest involvement of lumbar spine (L1) with radicular pain in line with a recently reported 42 cases of vertebral BT where pain, paraparesis, and paraplegia were presenting symptoms [3].

Treatment of BTs should be aimed primarily at its prevention by prompt treatment of HPTH with phosphate binders, vitamin D (analogues), calcimimetics, and prolonged dialysis sessions. Although not well studied, Mourad et al. reported improvement of BT lesion of secondary HPTH in a hemodialysis patient treated with high-dose intravenous calcimimetics. While, parathyroidectomy reserved as the rescue option in nonresponsive cases with secondary or tertiary HPTH [6, 9, 12]. In our patient, treatment was delayed by the misdiagnosis; thus, subtotal

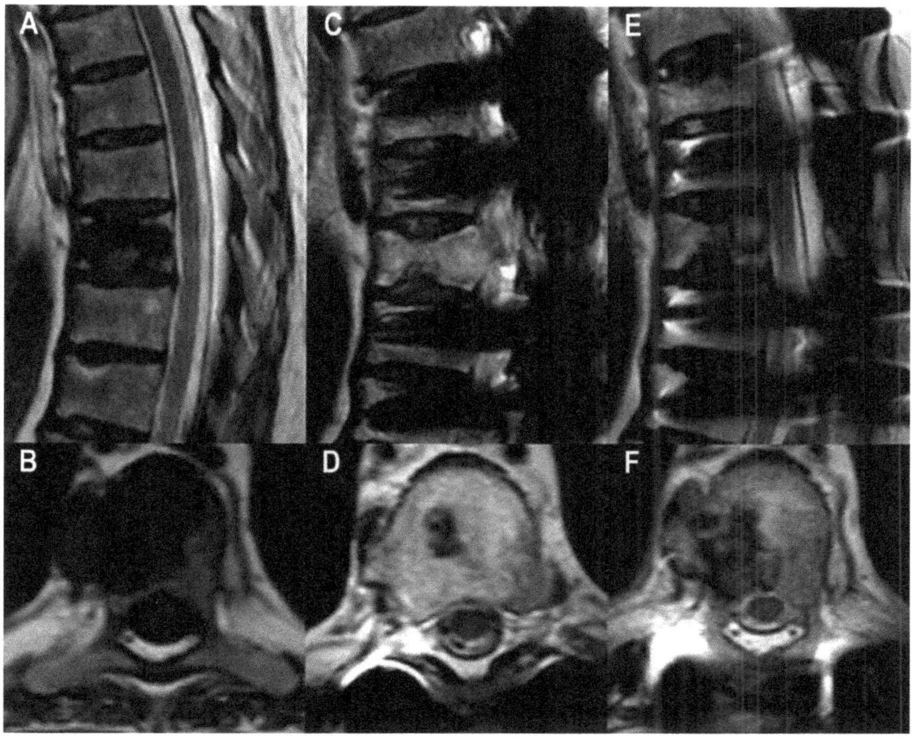

Figure 1: Spine MRI. (a, b) Sagittal T2 weighted Dixon in-phase and axial T1 weighted sequences from initial spine MRI showing tumor in the body of Th8. (c, d) Sagittal T2 weighted Dixon in-phase and axial T2 weighted sequences performed 19 months later showing spondylodesis and partial regression of tumor. (e, f) Sagittal and axial T2 weighted sequences performed additionally 33 months later showing progression of tumor.

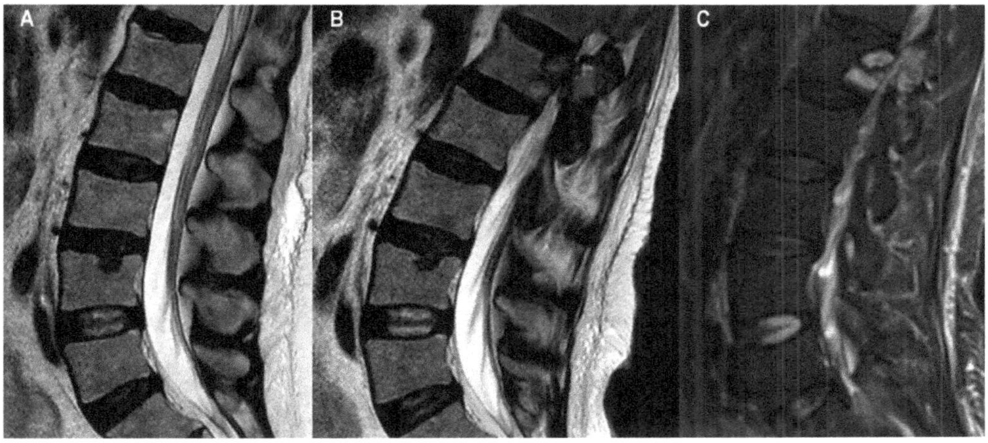

Figure 2: Sagittal spine MRI. (a) T2 weighted sequence from the same investigation as the latest thoracic image showing no lesions in L1. (b) T2 weighted sequence one year later showing tumor in the body and pedicle of L1. (c) T2 weighted Dixon fat suppressed sequence 9 months later showing no further progression of the tumor.

parathyroidectomy was chosen to be the appropriate treatment modality after review of her case. In review of 127 cases in 2015, Rafael et al. reported on a severe form of OFC and found that medical therapy was only offered to about 10% of cases. Parathyroidectomy was reported to be the most common treatment option, either alone (37%) or in combination with BT resection (22%) [2]. This choice can be debated, although parathyroidectomy is generally recognized as the gold standard for treatment of BTs. This decision was made after consultations with a multidisciplinary team of experts both nationally and internationally. However, our patient refused surgical intervention (resection of the tumor). Reviewing medical options, calcimimetics was ruled out due the longer response time. Denosumab is a neoadjuvant treatment modality in inoperable or locally advanced GCTB, approved by the US food and Drug Administration (FDA) on the basis of several nonrandomized phase 2 trials [13]. While both denosumab and

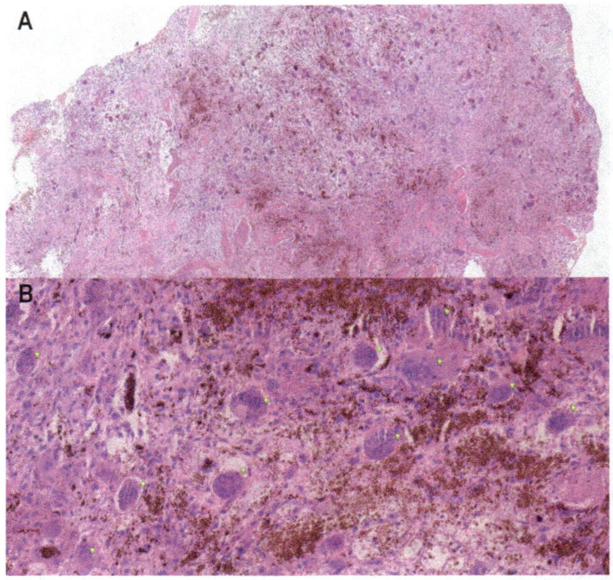

Figure 3: Brown tumor, located at Th12. (a) H&E, x5 histologic features of a giant cell reparative granuloma, in which stromal cells are admixed with osteoclastic giant cells, bone, and areas with hemorrhage. A zonal pattern is seen. Clusters of giant cells aggregate around red blood cells. The giant cells are surrounded by a zone of reactive fibrosis which, in turn, is bounded by the reactive bone. (b) H&E, x100 stromal cells admixed with osteoclast-like giant cells. The multinucleated giant cells, indicated by green dots, aggregate around red blood cells.

parathyroidectomy have the potential to result in severe hypocalcemia (hungry bone syndrome), denosumab was rejected due to its experimental nature and lack of experience of this treatment option by our local experts. Furthermore, our experts have ruled out GCTB and had the persuasion that our patient had BT.

4. Conclusion

Among patients with end-stage renal disease, including dialysis and renal transplant recipients with HPTH and skeletal pain, BT is a relevant differential diagnosis. Early suspicion is essential, and prevention should be the goal of treatment. Early intervention with noninvasive treatment options has good prognosis, as this usually leads to regression of the tumors. Likewise, it prevents the severe consequences such as destructive bone changes of these tumors and compression of adjacent structures.

References

[1] W. Watson Buchanan, G. R. Kraag, D. G. Palmer, Cockshott, and W. Peter, "The first recorded case of osteitis fibrosa cystica," *Canadian Medical Association Journal*, vol. 124, no. 6, pp. 812–815, 1981.

[2] R. M. Baracaldo, D. Bao, P. Iampornpipopchai, J. Fogel, and S. Rubinstein, "Facial disfigurement due to osteitis fibrosa cystica or brown tumor from secondary hyperparathyroidism in patients on dialysis: a systematic review and an illustrative case report," *Hemodialysis International*, vol. 19, no. 4, pp. 583–592, 2015.

[3] H. Tayfun, O. Metin, S. Hakan, B. Zafer, and A. Vardar, "Brown tumor as an unusual but preventable cause of spinal cord compression: case report and review of the literature," *Asian Journal of Neurosurgery*, vol. 9, no. 1, p. 40, 2014.

[4] A. Karagoz, K. Turkmen, R. Yazici et al., "An exceedingly rare localization of a brown tumor in a hemodialysis patient," *Hemodialysis International*, vol. 17, 2012.

[5] G. Campuzano-Zuluaga, W. Velasco-Pérez, and J. I. Marín-Zuluaga, "Case report A 60-year-old man with chronic renal failure and a costal mass: a case report and review of the literature," *Journal of Medical Case Reports*, vol. 3, no. 1, p. 7285, 2009.

[6] E. Eroglu, M. E. Kontas, I. Kocyigit et al., "Brown tumor of the thoracic spine presenting with paraplegia in a patient with peritoneal dialysis," *CEN Case Reports*, vol. 8, no. 4, pp. 227–232, 2019.

[7] K. M. Fargen, C. S. Lin, J. A. Jeung, A. T. Yachnis, R. P. Jacob, and G. J. Velat, "Vertebral brown tumors causing neurologic compromise," *World Neurosurgery*, vol. 79, pp. 208.e1–208.e6, 2013.

[8] S. Noman Zaheer, S. T. Byrne, S. I. Poonnoose, and N. J. Vrodos, "Brown tumour of the spine in a renal transplant patient," *Journal of Clinical Neuroscience*, vol. 16, no. 9, pp. 1230–1232, 2009.

[9] S. Moe, T. Drüeke, J. Cunningham et al., "Definition, evaluation, and classification of renal osteodystrophy: a position statement from Kidney Disease: improving Global Outcomes (KDIGO)," *Kidney International*, vol. 69, no. 11, pp. 1945–1953, 2006.

[10] KDIGO, "Clinical practice guideline for the diagnosis, evaluation, prevention and treatment of Chronic Kidney Disease-Mineral and Bone Disorder (CKD-MBD). Chapter 1: introduction and definition of CKD–MBD and the development of the guideline statements," *Kidney International*, vol. 76, 2009.

[11] H. L. Jaffe, "Hyperparathyroidism," *Bulletin of the New York Academy of Medicine*, vol. 16, pp. 291–311, 1940.

[12] G. Mourad, A. Argilés, C. Vela et al., "Control of severe hyperparathyroidism and regression of a brown tumour after

treatment with i. v. Alfacalcidol in a uraemic patient," *Nephrology Dialysis Transplantation*, vol. 10, no. 4, pp. 552–554, 1995.
[13] https://www.accessdata.fda.gov/drugsatfda_docs/label/2013/125320s094lbl.pdf.

Rapid Glomerulotubular Nephritis as an Initial Presentation of a Lethal Diquat Ingestion

Daniel Guck,[1] **Reynaldo Hernandez**,[2] **Steven Moore**,[2] **Andry Van de Louw**,[1] **and Philippe Haouzi**[1]

[1]*Division of Pulmonary and Critical Care Medicine, Department of Medicine, Pennsylvania State University, College of Medicine, Hershey, PA, USA*
[2]*Department of Emergency Medicine, Pennsylvania State University, College of Medicine, Hershey, PA, USA*

Correspondence should be addressed to Daniel Guck; dguck@pennstatehealth.psu.edu

Academic Editor: Yoshihide Fujigaki

Introduction. Diquat is an herbicide that can lead to rapid multiorgan system failure upon toxic ingestion. Although Diquat shares a similar chemical structure with paraquat, diquat is still readily available to the general population, and in contrast to paraquat, it is not regulated. We present a case of an intentional diquat poisoning which emphasizes the necessity of the early recognition due to atypical symptoms within the first 24 hours and certainly enhanced regulatory restrictions on this very toxic compound. *Case.* A 60-year-old male with a history of severe depression presented to the emergency department after intentional ingestion of a commercial herbicide containing diquat dibromide 2.30%. The earliest manifestations of this acute diquat intoxication comprised a glomerulonephritis and proximal tubular dysfunction. Progressive multiorgan system failure then developed with a significant delay (24–38 hours) including acute renal, liver failure, and then respiratory failure with refractory hypoxemia. Despite maximal supportive care, the end organ failure was lethal. *Discussion.* Diquat intoxication should be suspected in patient presenting an acute glomerulonephritis with coma. Diquat should undergo the same regulatory restrictions as paraquat-containing compounds.

1. Introduction

Diquat (1, 1′-ethylene-2, 2′-bipyridylium) is an herbicide used commercially to treat terrestrial and aquatic vegetation [1]. The toxidrome of diquat intoxication is usually considered to be very similar to that of paraquat, since both agents share a similar chemical structure. However, their mechanisms of toxicity remain poorly understood but seem to involve a rapid oxidative stress and superoxide radical production [2]. The resultant clinical toxic manifestations range from mild local irritative effects to multiorgan system failure and death, in keeping with the dose ingested [2]. We present a case of an intentional diquat ingestion leading to early neurological and renal toxicity which developed into a delayed fatal multiorgan failure. This emphasizes important recognizing the timeline of the symptoms of an acute diquat intoxication and the necessity to apply early aggressive interventions to reduce gastrointestinal absorption. Last, the regulatory restrictions currently in place for paraquat should be applied to diquat.

2. Case Presentation

A 60-year-old male with a history of severe depression presented to the emergency department two hours after an intentional ingestion of ~500 milliliters of a commercial herbicide containing diquat dibromide 2.30%. On initial examination, the patient did not show any hypoxemia, circulatory, or renal failure, but had depressed mental status. Within thirty minutes, a rapid decline in mental status prompted intubation for airway protection. Direct laryngoscopy during the intubation revealed mucus membrane erosion in the posterior pharynx. The orogastric tube was placed after intubation, and 400 ml of green liquid was suctioned from the patient's stomach. Activated charcoal was not administered per recommendation of our

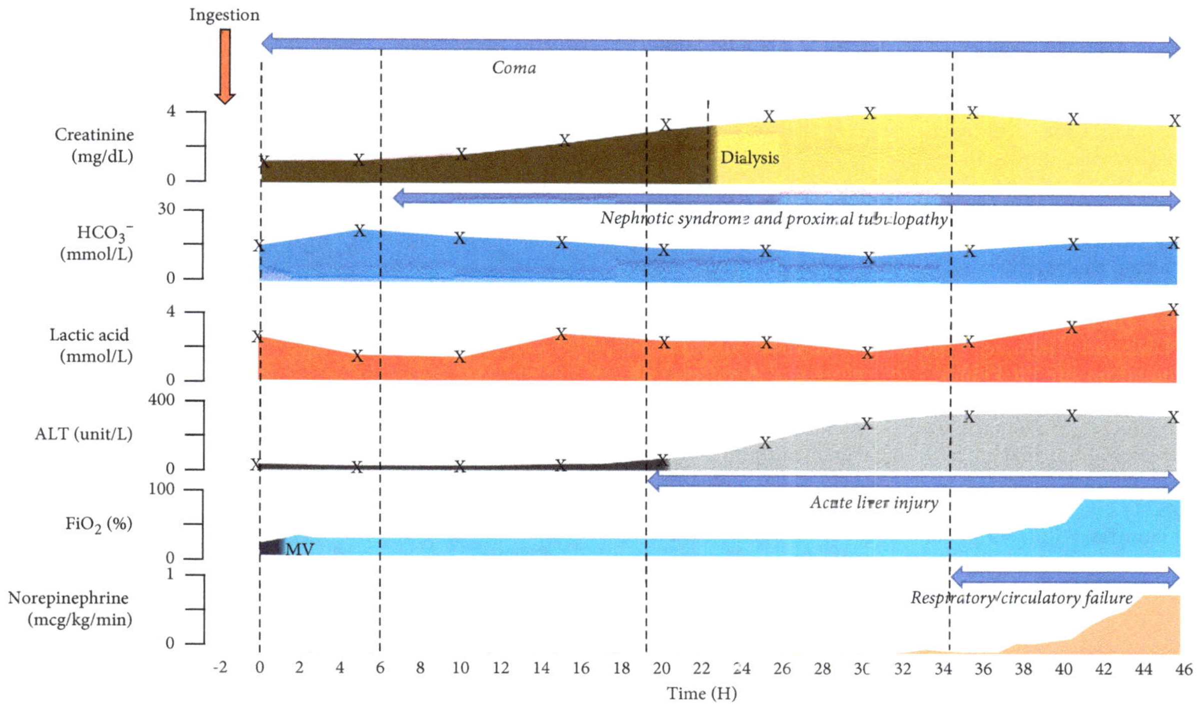

FIGURE 1: Schematic presentation of the clinical course presented by the patient from admission to the fatal outcome. Trends of the most relevant blood tests, the inspired fraction of O_2 required to maintained $SaO_2 > 90\%$, and the level of vasopressor (norepinephrine) support after diquat ingestion are displayed. ALT, alanine aminotransferase; HCO_3^-, bicarbonate; MV, mechanical ventilation.

poison control center due to the delayed arrival of the patient to the emergency department after ingestion. Blood diquat levels determined within 4 hours following the ingestion reached 9.9 μg/ml (a concentration typically associated with a lethal outcome [3]). After transfer to the medical intensive care unit, the patient was started on a combination of N-acetylcysteine, ascorbic acid, vitamin E, and dexamethasone. Within twenty-four hours following the ingestion, the patient presented a nephrotic range proteinuria (urine protein: creatinine >32 g/day) along with marker of proximal tubular dysfunction including glycosuria, phosphaturia, and increased bicarbonaturia. An acute kidney injury later developed (GFR 17 mL/min/ 1.73 m^2) with worsening anion gap metabolic acidosis requiring continuous renal replacement therapy as illustrated in Figure 1. At the same time, a rapid elevation in transaminases and signs of hepatic failure developed (INR 1.4). The respiratory status deteriorated 36 hours only after ingestion with a refractory hypoxemia and imaging of the chest compatible with ARDS. While transthoracic echocardiogram performed and the circulatory status remain within the normal range at 24 hours, an irreversible shock with hyperlactacidemia requiring vasopressor support developed around 36 hours. Despite maximal medical therapy, multiorgan system failure was fatal.

3. Discussion

There is limited understanding of the mechanisms of diquat toxicity and no clear rationale for an effective strategy of treatment. Diquat ingestion, in contrast to paraquat, appears to produce very early adverse neurological syndromes (depressed mental status) due to either direct or secondary neurologic injury after ingestion [4]. As diquat is renally excreted, tubular damage results in glomerulonephritis with proximal tubular necrosis developing within 24 hours and resulting in glucosuria and proteinuria, often without diuresis [5]. This is often accompanied by liver injury [6]. Only much later, acute hypoxic respiratory failure and refractory shock can develop. This sequence differs from that produced by paraquat which produces an early pulmonary toxicity and delayed neurological symptoms. Agents counteracting the oxidative stress have been proposed for treating paraquat intoxication [7], but we have currently no standard of care for diquat poisoning. The primary treatment goal is to prevent gastrointestinal absorption either by gastric suctioning and administration of activated charcoal or Fullers earth [8]. More research on the mechanisms of toxicity and treatments of poisoning by this family on compounds is certainly warranted. Finally, it is unclear why diquat is still a readily available herbicide, while paraquat usage is tightly regulated, as both chemicals, despite some differences, are extremely toxic.

References

[1] N. Magalhães, F. Carvalho, and R. J. Dinis-Oliveira, "Human and experimental toxicology of diquat poisoning: toxicokinetics, mechanisms of toxicity, clinical features, and treatment," *Human and Experimental Toxicology*, vol. 37, pp. 1131–1160, 2018.

[2] G. M. Jones and J. A. Vale, "Mechanisms of toxicity, clinical features, and management of diquat poisoning: a review," *Journal of Toxicology—Clinical Toxicology*, vol. 38, no. 2, pp. 123–128, 2000.

[3] K. Ameno, C. Fuke, Y. Shirakawa et al., "Different distribution of paraquat and diquat in human poisoning cases after ingestion of a combined herbicide," *Archives of Toxicology*, vol. 68, no. 2, pp. 134–137, 1994.

[4] J. Xing, Z. Chu, D. Han et al., "Lethal diquat poisoning manifesting as central pontine myelinolysis and acute kidney injury: a case report and literature review," *Journal of International Medical Research*, vol. 48, no. 7, 2020.

[5] E. A. Lock and J. Ishmael, "The acute toxic effects of paraquat and diquat on the rat kidney," *Toxicology and Applied Pharmacology*, vol. 50, no. 1, pp. 67–76, 1979.

[6] P. Hantson, P. Wallemacq, and P. Mahieu, "A case of fatal diquat poisoning: toxicokinetic data and autopsy findings," *Journal of Toxicology—Clinical Toxicology*, vol. 38, no. 2, pp. 149–152, 2000.

[7] Z. E. Suntres, "Role of antioxidants in paraquat toxicity," *Toxicology*, vol. 180, no. 1, pp. 65–77, 2002.

[8] J. Reigart and J. Roberts, *Recognition and Management of Pesticide Poisonings*, J. Reigart and J. Robert, Eds., , US Environmental Protection Agency, Washington, DC, USA, 6th edition, 2013.

Mutation in the *SLC2A9* Gene: A New Family with Familial Renal Hypouricemia Type 2

Christian Maalouli,[1] **Karin Dahan**,[2,3] **Arnaud Devresse**,[1] **and Valentine Gillion**[1]

[1]*Division of Nephrology, Cliniques Universitaires Saint-Luc, Université Catholique de Louvain, Brussels, Belgium*
[2]*Division of Human Genetics, Cliniques Universitaires Saint-Luc, Université Catholique de Louvain, Brussels, Belgium*
[3]*Center of Human Genetics, Institut de Pathologie et de Génétique, Charleroi, Belgium*

Correspondence should be addressed to Valentine Gillion; valentine.gillion@uclouvain.be

Academic Editor: Salih Kavukcu

Familial renal hypouricemia is a rare genetic disorder characterized by a defect in renal tubular urate reabsorption. Some patients present with exercise-induced acute kidney injury and nephrolithiasis. Type II is caused by mutations in the *SLC2A9* gene. Here, we report the case of a young patient who developed acute kidney injury after exercise secondary to familial renal hypouricemia type II. The same mutation was found in other asymptomatic members of his family. We review the medical literature on this condition. This case highlights the importance of considering uric acid disorders in the work-up of acute kidney injury after exercise.

1. Introduction

Hypouricemia may be caused by decreased uric acid production or increased uric acid clearance [1–4]. The latter may be due decreased renal tubular reabsorption secondary to acquired disorders such as Fanconi syndrome or inherited disorders such as familial renal hypouricemia (RHUC) [1–6]. Unlike hyperuricemia and gout, hypouricemia has been thought as a disorder with no clinical significance. However, individuals with RHUC may present with exercise-induced acute kidney injury and nephrolithiasis [1–10]. Here, we report the case of a patient who developed acute kidney injury after strenuous exercise. The work-up has led to the discovery of a new family with RHUC type II.

2. Case Presentation

A 20-year-old man presented to the nephrology department with acute pain of both flanks which started after a physical exercise at school. His past medical history was unremarkable. He was not taking any medications or illicit drugs, and he denied smoking and consuming alcohol.

There was no abnormal finding in his physical examination. Vital signs were normal. Laboratory tests on admission showed acute kidney injury with a creatine kinase level of only twice the upper limit of the normal (Table 1). Urinalysis was bland, and the proteinuria was within the range (Table 1). Contrast-enhanced computed tomography showed decreased enhancement of the kidneys without any abnormality of the vessels and showed no urolithiasis. After conservative therapy including intravenous fluid administration, the renal function recovered gradually and returned to the normal at the fourth day after admission.

The patient reported that he was admitted 4 months ago in the emergency room of another hospital for a similar pain which occurred also after a strenuous exercise. Although laboratory tests showed acute kidney injury, he was discharged without any further investigation.

Laboratory tests were marked by severe hypouricemia. The elevated fractional excretion of urate (119%; $N < 10\%$) suggested a highly increased urinary excretion of uric acid with tubular secretion. Blood and urinary tests showed no argument for Fanconi syndrome or syndrome of inappropriate antidiuretic hormone. Interesting enough, severe

Table 1: Laboratory findings.

Test		Unit	Value at presentation	Normal range
	CRP	mg/l	3.3	<5
	Creatinine	mg/dl	1.9	0.6–1.3
	Urea	mg/dl	60	17–48
	Uric acid	mg/dl	0.2	3.5–7.2
	Sodium	mmol/l	139	135–145
	Potassium	mmol/l	5.2	3.5–5.0
	Bicarbonate	mmol/l	22	23–29
Serum	Calcium	mmol/l	2.3	2.2–2.5
	Phosphate	mmol/l	0.9	0.8–1.45
	Hemoglobin	g/dl	15.3	13–18
	WBC	/μl	12310	3500–11000
	Neutrophils	/μl	9630	1500–6700
	Platelets	/μl	170000	150000–450000
	LDH	U/l	262	135–225
	CK	U/l	640	40–300
	RBC	/μl	2	<25
	WBC	/μl	20	<25
	Creatinine	g/24h	0.98	0.8–2.5
Urine	Protein	g/24h	0.08	<0.15
	Sodium	mmol/24h	216	40–220
	Potassium	mmol/24h	34	25–125
	Uric acid	mg/24h	234	250–750

Abbreviations: CRP, C-reactive protein; WBC, white blood cell; RBC, red blood cell; LDH, lactate dehydrogenase; CK, creatine kinase.

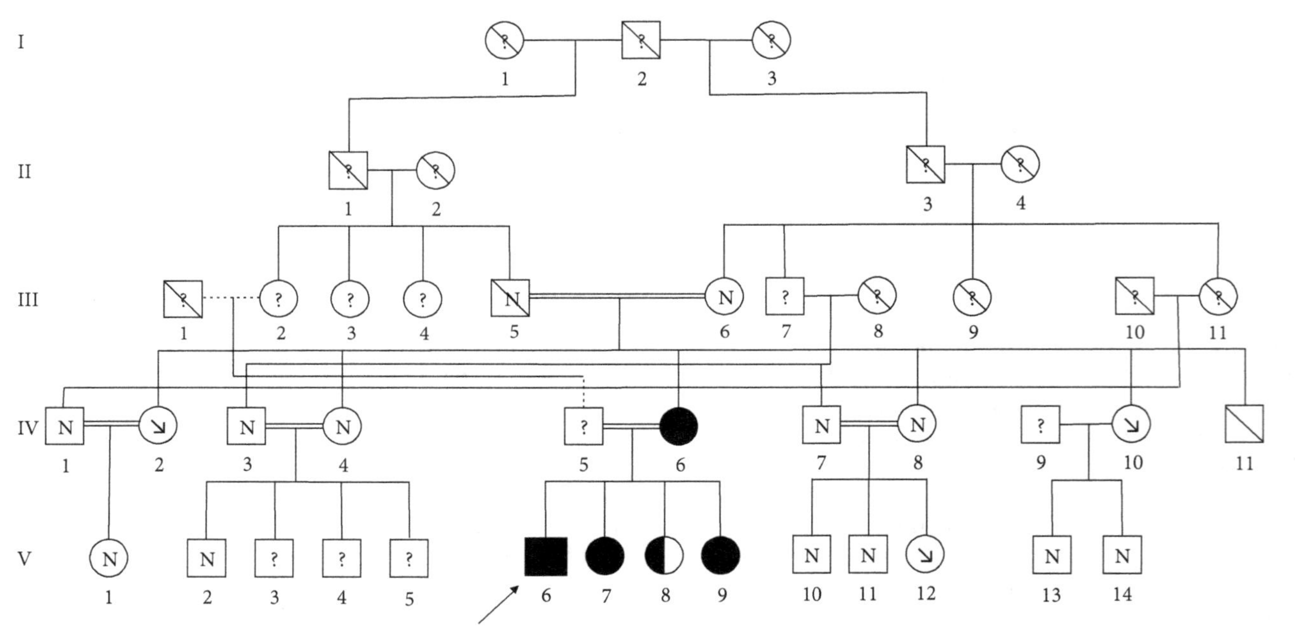

Figure 1: Pedigree of the patient. Solid symbols denote family members with homozygous mutation; half-solid denote heterozygous mutation. "N" denotes family members with normal uric acid level; "↘" denotes severe hypouricemia. "?" denotes family members with no laboratory data. Circles represent female family members, squares represent male family members, and crosses represent dead family members. Double lines indicate consanguineous marriage. Arrow indicates the index patient.

hypouricemia was also found in the laboratory tests of his mother and one of his maternal aunts. The occurrence of two episodes of acute kidney injury following intense exercise with the presence of hereditary severe hypouricemia highly suggested exercise-induced acute kidney injury due to familial renal hypouricemia.

This index patient (V6) is a member of a highly consanguineous Pakistani family with cousin marriages over two successive generations (Figure 1). DNA sequencing by next-generation sequencing identified an homozygosity for a class 5 variant of the *SLC2A9* gene (NM_020041.3): c.646G > A, p.(Gly216Arg) confirmed by the Sanger technique [5]. Genetic testing of the patient's mother revealed the same homozygous mutation. Severe hypouricemia with the familial homozygous mutation was found in two of his clinically unaffected sisters (V7 and V9). The third sister (V8) is heterozygous for the mutation and is presenting with normal uric acid level. Profound hypouricemia was also measured in one of his aunts (IV2) and one of his cousins (V12). All of these analyses confirmed an autosomal recessive mode of inheritance. Besides the index patient, no medical history was known in all of the family members except his grandfather (III5) who suffered from kidney stones.

3. Discussion

RHUC is a rare autosomal recessive genetic disease caused by impaired renal tubular urate transport [1–10]. Less common than type 1 caused by mutations in the *SLC22A12* gene encoding the major uric acid transporter URAT1 (OMIM #220150), type 2 (RHUC2, OMIM #612076) is caused by mutations in the *SLC2A9* gene which encodes GLUT9 [1–5, 7–10]. Its long variant GLUT9L is the only major urate efflux transporter at the basolateral membrane, explaining why homozygous loss-of-function mutations of GLUT9 cause a total defect of uric acid tubular absorption [1, 4, 7–9]. To date, no more than 15 families have been described [1–4, 8, 9]. Although most patients are asymptomatic, the major complications are exercise-induced acute kidney injury (EIAKI) and urolithiasis [1–10]. EIAKI often follows intense exercise and is mostly described in males [4, 8, 10]. It may be secondary to excessive oxidative stress leading to renal vasoconstriction or precipitation of uric acid in the tubules [1, 3, 4, 8, 10]. When compared to type 1, patients with type 2 appear to have much higher renal excretion of uric acid and to be more vulnerable for EIAKI and nephrolithiasis [1, 9]. Measures to prevent these complications include limiting anaerobic physical exercise and maintaining adequate fluid intake [8–10]. Allopurinol may be proposed in specific cases [2–4, 9, 10].

Consent

Informed consent was obtained from the patient.

References

[1] D. Dinour, N. K. Gray, S. Campbell et al., "Homozygous SLC2A9 mutations cause severe renal hypouricemia," *Journal of the American Society of Nephrology*, vol. 21, no. 1, pp. 64–72, 2010.

[2] H. Shen, C. Feng, X. Jin et al., "Recurrent exercise-induced acute kidney injury by idiopathic renal hypouricemia with a novel mutation in the SLC2A9 gene and literature review," *BMC Pediatrics*, vol. 14, no. 1, p. 73, 2014.

[3] M. Windpessl, M. Ritelli, M. Wallner, and M. Colombi, "A Novel homozygous SLC2A9 mutation associated with renal-induced hypouricemia," *American Journal of Nephrology*, vol. 43, no. 4, pp. 245–250, 2016.

[4] C. Wang, J. Wang, S. Liu et al., "Idiopathic renal hypouricemia: a case report and literature review," *Molecular Medicine Reports*, vol. 20, no. 6, pp. 5118–5124, 2019.

[5] B. Stiburkova, J. Taylor, A. M. Marinaki, and I. Sebesta, "Acute kidney injury in two children caused by renal hypouricaemia type 2," *Pediatric Nephrology*, vol. 27, no. 8, pp. 1411–1415, 2012.

[6] H. O. Kim, C.-G. Ihm, K. H. Jeong et al., "A case report of familial renal hypouricemia confirmed by genotyping ofSLC22A12, and a literature review," *Electrolytes & Blood Pressure*, vol. 13, no. 2, pp. 52–57, 2015.

[7] H. Matsuo, T. Chiba, S. Nagamori et al., "Mutations in glucose transporter 9 gene SLC2A9 cause renal hypouricemia," *The American Journal of Human Genetics*, vol. 83, no. 6, pp. 744–751, 2008.

[8] G. Jeannin, N. Chiarelli, M. Gaggiotti et al., "Recurrent exercise-induced acute renal failure in a young Pakistani man with severe renal hypouricemia and SLC2A9compound heterozygosity," *BMC Medical Genetics*, vol. 15, no. 1, p. 3, 2014.

[9] A. Peris Vidal, J. Marin Serra, E. Lucas Sáez et al., "Hereditary renal hypouricaemia type 1 and 2 in three Spanish children. Review of published paediatric cases," *Nefrologia*, vol. 39, no. 4, pp. 355–361, 2019.

[10] Y. Shimizu, K. Wakabayashi, A. Totsuka et al., "Exercise-induced acute kidney injury in a police officer with hereditary renal hypouricemia," *Case Reports in Nephrology and Dialysis*, vol. 9, no. 2, pp. 92–101, 2019.

36

Acute Esophageal Necrosis Early after Renal Transplantation

Ahmad Makeen,[1] Faisal Al-Husayni ,[1,2] and Turki Banamah [2,3,4]

[1]*Department of Internal Medicine, National Guard Hospital, Jeddah, Saudi Arabia*
[2]*King Abdullah International Medical Research Center, Jeddah, Saudi Arabia*
[3]*Department of Nephrology, National Guard Hospital, Jeddah, Saudi Arabia*
[4]*King Saud bin Abdulaziz University for Health Sciences, Jeddah, Saudi Arabia*

Correspondence should be addressed to Turki Banamah; banamahtu@ngha.med.sa

Academic Editor: Phuong Chi Pham

Background. Acute esophageal necrosis (AEN) is defined as a diffused black discoloration of the esophageal mucosa involving mainly the distal part of the esophagus. It is considered a rare clinical entity with a high mortality rate. The etiology of AEN is unknown, but it has been correlated to many causes such as malignancies, infections, and hemodynamics instability. Here, we report a case of a patient developing AEN a few days after kidney transplantation. *Case Presentation.* A 57-year-old male was admitted electively for kidney transplantation that he received from his son. The surgery was complicated with a significant drop in blood pressure but otherwise was uneventful. The patient was showing good signs of recovery but then suffered from significant hematemesis. An urgent upper esophagogastroduodenoscopy revealed black discoloration of the esophageal mucosa in keeping with AEN. The patient was treated with proton pump inhibitors infusion and started empirically on antivirals and antifungals. The patient's condition improved in regards to the AEN; nonetheless, the complications resulted in graft loss, and the patient returned to hemodialysis. *Conclusion.* AEN is a critical condition that mandates early intervention. Identifying high-risk populations may aid in early anticipation and diagnosis. Patients with chronic kidney disease are at risk of atherosclerosis leading to a low flow state which is exacerbated during renal transplantation surgery, especially if the procedure was complicated with a drop in blood pressure.

1. Background

Acute esophageal necrosis (AEN) is a rare disease most commonly involved in the lower third of the esophagus with upper gastrointestinal bleeding (UGIB) representing the most widely manifesting symptom. Several retrospective and prospective trials reported an incidence ranging between 0.01–0.28% [1, 2]. Men tend to have a higher prevalence compared with women. Gurvits et al. were the first to describe AEN as a distinct clinical syndrome with a structured approach to defining associated risk factors and pathogenesis [3]. Patients are usually elderly and have multiple comorbidities, commonly diabetes and hypertension [4]. The underlying pathogenesis is not fully understood; however, the development of AEN is believed to be a result of a combination of variables rather than a single cause.

The previous literature defined many events that repetitively noted to accompany cases of AEN including acute ischemia and hemodynamic instability, diabetic ketoacidosis, infection, and poor nutritional status [5–7]. This disease was diagnosed by upper esophagogastroduodenoscopy (EGD) finding of circumferential mucosal necrosis with black discoloration of the distal esophagus. No specific therapy for AEN and treatment is mainly supportive.

Among options offered to patients with ESKD, kidney transplantation represents the best survival benefit, and it improves the quality of life when compared to other alternatives of kidney replacement therapy [8, 9]. Renal transplant recipients are immunocompromised which increases the risk of opportunistic infection, and the use of immunosuppressive medications such as glucocorticoid also plays a role in the disruption of the normal gastric mucosa.

AEN has been reported in renal transplant recipients in few reported cases [10–13], which is thought to be secondary to multiple factors.

Herein, we are presenting a case of an adult male who develops AEN early after renal transplantation surgery.

2. Case Presentation

A 57-year-old gentleman who is known to have an end-stage kidney disease (ESKD) on intermittent hemodialysis (HD) through left arteriovenous fistula for two years. The reason for his kidney failure was attributed to long-standing hypertension. After a shared discussion and full clinical and laboratory assessment, the patient opted to undergo renal transplantation as a recipient from his son.

As part of the pretransplantation workup, human leukocyte antigen (HLA) tissue typing was compatible with his donor son. Two weeks before transplant, the crossmatch with his son was completely negative for T- and B-cells. Serological results are shown in Table 1. His urine microscopy revealed no white blood cells (WBCs), only a few red blood cells (RBCs), and epithelial cells. The stool was negative for occult blood, and no WBCs were observed in microscopy. Chest X-ray was unremarkable. His electrocardiography (ECG) was within normal limits, and echocardiography demonstrated a normal left ventricular function with an ejection fraction of 60% and grade 1 diastolic dysfunction most likely secondary to his long-standing hypertension. An ultrasound of the abdomen and pelvis showed a bilateral echogenic kidney with multiple left renal cysts. Ultrasound Doppler of iliac vessels appears unremarkable, and voiding cystourethrogram was normal.

The patient was admitted one day before surgery, and induction with basiliximab was carried as the patient was considered low immunological risk based on pretransplantation workup. He was started on usual maintenance therapy which included tacrolimus, mycophenolate (MMF), and prednisone along with valganciclovir and trimethoprim/sulfamethoxazole as prophylaxis for both *Cytomegalovirus* (CMV) and *Pneumocystis* pneumonia.

The next day, surgery commenced which went smoothly with no bleeding or major complications except a significant drop in his systolic blood pressure at the beginning of surgery during anesthesia induction from 225/115 to 100/55 for almost 2-3 hours. By the end of the surgery, the patient's vital signs were stable, with good urine output. Creatinine level improved from 774 μmol/L before the operation to 149 μmol/L on the second day after the transplantation.

On the third day, the patient vomited blood of moderate amount with a drop in Hb to 7.1 g/L from 8.3 g/L. He never had a previous history of gastroesophageal reflux disease, cholelithiasis, or alcohol intake. An upper esophagogastroduodenoscopy (EGD) was arranged on the same day which showed an area of necrosis with black esophagus in the lower third which attributed to possible fungal infection or secondary to a major drop in blood pressure during surgery (Figure 1). The CT angiogram conveyed thickened wall of the esophagus with a good enhancement of the esophageal mucosa and no evidence of bowel ischemia.

Table 1: Patient's laboratory results prior to renal transplantation.

Serology	Result
CMV IgM	Negative
CMV IgG	Positive
CMV PCR	Not detected
EBV IgM	Negative
HSV	Negative
VZV	Negative
Hepatitis B surface Ag	Negative
Anti-hepatitis B core	Negative
Anti-hepatitis B surface Ab	>1000
Hepatitis C	Negative
HIV	Negative
ANA	2.1
Complement (C3/C4)	Negative

The patient was started on esomeprazole infusion, caspofungin for possible fungal infection, and ganciclovir instead of oral valganciclovir. Moreover, intravenous (IV) tacrolimus was not available; thus, oral tacrolimus was replaced by IV cyclosporin. Also, he was started on IV methylprednisone.

The esophageal brushing showed predominantly necrotic debris and acute/chronic inflammatory cells with few reactive squamous cells with no prominence in cytologic atypia. In addition, no definite candida organisms or nuclear changes of herpes infection or other viral infections were identified.

Three days later, the patient started to gain weight of around 20 kg compared to admission weight with clinical evidence of volume overload. He was shifted to the intensive care unit (ICU) and intubated. His stay was complicated by a central line infection with pseudomonas bacteremia. The patient reached the maximum dose of diuretics without achieving sufficient diuresis and with worsening in his creatinine; thus, he was started on hemodialysis (HD) with ultrafiltration.

The patient's condition improved without signs of gastrointestinal bleeding. EGD was repeated showing a complete resolution of the black esophagus and some stricture at the lower part which is a complication of the necrosis. The patient was discharged in a good condition but remained on HD for the following two years.

3. Discussion

AEN is a catastrophic rare clinical syndrome which is present usually with a UGIB in patients with multiple underlying medical conditions and poor general health status. Although mortality associated with AEN is reported to reach around 30% [4], the disease is thought to be underdiagnosed [14]. The mechanism that explains the development of AEN is complex and necessitates a combination of underlying risk factors with a triggering event.

The patient's general condition and presence of DM, hypertension, chronic kidney disease (CKD), and nutritional status may cause atherosclerosis, which leads to a low flow state precipitating AEN [15–19]. The occurrence of the AEN in most cases also requires an acute event enhancing the progression to the full disease picture. Hypotension in case of shock state, inflammatory condition, esophageal CMV

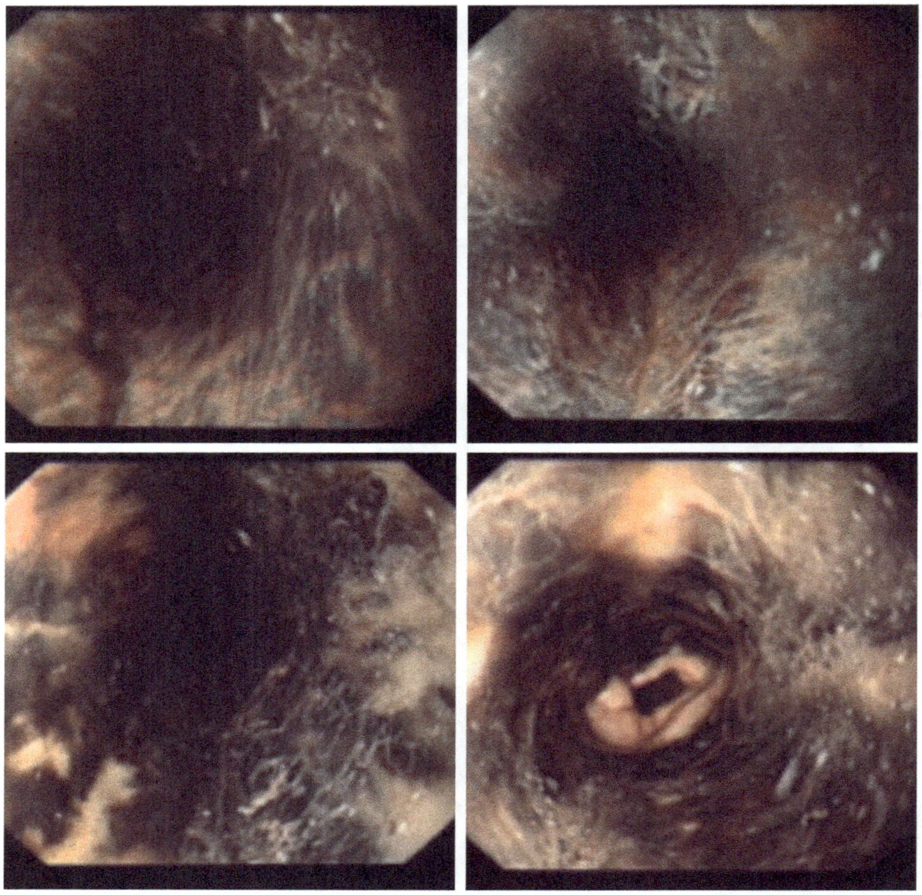

FIGURE 1: A view of the patient's esophagus showing black discoloration confirming the diagnosis of acute esophageal necrosis.

infection, malignancy, and medications has been reported to be a primary cause of AEN [15–20].

Cases of AEN following organ transplantation have been reported previously [21]. The fact that those patients are immunocompromised explains CMV and *Candida*-related AEN in such patients. In addition, graft versus host disease has been associated with AEN in renal transplant recipients [22]. Even though a low flow state and a hemodynamic compromise were associated with few cases of AEN following surgery, AEN can occur while the patient maintains normal blood pressure [11]. Steroids and MMF are used as maintenance therapy after transplant; such therapy might play a role in the development of AEN by interfering with a normal esophageal mucosal barrier. Calcineurin inhibitors are vasoconstrictors that may also enhance hypoperfusion and esophageal ischemia in patients with risk factors.

We are presenting a case of a renal transplant recipient who developed AEN early after surgery. The reason is most likely attributed to a significant drop in his systolic pressure during operation due to anesthesia induction, which led to hypoperfusion and ischemia. His history of long-standing hypertension and CKD with subsequent probable atherosclerosis has exacerbated his low flow state. No evidence of infection was detected. Unfortunately, our patient's hospital course was complicated by acute pulmonary edema, intubation, and ICU admission. His kidney function deteriorates most likely secondary to acute tubular necrosis related to central line infection. However, underlying graft rejection is another possibility. The patient underwent another EGD three weeks after the first one which showed complete resolution of the black esophagus with stricture over the distal esophagus as a result of previous inflammation.

4. Conclusions

AEN is a rare lethal disease with a significant mortality rate. Diagnosis requires a high index of suspicion with attention to the risk factors. Renal transplant recipients may be considered as a risk group in which achieving sustainable normal hemodynamics and closely observing for any signs of opportunistic infection might be protective.

References

[1] M. Moretó, E. Ojembarrena, M. Zaballa, J. G. Tánago, and S. Ibáñez, "Idiopathic acute esophageal necrosis: not necessarily a terminal event," *Endoscopy*, vol. 25, no. 8, pp. 534–538, 1993.

[2] R. Ramos, J. Mascarenhas, P. Duarte, C. Vicente, and C. Casteleiro, "[Acute esophageal necrosis:a retrospective case series]," *Revista Española de Enfermedades Digestivas*, vol. 100, pp. 583–585, 2008.

[3] G. E. Gurvits, A. Shapsis, N. Lau, N. Gualtieri, and J. G. Robilotti, "Acute esophageal necrosis: a rare syndrome," *Journal of Gastroenterology*, vol. 42, no. 1, pp. 29–38, 2007.

[4] H. M. Abdullah, W. Ullah, M. Abdallah, U. Khan, A. Hurairah, and M. Atiq, "Clinical presentations, management, and outcomes of acute esophageal necrosis: a systemic review," *Expert Review of Gastroenterology & Hepatology*, vol. 13, no. 5, pp. 507–514, 2019.

[5] N. R. Kalva, M. R. Tokala, S. Dhillon et al., "An unusual cause of acute upper gastrointestinal bleeding: acute esophageal necrosis," *Case Reports in Gastrointestinal Medicine*, vol. 2016, Article ID 6584363, 4 pages, 2016.

[6] M. Talebi-Bakhshayesh, F. Samiee-Rad, H. Zohrenia, and A. Zargar, "Acute esophageal necrosis:a case of black esophagus with DKA," *Archives of Iranian Medicine*, vol. 18, pp. 384-385, 2015.

[7] V. Sharma, A. De, A. Ahuja, S. Lamoria, and B. M. S. Lamba, "Acute esophageal necrosis caused by candidiasis in a patient with systemic lupus erythematosus," *Journal of Emergency Medicine*, vol. 51, no. 1, pp. 77–79, 2016.

[8] T. E. Pesavento, "Kidney transplantation in the context of renal replacement therapy," *Clinical Journal of the American Society of Nephrology*, vol. 4, no. 12, pp. 2035–2039, 2009.

[9] W. Fiebiger, C. Mitterbauer, and R. Oberbauer, "Health-related quality of life outcomes after kidney transplantation," *Health and Quality of Life Outcomes*, vol. 2, no. 1, p. 2, 2004.

[10] D. Mealiea, D. Greenhouse, M. Velez, P. Moses, and C. E. Marroquin, "Acute esophageal necrosis in an immunosuppressed kidney transplant recipient: a case report," *Transplantation Proceedings*, vol. 50, no. 10, pp. 3968–3972, 2018.

[11] A. M. Kesler, P. T. Kröner, and H. M. Wadei, "Acute esophageal necrosis following kidney transplantation," *American Journal of Gastroenterology*, vol. 113, p. S1038, 2018.

[12] F. Caravaca-Fontán, S. Jimenez, A. Fernández-Rodríguez, R. Marcén, and C. Quereda, "Black esophagus in the early kidney post-transplant period," *Clinical Kidney Journal*, vol. 7, no. 6, pp. 613-614, 2014.

[13] M. A. Yu, R. Mulki, and J. Massaad, "The black esophagus in the renal transplant patient," *Case Reports in Nephrology*, vol. 2019, Article ID 5085670, 3 pages, 2019.

[14] L. Julián Gómez, J. Barrio, R. Atienza et al., "[Acute esophageal necrosis: an underdiagnosed disease]," *Revista Espanola de Enfermedades Digestivas*, vol. 100, pp. 701–705, 2008.

[15] M. Lahbabi, A. Ibrahimi, and N. Aqodad, "Acute esophageal necrosis: a case report and review," *The Pan African Medical Journal*, vol. 14, p. 109, 2013.

[16] D. A. Neumann II, D. L. Francis, and T. H. Baron, "Proximal black esophagus: a case report and review of the literature," *Gastrointestinal Endoscopy*, vol. 70, no. 1, pp. 180-181, 2009.

[17] C. de la Serna-Higuera, J. Martínez, M.-I. Martín-Arribas, S. Rodríquez-Gómez, A. Pérez-Villoria, and A. Betancourt, "Acute necrotizing esophagitis," *Gastrointestinal Endoscopy*, vol. 54, no. 2, p. 225, 2001.

[18] R. Trappe, H. Pohl, A. Forberger, R. Schindler, and P. Reinke, "Acute esophageal necrosis (black esophagus) in the renal transplant recipient: manifestation of primary cytomegalovirus infection," *Transplant Infectious Disease*, vol. 9, no. 1, pp. 42–45, 2007.

[19] J. W. Mall, H. Zuckermann-Becker, C. Pollmann, I. Opitz, P. Rogalla, and M. Walter, "Esophageal necrosis and perforation of the left main bronchus following photodynamic therapy of esophageal carcinoma," *The Thoracic and Cardiovascular Surgeon*, vol. 50, no. 2, pp. 111–113, 2002.

[20] W. Ullah, H. M. A. Abdullah, A. Rauf, and K. Saleem, "Acute oesophageal necrosis: a rare but potentially fatal association of cocaine use," *BMJ Case Reports*, vol. 2018, 2018.

[21] J. A. Planchard, A. F. Dikstein, J. Koveleskie, A. Cohen, and G. E. Gurvits, "Acute esophageal necrosis following orthotopic liver transplantation," *Cureus*, vol. 11, p. e4090, 2019.

[22] D. Singh, R. Singh, and A. S. Laya, "Acute esophageal necrosis: a case series of five patients presenting with "black esophagus"," *Indian Journal of Gastroenterology*, vol. 30, no. 1, pp. 41–45, 2011.

A Rare Case of Immunotactoid Glomerulopathy Associated with Hodgkin Lymphoma

Keiki Nagaharu,[1,2] **Yuka Sugimoto**,[2] **and Keiki Kawakami**[1]

[1]*Department of Hematology and Oncology, Suzuka General Hospital, Yamanohana 1275-53, Suzuka 513-8630, Mie Prefecture, Japan*
[2]*Department of Hematology and Oncology, Mie University Graduate School of Medicine, Edobashi 2-174, Tsu 514-8507, Mie Prefecture, Japan*

Correspondence should be addressed to Keiki Nagaharu; keiki.nagaharu@gmail.com

Academic Editor: Yoshihide Fujigaki

Immunotactoid glomerulopathy (ITG) is characterized by Congo red-negative microtubular deposits, and it has been reported as a rare paraneoplastic syndrome due to hematologic malignancies, viral infections, or autoimmune diseases. In hematologic malignancies, multiple myeloma and other mature B-cell malignancies are the most common hematologic malignancies, and Hodgkin lymphoma (HL) is extremely rare. A 59-year-old woman was admitted to our hospital because of a pulmonary mass and proteinuria. Computed tomography-guided lung biopsy confirmed the presence of HL stage IIA. Immunofixation of peripheral blood was positive for immunoglobulin G (IgG) kappa. Renal biopsy showed mesangial proliferation with deposits in the subendothelial lesion and no invasion of the HL. These deposits were positive for IgG3, C3, and kappa light chain but negative for C1q and lambda light chain. Electron microscopy showed randomly aligned tubular structures with a diameter of approximately 50 nm. We diagnosed the patient with immunotactoid nephropathy and HL. After systemic chemotherapy, the patient achieved a complete response and loss of proteinuria. On the contrary, her serum monoclonal gammopathy was observed after chemotherapy. The existence of a monoclonal antibody itself might not be a sufficient factor for ITG in some cases, and an additive trigger is necessary for development.

1. Introduction

Immunotactoid glomerulopathy (ITG) is an extremely rare condition (approximately less than 1% of renal biopsies [1]) and was first introduced by Schwartz and Lewis [2]. ITG is defined by Congo red-negative microtubular deposits and has been reported as a rare paraneoplastic syndrome due to B-cell lymphoma or multiple myeloma.

Hodgkin lymphoma (HL) is the most common lymphoma in Western countries. Approximately 0.4% of HL cases show glomerular dysfunction, which is mainly diagnosed as minimal change nephrotic syndrome (MCNS) [3]. Serum monoclonal antibodies are normally undetected, but a few cases have been reported as HL with monoclonal gamma globulin [4]. We encountered a case of HL presenting with ITG, and renal biopsy revealed immunotactoid nephropathy (ITG).

2. Case Presentation

A 59-year-old woman was admitted to our hospital with chronic cough. Her medical history included glaucoma without medication and a resected benign ovarian cyst. In addition, she had been diagnosed with elevated immunoglobulin G (IgG) levels 3 years prior to admission. Three months before her admission, she noticed a sore throat and cough without sputum. She had been diagnosed with pneumonia because of pulmonary infiltration on chest radiography, and levofloxacin was prescribed in another clinic. However, her symptoms did not resolve, and she was referred to our hospital.

On admission, chest auscultation revealed attenuated respiratory sounds in the left upper lung. Complete blood counts revealed leukocytosis with predominant neutrophils (12,300/μL (normal, <9,000); neutrophil, 93%). Blood

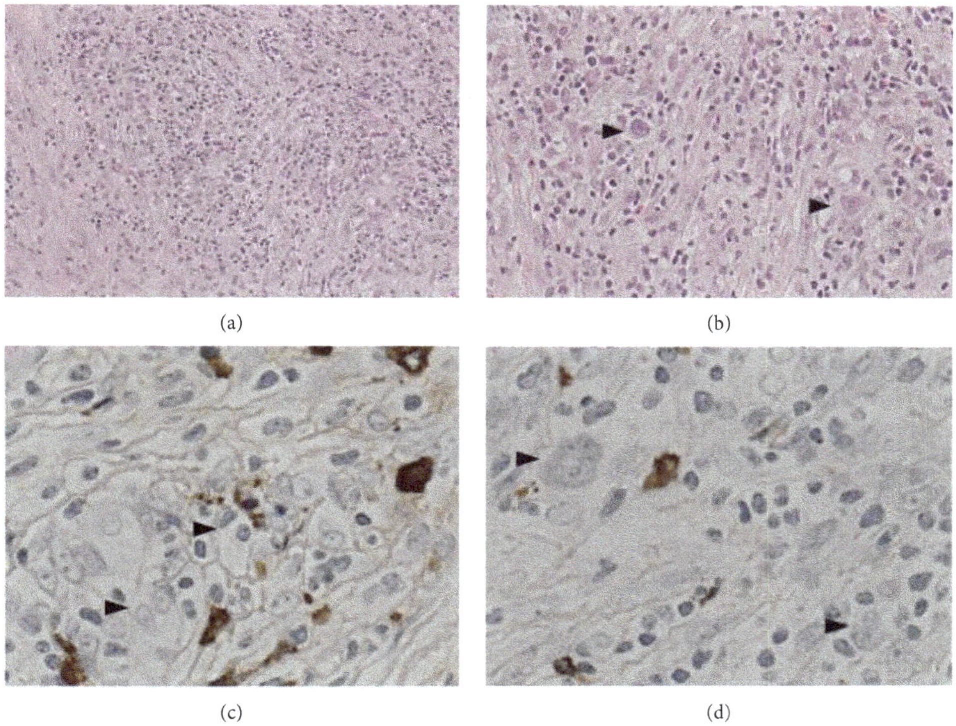

Figure 1: Histopathological evaluation of pulmonary biopsy. (a) HE (×40). (b) PAS (×100). Stained pulmonary biopsy reveals "Hodgkin cells." Immunofluorescence staining of these Hodgkin cells is negative for kappa (c) and lambda (d).

biochemistry revealed hypoalbuminemia (3.3 g/dL), elevated C-reactive protein (10.4 mg/dL), high-soluble interleukin-2 receptor (3,940 IU/dL (normal, <550 IU/dL)), and normal IgG (1,392 mg/dL (normal, <1,700 mg/dL)). However, immunofixation of the serum revealed a low amount of monoclonal IgG kappa. Others including serum electrolytes, blood urea (9.2 mg/dL), creatinine (0.60 mg/dL), IgA (271 mg/dL), IgM (103 mg/dL), C3 (106 mg/dL), and C4 (34 mg/dL) were within normal limits. Serum tests for PR3-ANCA, MPO-ANCA, anti-Ri antibody, anti-Hu antibody, anti-Yo antibody, anti-dsDNA IgG antibody, and anti-dsDNA IgM were all negative. Despite repetitive evaluations, the patient tested negative for cryoglobulin. Antibody tests for hepatitis B virus, hepatitis C virus, and human immunodeficiency virus (HIV) were also negative. Computed tomography (CT) showed a tumor combined with infiltration in the left lower lobe. Pathological findings of CT-guided biopsy of the tumor confirmed stage IIB nodular sclerosis classical HL (Figure 1). Bone marrow specimens revealed a normal population without the proliferation of plasma cells.

Despite normal eGFR, her urine was positive for protein, and the estimated daily urine protein amount was 1.36 g/g. Urinary protein was mainly albumin, and urinary monoclonal gamma globulin was absent. Renal biopsy revealed mesangial proliferation and a thickened glomerular basal membrane. PAS-positive and Congo red-negative deposits were observed in the glomerular capillary walls (Figures 2(a) and 2(b)). Immunofluorescence staining was positive for IgG and C3 in the deposits (Figures 2(c) and 2(d)). Immunohistochemistry showed positivity for kappa light chain (Figure 2(e)) and IgG3 (Figure 2(g)) and negative for lambda light chain (Figure 2(f)), IgG1, IgG2, IgG4, and C1q (data not shown). Electron microscopy indicated randomly aligned tubular structures located in the subendothelial and mesangial areas of the glomeruli (Figures 2(h) and 2(i)). The diameter of these tubular structures was approximately 50 nm. We finally diagnosed her renal findings as ITG.

She was treated with six courses of ABVD (Adriamycin 25 mg/m^2, bleomycin 10 IU/m^2, vinblastine 6 mg/m^2, and dacarbazine 375 mg/m^2 on days 1 and 15, every 4 weeks) without significant adverse events, and the pulmonary lesion disappeared quickly. Urinary protein was negative after two courses of ABVD. However, her serum monoclonal IgG kappa light chain was detected.

3. Discussion

The association between HL and nephrotic syndrome is rare (approximately 0.4% in adults) [3]. Among patients with HL with nephrotic syndrome, MCNS is observed as a paraneoplastic manifestation [5]. However, renal pathological findings in our case confirmed membranoproliferative glomerulonephritis with nonamyloid deposits, which was finally diagnosed as ITG. The distinction between ITG, fibrillary glomerulonephritis, and type I cryoglobulin nephropathy has been controversial because of their similar clinical and pathological features. In fact, some ITG cases are not distinguished from the others. Our case is compatible with ITG in view of the restricted light chain and tubular

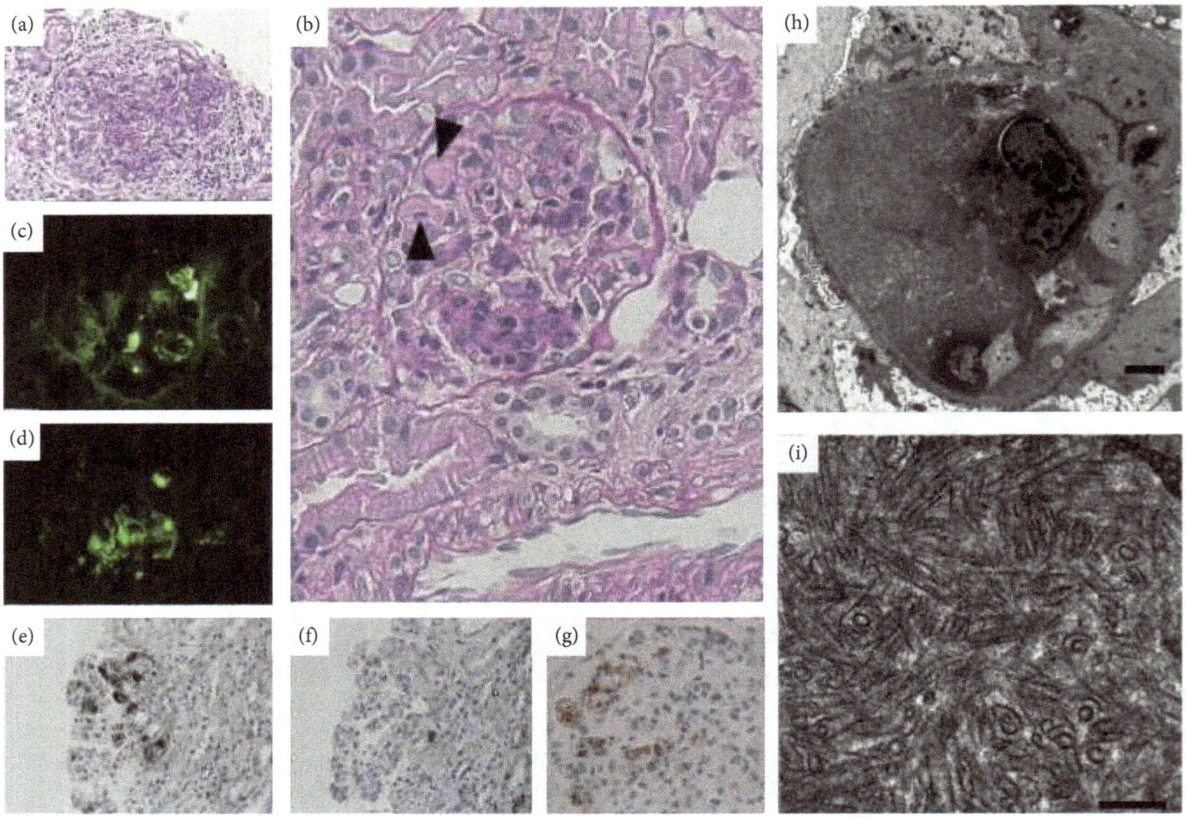

FIGURE 2: Histopathological evaluation of renal biopsy. (a) PAS (×40). (b) PAS (×100). Stained renal biopsy sections at diagnosis reveal mesangial proliferation and subendothelial deposits (arrowheads). Immunofluorescence staining of these deposits is positive for IgG (c) (×40) and C3 (d) (×40). Immunostaining of the light chain is positive for kappa light chain (e) (×40), negative for lambda light chain (f) (×40), and positive for IgG3 (g) (×40). Using electric microscopy ((h) (×2,500), (i) (×25,000)), these deposits are composed of a tubular structure with a diameter of 50 nm. Black bars in (h) and (i) represent 2.5 μm and 500 nm, respectively.

TABLE 1: Literature review of previous ITG case reports (available 39 cases).

	Age and sex	Hematologic underlying disease	No.
Age	Median 60 (6–79)	Multiple myeloma	5
Sex	Male, 56%; female, 44%	Lymphoplasmacytic leukemia	4
		Chronic lymphocytic leukemia	3
	Component of deposits	Mycosis fungoides	1
IgG	69%	POEMS	1
IgM	30%	AITL	1
IgA	7%	HES	1

The literature search was performed using PubMed with the following medical keywords: {immunotactoid nephropathy} or {immunotactoid glomerulopathy}. Among 136 articles, we adapted the reports with at least one of the following data: age and sex, deposit immunoglobulin, and hematologic underlying diseases.

diameter of the deposit. On the contrary, random alignment of tubular deposits and small-vessel thrombosis in renal biopsy were characteristics of cryoglobulin nephropathy. However, there were no cryoglobulin-related peripheral symptoms, and serum cryoglobulin was repetitively negative. We diagnosed ITG rather than cryoglobulin nephropathy.

ITG is a rare disease that accounts for only 0.06% of all kidney biopsies [6]. To date, at least 39 patients have been published as case reports (Table 1). The peak of occurrence is at 60 years of age, and deposits are IgG dominant (approximately 70%), which is compatible with a previous report [7]. Hematologic malignancies, including multiple myeloma, lymphoplasmacytic lymphoma, and diffuse large B-cell lymphoma, have been reported. These cases were also positive for serum monoclonal immunoglobulins. However, T-cell lymphoma [8] and mycosis fungoides [9] have been reported as ITG cases. Monoclonal gammopathy was negative in these cases. In addition, several types of underlying diseases other than hematologic malignancies include tuberculosis [10], HIV infection [11–13], and hepatitis C virus infection [14, 15]. To the best of our knowledge, this is the first reported case of HL with ITG.

In our case, we suspected that ITG nephropathy was induced as a paraneoplastic syndrome. Hudnall et al. [4] described a case of HL with heavy chain monoclonal gammopathy, and they suggested three possible pathogeneses of monoclonal gammopathy in HL: (1) two distinct neoplastic processes, (2) produced by Hodgkin cells, or (3) a single neoplastic process leading to two subclones (one producing HL and the other producing gammopathy). As for the second possibility, we performed additional immunohistochemical staining of HL cells in pulmonary lesions, which was negative for light chain expression (Figures 1(c) and 1(d)). As for the first and third Hudnall et al.'s hypotheses, our patient's medical history included elevated IgG, but the etiology was unknown. As HL itself generally does not accompany monoclonal gammopathy, our case might have underlying monoclonal gammopathy before the onset of HL. The exact mechanism is uncertain, but HL may produce some trigger substances for the development of ITG. In conclusion, we encountered a rare case of HL presenting with ITG. We could not reveal the exact mechanism, and further development of the pathological elucidation of ITG is desired.

Acknowledgments

The authors would like to thank Dr. Shinichi Mizuno, Dr. Mika Goto, and Dr. Kensuke Joh for their helpful suggestions. They would like to thank Editage (http://www.editage.com) for English language editing.

References

[1] S. H. Nasr, A. M. Valeri, L. D. Cornell et al., "Renal monoclonal immunoglobulin deposition disease: a report of 64 patients from a single institution," *Clinical Journal of the American Society of Nephrology*, vol. 7, no. 2, pp. 231–239, 2012.

[2] M. M. Schwartz and E. J. Lewis, "The quarterly case: nephrotic syndrome in a middle-aged man," *Ultrastructural Pathology*, vol. 1, no. 4, pp. 575–582, 1980.

[3] C. E. Alpers and R. S. Cotran, "Neoplasia and glomerular injury," *Kidney International*, vol. 30, no. 4, pp. 465–473, 1986.

[4] S. D. Hudnall, J. B. Alperin, and J. R. Petersen, "Composite nodular lymphocyte-predominance Hodgkin disease and γ-heavy-chain disease," *Archives of Pathology & Laboratory Medicine*, vol. 125, no. 6, pp. 803–807, 2001.

[5] V. Audard, F. Larousserie, P. Grimbert et al., "Minimal change nephrotic syndrome and classical Hodgkin's lymphoma: report of 21 cases and review of the literature," *Kidney International*, vol. 69, no. 12, pp. 2251–2260, 2006.

[6] A. B. Fogo, M. A. Lusco, B. Najafian, and C. E. Alpers, "AJKD atlas of renal pathology: immunotactoid glomerulopathy," *American Journal of Kidney Diseases*, vol. 66, no. 4, pp. e29–e30, 2015.

[7] J. L. Rosenstock, G. S. Markowitz, A. M. Valeri, G. Sacchi, G. B. Appel, and V. D. D'Agati, "Fibrillary and immunotactoid glomerulonephritis: distinct entities with different clinical and pathologic features," *Kidney International*, vol. 63, no. 4, pp. 1450–1461, 2003.

[8] M. S. Duwaji, D. G. Shemin, L. J. Medeiros, and A. R. Esparza, "Proliferative glomerulonephritis with unusual, organized, cylindrical deposits associated with angioimmunoblastic lymphadenopathy-like T-cell lymphoma," *Archives of Pathology & Laboratory Medicine*, vol. 119, no. 4, pp. 377–380, 1995.

[9] A. Torrelo, M. T. Rivera, F. Mampaso et al., "Immunotactoid glomerulopathy associated with mycosis fungoides," *Postgraduate Medical Journal*, vol. 66, no. 779, pp. 773–775, 1990.

[10] A. Gupta and A. Khaira, "Immunotactoid glomerulopathy and tuberculosis: a novel association," *Nefrologia: Publicacion Oficial de la Sociedad Espanola Nefrologia*, vol. 31, no. 3, pp. 369–371, 2011.

[11] C. Chen, K. D. Jhaveri, C. Hartono, and S. V. Seshan, "An uncommon glomerular disease in an HIV patient: value of renal biopsy and review of the literature," *Clinical Nephrology*, vol. 75, no. 1, pp. 80–88, 2011.

[12] M. Haas, S. Rajaraman, T. Ahuja, M. Kittaka, and T. Cavallo, "Fibrillary/immunotactoid glomerulonephritis in HIV-positive patients: a report of three cases," *Nephrology Dialysis Transplantation*, vol. 15, no. 10, pp. 1679–1683, 2000.

[13] J. L. Martin, D. Thomas, and R. E. Colindres, "Immunotactoid glomerulopathy in an HIV-positive African-American man," *American Journal of Kidney Diseases: The Official Journal of the National Kidney Foundation*, vol. 42, no. 6, pp. E6–E10, 2003.

[14] M. B. Stokes, "Immune complex glomerulonephritis in patients with hepatitis C. Saudi journal of kidney diseases and transplantation: an official publication of the Saudi Center for Organ Transplantation," *Saudi Arabia*, vol. 11, no. 3, pp. 396–404, 2000.

[15] L. Maldonado, A. Das, A. G. Kahn, and D. Howell, "Immunotactoid glomerulopathy in a patient with hepatitis C viral infection," *Ultrastructural Pathology*, vol. 41, no. 1, pp. 98-99, 2017.

38

Acute Kidney Injury Secondary to Rhabdomyolysis and COVID-19: A Case Report and Literature Review

Vishaka K. Chetram, Akram I. Ahmad, Saira Farid, and Tanuj Sood

Department of Internal Medicine, Washington Hospital Center, Washington, DC 20010, USA

Correspondence should be addressed to Vishaka K. Chetram; vishaka.k.chetram@gunet.georgetown.edu

Academic Editor: Bernard G Jaar

The viral infection causing COVID-19 most notably affects the respiratory system but can result in extrapulmonary clinical manifestations as well. Rhabdomyolysis-associated acute kidney injury (AKI) in the setting of COVID-19 is an uncommon complication of the infection. There is significant interest in this viral infection given its global spread, ease of transmission, and varied clinical manifestations and outcomes. This case report and literature review describes the symptoms, laboratory findings, and clinical course of a patient who developed AKI secondary to rhabdomyolysis and COVID-19, which will help clinicians recognize and treat this condition.

1. Introduction

The novel coronavirus which emerged in late 2019, designated as severe acute respiratory syndrome coronavirus 2 (SARS-CoV-2) and responsible for COVID-19, has infected more than 85 million people worldwide and has grown into a global pandemic. The incubation period, disease severity, initial presentation, and laboratory findings are varied [1–4]. Multiorgan complications include respiratory failure, cardiac arrhythmias, cardiomyopathy, encephalopathy, thromboembolic events, and acute kidney injury (AKI) [5–7].

Kidney involvement in the setting of COVID-19 manifests as hematuria, proteinuria, and/or an AKI, which is associated with increased mortality and more severe infections [8, 9]. Estimates of the incidence of AKI range from 17% to 37% and between 5–15% require kidney replacement therapy [8, 10]. The etiology of kidney dysfunction remains unexplored and may be the result of direct viral infection, cytokine release, altered hemodynamics, or multifactorial, including rhabdomyolysis. Characterized as a clinical syndrome of muscle weakness, myalgia, tea-coloured urine, and muscle swelling, rhabdomyolysis is defined with a creatine kinase value greater than 1000 IU/L or higher than 5 times the upper limit of normal [11]. Rhabdomyolysis occurs due to trauma, drugs, electrolyte abnormalities, and also rarely, viral infections such as influenza A and B, coxsackievirus, Epstein–Barr, herpes simplex, parainfluenza, adenovirus, echovirus, HIV, cytomegalovirus, and most recently, COVID-19 [12, 13]. Thus, our aim in this case report is to present the symptoms, laboratory findings, and clinical course of a patient who presented with AKI secondary to rhabdomyolysis and COVID-19 and provide a literature review of the reported cases.

2. Case Report

A 62 year-old-African American male patient presented to the emergency department with a 3-day history of general feeling of malaise, poor appetite, decreased urine output, and blood in his urine. His comorbidities include hypertension, morbid obesity (BMI of 39.6), and suboptimally controlled type II diabetes. He was socially distancing alone at home and reported no known sick contacts. He denied taking any anticoagulation medication and had no symptoms of urinary urgency or dysuria. He also denied recent strenuous activity, alcohol ingestion, or taking any over-the-counter supplements. Home medications included aspirin 81 mg, glargine 25 units daily, hydrochlorothiazide-lisinopril 12.5mg–20 mg daily, pioglitazone 30 mg, and simvastatin 20 mg daily.

On presentation, he was febrile to 38.1°C with a heart rate of 103, respiratory rate of 20, blood pressure of 91/58 mmHg, and saturating well on room air. Physical examination yielded a patient with a large body habitus and mild respiratory distress. Pertinent initial laboratory findings revealed a sodium of 132 mmol/L, potassium 4.5 mmol/L, magnesium 2.0 mg/dL, phosphorus 8.9 mg/dL, corrected calcium 4.4 mg/dL, BUN 54 mg/dL, creatinine 4.90 mg/dL (baseline of 1.1 mg/dL), glucose 372 mg/dL, aspartate aminotransferase (AST) 1077 units/L (baseline of 16 units/L), alanine aminotransferase (ALT) of 158 units/L (baseline of 24 units/L), alkaline phosphatase 45 units/L, total bilirubin 0.4 mg/dL, glomerular filtration rate (GFR) 14 mL/min, and lactic acid of 2.1 mmol/L. Urine albumin-to-creatinine ratio one month prior to presentation was 30 mg/g. Creatinine kinase was 327, 629 units/L, and peaked on presentation. Hemoglobin A1C glycosylated was 12.9%. D-dimer was 2.01 mcg/mL FEU. Arterial blood gas showed a pH of 7.35, CO2 of 31 mmHg, and bicarbonate of 17.1 mmol/L. C-reactive protein (CRP) was 136.39 mg/L, and thyroid-stimulating hormone (TSH) was 1.397 uIU/mL. Hepatitis viral panel was obtained and negative. Urine toxicology was negative. Urine analysis showed a moderate amount of blood and 19/hpf red blood cells. The progression of creatinine and creatinine kinase is depicted in Figure 1, respectively.

Point-of-care ultrasound of the bladder showed <100 mL of urine. Ultrasound of the abdomen showed hepatomegaly with fatty infiltration and no acute cholecystitis or choledocholithiasis, as well as no hydronephrosis. The initial chest radiograph was significant for multifocal patchy airspace disease suggestive of atypical pneumonia or viral infection including COVID-19 (Figure 2).

Initial COVID-19 RNA PCR was negative. Respiratory viral panel for influenza and respiratory syncytial virus (RSV) was also negative. He was given a bolus of 2 L lactated ringer (LR) and started on maintenance LR at 200 mL/hour as well as sevelamer 2400 mg three times a day. For the first 48 hours, he was anuric. He also received ceftriaxone and azithromycin for community-acquired pneumonia coverage. His anion gap and metabolic acidosis resolved shortly after administration of IV fluids. Following the first 48 hours, his urine output increased to 600 mL over 24 hours on the third day and was red tinged. Urine output decreased to 210 mL and 150 mL per 24 hours on hospitalization days four and five, respectively. On the third day of his hospitalization, given the elevated D-dimer and concerning chest radiograph findings, COVID-19 PCR was repeated and found to be positive.

Despite his positive test, the patient did not have respiratory symptoms and continued to oxygenate well on room air. On day 3, continuous renal replacement therapy (CRRT) was initiated due to persistent low urine output, worsening kidney indices, and volume overload. He received 3 consecutive days of CRRT while maintenance fluids were continued at 100 mL per hour. His urine output gradually increased, and CRRT was interrupted. By day 5, his creatine kinase downtrended to 57, 074 units/L with improved serum creatinine to 5.46 mg/dL. At the end of the first week of his hospitalization, his urine appeared clear and total 24-hour output was 700 mL. Given his improvement in urine output and downward trend in creatinine, CRRT was stopped.

On day 8 of his hospitalization, his oxygen levels desaturated to 87% while walking to the bathroom and he was placed on 2 L supplemental oxygen via a nasal cannula. Maintenance fluids were also discontinued at this time, and he developed a fever to 38.1°C. Chest X-ray showed worsening bilateral infiltrates (Figure 3).

At this point in his clinical course, his blood pressures remained elevated, ranging from 170/80 to 200/90, and antihypertensive medication doses were progressively increased up to amlodipine 10 mg daily and hydralazine 100 mg thrice a day. On day 12, the patient went into acute hypoxic respiratory failure, developed tachycardia with a heart rate of 120s beats per minute and tachypnea with a respiratory rate of 30. An arterial blood gas (ABG) was obtained which showed a pH of 7.41, CO_2 29 mmHg, bicarbonate 18.4 mmol/L and PaO_2 of 82 mmHg. He was placed on BiPAP at 60% FiO_2, broad-spectrum antibiotics for pneumonia coverage, and heparin drip for suspected pulmonary embolism and was transferred to the intensive care unit (ICU).

In the ICU, he was started on a 10-day course of dexamethasone and weaned to a high-flow nasal cannula after 2 days. Remdesevir was never given due to kidney dysfunction. He was also intermittently treated with diuretics. By day 14 of his hospitalization, his daily urine output was 2.9 L and clear in color. He received an echocardiogram which showed an ejection fraction of 65–70% with no valvular or diastolic dysfunction. Ultrasound of the lower extremities was negative for deep vein thrombosis. As his respiratory status improved, he was weaned to 6 L supplemental oxygen via a nasal cannula and was transferred out of the ICU. The patient gradually improved as he completed the 10-day course of dexamethasone, and at the time of discharge, 26 days after his presentation, his creatinine gradually decreased to 1.16 mg/dL and he was sent home, on room air.

3. Discussion

COVID-19-related kidney dysfunction occurs in a number of ways [14] and can manifest as (1) prerenal AKI from volume depletion or cardiorenal syndrome, (2) acute tubular injury in the setting of circulatory collapse, (3) thrombotic microangiopathy secondary to hypercoagulation, (4) collapsing glomerulopathy in APOL1 gene variants, and (5) myoglobin cast nephropathy due to rhabdomyolysis. Emerging literature has connected COVID-19 to the development of rhabdomyolysis and acute kidney injury, but only few cases have been reported (Table 1) and the physiology link remains unknown.

The proposed hypotheses include direct invasion of muscle tissue, release of toxic cytokines, namely, TNF-alpha, and destruction of muscle cell membranes by circulating toxins [25]. Approximately 5% of hospitalized COVID-19

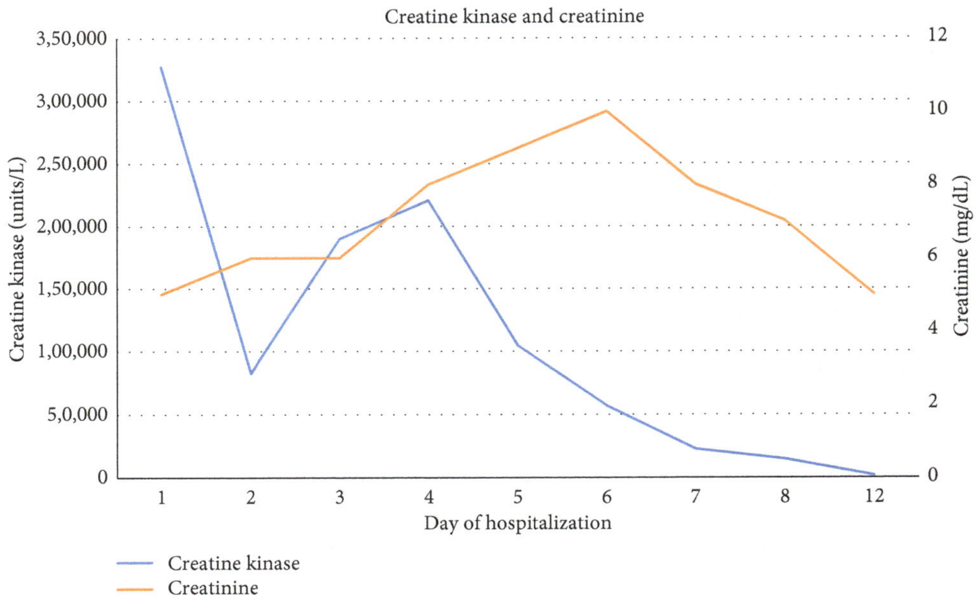

Figure 1: Trend of creatinine kinase and creatinine.

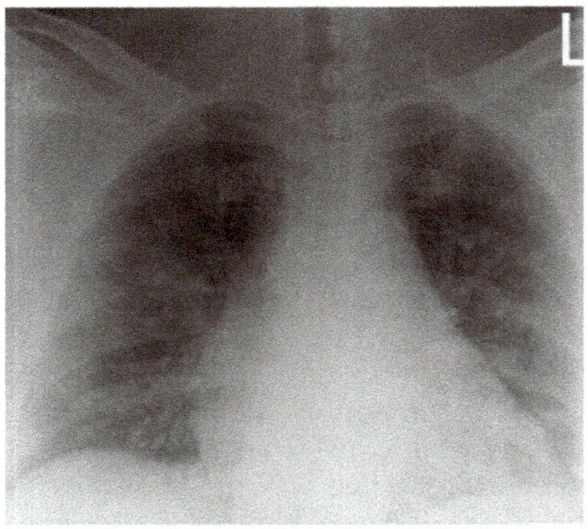

Figure 2: Chest X-ray showing multifocal patchy airspace disease, COVID-19.

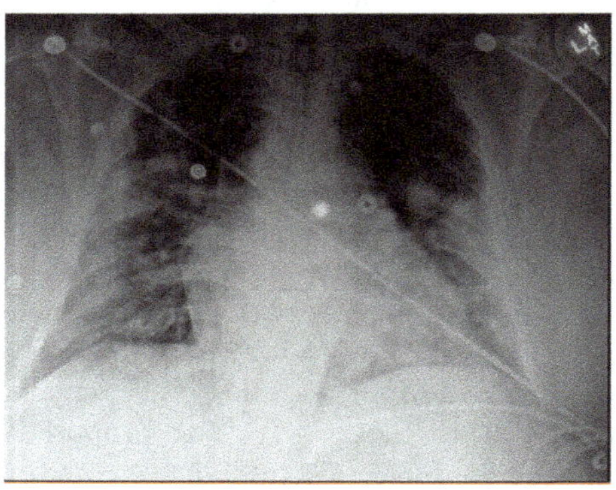

Figure 3: Chest X-ray on day 14 showing worsening bilateral infiltrates.

Table 1: Summary of the reported cases.

	Demographics	Clinical Presentation	Comorbidities	Pertinent labs	Clinical course and outcome
Taxbro et al. [15]	38-year-old male	1 week of fever, myalgia, nausea, emesis, dry cough, dyspnea, and abdominal pain	Type 2 diabetes Gout	CRP: 145 mg/dL Creatinine: 51 mmol/L D-dimer: 0.19 mg/dL No reported CK	Complete recovery after ICU admission requiring intubation LOS: 23 days
Valente-Acosta et al. [16]	71-year-old male	1 week of dry coughing, mild dyspnoea and fever, and myalgia and arthralgia, predominantly in his legs	Benign prostatic hyperplasia	CRP: 2.9 mg/dL Creatinine: 1.68 mg/dL LDH: 541 U/L D-dimer: 983 ng/mL CK peak: 8,720 U/L	Complete recovery after ICU admission requiring intubation LOS: 16 days
	34-year-old male	Fever, cough, dyspnea, and weakness	Prediabetes	— Creatinine 0.89 mg\dl — — CK peak: 5,454 U/L	Died in hospital LOS: not reported
	71-year-old male	Fever, cough, and dyspnea	Hypertension Schizophrenia Seizures	— Creatinine: 4.1 mg/dL — — CK peak: 10,247 U/L	Died in hospital LOS: not reported
Singh et al. [17]	88-year-old male	Confusion	Diabetes Hypertension	— Creatinine: 2.25 mg/dL — — CK peak: 2,628 U/L	Died in hospital LOS: not reported
	36-year-old male	Fever, cough, and dyspnea	None	— Creatinine: 1.03 mg/dL — — CK peak: 5,531 U\L	Died in hospital LOS: not reported
	39-year-old male	Myalgias, fever, cough, and dyspnea	Hypertension	— Creatinine: 3.8 mg/dL — — CK peak: 4,330 U/L	Died in hospital LOS: not reported

Table 1: Continued.

	Demographics	Clinical Presentation	Comorbidities	Pertinent labs	Clinical course and outcome
Husain et al. [18]	38-year-old male	Sever, cough, dyspnea, and myalgia	Not reported	CRP: 98.3 mg/dL Creatinine: 1.5 mg/dL LDH: 398 U/L — CK peak: 33,000 U/L	Complete recovery after ICU admission LOS: 3 months
Chedid et al. [19]	51-year-old male	2 days of diffuse myalgias, dry cough, and mild chills	Hypertension Type 2 diabetes OSA CKD II	CRP: 98.3 mg/dL Creatinine: 2.48 mg/dL LDH: 2150 U/L — CK peak: 464,000 U/L	Dialysis as outpatient LOS: not reported
Singh et al. [20]	67-year-old male	Fever and dyspnea	Hypertension	— Creatinine: 1.16 mg/dL LDH: 459 U/L D-dimer: 0.62 ng/mL CK peak: 19,773 U/L	Died in hospital LOS: 21 days
	39-year-old male	Fever, myalgia, dyspnea, and altered mental status	Hypertension	CRP: 98.3 mg/dL Creatinine: 3.8 mg/dL LDH: 907 U/L D-dimer: 1.92 ng/mL CK: 4,330 U/L	Died in hospital LOS: 1 day
Alejandro et al. [21]	89-year-old male	Dyspnea, fever, cough, and malaise	Hypertension, coronary artery disease, and heart failure with preserved ejection fraction	Creatinine: 2.0 mg/dL LDH: 805 U/L — CK: 2,751 U/L	Complete recovery LOS: 12 days
Pellegrini et al. [22]	34-year-old male	2 days of emesis, sore throat, nonproductive cough, and dyspnea	Not reported	CRP: 3.3 mg/dL Creatinine: 1.4 mg/dL LDH: 854 U/L — CK: 73,922 U/L	Complete recovery LOS: 8 days

Table 1: Continued.

	Demographics	Clinical Presentation	Comorbidities	Pertinent labs	Clinical course and outcome
Chong and Saha [23]	37-year-old male	2 days of dyspnea and fatigue	Not reported	— Creatinine: 5.0 mg/dL — — CK peak: 35,000 U/L	Died in hospital LOS: 12 day
Chan et al. [24]	75-year-old female	4 days of weakness and decrease in appetite	Coronary artery disease, hypertension, and GERD	— Creatinine: 1.2 mg/dL — — CK: 2,767 U/L	Complete recovery LOS: not reported
	71-year-old male	Generalized weakness and leg twitching	Hypertension, seizure, CKD, and overactive bladder	— Creatinine: 5.6 mg/dL — — CK: 1,859 U/L	Hospitalized as inpatient LOS: undetermined
Chetram et al., 2021 (this manuscript)	62-year-old male	3-day history of general feeling of malaise, poor appetite, decreased urine output, and blood in his urine	Hypertension, type II diabetes, obesity	CRP: 136.39 mg/L Creatinine: 4.9 mg/dL — D-dimer: 2.01 mcg/dL CK peak: 327,629 U/L	Complete recovery LOS: 26 days

patients develop an AKI [26], and up to 40% of those are admitted to the ICU [27]. Studies have indicated that the development of stage II or III AKI incurs a poor prognosis with mortality rates as high as 70% in those requiring kidney replacement therapy [26, 28, 29]. The patient in this case report developed stage III AKI secondary to his rhabdomyolysis which was the presenting symptom of COVID-19. Although he required kidney replacement therapy, he fortunately obtained complete recovery despite a prolonged hospital course and also requiring ICU level of care.

Rhabdomyolysis has been described as a late complication of COVID-19 [30], but in our case, it was the presenting clinical manifestation even before respiratory symptoms developed and in light of a negative initial COVID-19 test. Of the reported cases, the classic triad of weakness, myalgia, and tea-coloured urine was not seen in any patients and only 7 of 16 reported one symptom, most commonly myalgia. In this case report, the patient presented with tea-coloured urine, decreased urine output, and general malaise and weakness. Myalgia is a common complaint of viral infections, including influenza. Thus, in patients presenting with myalgia and respiratory symptoms or high suspicion of COVID-19, we recommend evaluating serum creatine kinase and serum creatinine and closely monitoring urine output. The development of rhabdomyolysis and AKI does not appear to have a predilection in patients with certain comorbidities or age. Additionally, it appears that peak creatinine kinase is not associated with in-hospital mortality. In this case, peak creatine kinase was 327, 629 units/L, the second highest of the reported cases, and the patient recovered completely. This contrasts with the cases reported by Singh et al. where peak creatinine kinase was less than <10,000 units/L and patients died during their hospitalization.

The favourable outcome of our patient may be linked to early identification and IV fluid therapy.

Regarding management of rhabdomyolysis, the mainstay continues to be correction of intravascular volume depletion and prevention of intratubular cast formation with fluid resuscitation. The initial recommended rate is 1 L/hour followed by 500 mL/hour thereafter with either isotonic saline or lactate ringers, although there is no strong evidence supporting either of these IV fluid formulations [31]. The goal of therapy is increased urine output; however, clinicians should be cognizant of volume overload in the setting of oliguria [32]. Additionally, electrolyte abnormalities such as hyperkalemia, hyperphosphatemia, and hypercalcemia or hypocalcaemia should be monitored closely and addressed quickly. Further evidence is needed on target therapies to prevent rhabdomyolysis-associated AKI [33].

A potential limitation to this report is that the patient was taking 20 mg simvastatin as a home medication, a notable cause of myopathy and rhabdomyolysis. Statin-induced rhabdomyolysis is rare and occurs in <0.1% of cases [34]. Furthermore, in larger, follow-up studies, rhabdomyolysis-associated acute kidney failure only developed when statins were used in combination with cyclosporine, gemfibrozil, protease inhibitors, niacin, digoxin, and some antimicrobials [35], none of which this patient was taking at the time. Lastly, although myopathy can occur at any time during treatment with a statin, the onset of symptoms is usually within months of initiation of therapy. Approximately 2/3 of patients experience myopathy in the first six months of starting therapy [36], and the patient in this case report had been on statin therapy for eighteen months without changes in dose. Pioglitazone has been associated with rhabdomyolysis [37], although it appears to be at higher doses (75 mg/day) and rare. Risk factors for thiazolidinedione-induced rhabdomyolysis include concomitant therapy with fibrate, alcohol abuse, and asymptomatic mild creatinine phosphokinase elevation prior to initiating therapy. The patient in this report was on a lower dose of pioglitazone (30 mg/day) and had no further additional risk factors. Other causes of rhabdomyolysis were excluded with thyroid function tests and urine toxicology.

In summary, this is a unique presentation and complication of COVID-19 in a patient who initially tested negative for the virus. This case was unique in that the patient had a favourable prognosis and although being being admitted to the ICU, recovered completely. Most described cases presented with respiratory symptoms or were diagnosed with COVID-19 and were subsequently found to have rhabdomyolysis and kidney dysfunction, unlike the case in this report. This case report also details the clinical presentation, hospital course, and treatment which adds to the existing literature on the phenomenon. It is imperative for clinicians to be aware of the potential for COVID-19 patients to develop rhabdomyolysis, initiate early treatment, and minimize the kidney dysfunction.

Consent

Written informed consent was obtained prior to the preparation of this manuscript.

Disclosure

The funder was not involved in the manuscript writing, editing, approval, or decision to publish.

Acknowledgments

This work was funded by MedStar Health.

References

[1] Z. Wu and J. M. McGoogan, "Characteristics of and important lessons from the coronavirus disease 2019 (COVID-19) outbreak in China," *JAMA*, vol. 323, no. 13, p. 1239, 2020.

[2] F. Zhou, T. Yu, R. Du et al., "Clinical course and risk factors for mortality of adult inpatients with COVID-19 in Wuhan, China: a retrospective cohort study," *The Lancet*, vol. 395, no. 10229, pp. 1054–1062, 2020.

[3] E. K. Stokes, L. D. Zambrano, K. N. Anderson et al., "Coronavirus disease 2019 case surveillance-United States, january 22-may 30, 2020," *MMWR. Morbidity and Mortality Weekly Report*, vol. 69, no. 24, pp. 759–765, 2020.

[4] W.-J. Guan, Z.-Y. Ni, Y. Hu et al., "Clinical characteristics of coronavirus disease 2019 in China," *New England Journal Of Medicine*, vol. 382, no. 18, pp. 1708–1720, 2020.

[5] D. Wang, B. Hu, C. Hu et al., "Clinical characteristics of 138 hospitalized patients with 2019 novel coronavirus-infected pneumonia in wuhan, China," *JAMA*, vol. 323, no. 11, p. 1061, 2020.

[6] E. M. Liotta, A. Batra, J. R. Clark et al., "Frequent neurologic manifestations and encephalopathy-associated morbidity in Covid-19 patients," *Annals Of Clinical And Translational Neurology*, vol. 7, no. 11, pp. 2221–2230, 2020.

[7] N. V. Kolhe, R. J. Fluck, N. M. Selby, and M. W. Taal, "Acute kidney injury associated with COVID-19: a retrospective cohort study," *PLOS Medicine*, vol. 17, no. 10, Article ID e1003406, 2020.

[8] S. Y. Robbins-Juarez, L. Qian, K. L. King et al., "Outcomes for patients with COVID-19 and acute kidney injury: a systematic review and meta-analysis," *Kidney International Reports*, vol. 5, no. 8, pp. 1149–1160, 2020.

[9] L. He, Q. Zhang, Z. Li et al., "Incorporation of urinary neutrophil gelatinase-associated lipocalin and computed tomography quantification to predict acute kidney injury and in-hospital death in COVID-19 patients," *Kidney Diseases*, vol. 7, pp. 1–11, 2020.

[10] J. S. Hirsch, J. H. Ng, D. W. Ross et al., "Acute kidney injury in patients hospitalized with COVID-19," *Kidney International*, vol. 98, no. 1, pp. 209–218, 2020.

[11] K. Stahl, E. Rastelli, and B. Schoser, "A systematic review on the definition of rhabdomyolysis," *Journal Of Neurology*, vol. 267, no. 4, pp. 877–882, 2019.

[12] U. Singh and W. M. Scheld, "Infectious etiologies of rhabdomyolysis: three case reports and review," *Clinical Infectious Diseases*, vol. 22, no. 4, pp. 642–649, 1996.

[13] M. D. Nauss, E. L. Schmidt, and A. M. Pancioli, "Viral myositis leading to rhabdomyolysis: a case report and literature review," *The American Journal Of Emergency Medicine*, vol. 27, no. 3, 2009.

[14] J. H. Ng, V. Bijol, M. A. Sparks, M. E. Sise, H. Izzedine, and K. D. Jhaveri, "Pathophysiology and pathology of acute kidney injury in patients with COVID-19," *Advances In Chronic Kidney Disease*, vol. 27, no. 5, pp. 365–376, 2020.

[15] K. Taxbro, H. Kahlow, H. Wulcan, and A. Fornarve, "Rhabdomyolysis and acute kidney injury in severe COVID-19 infection," *BMJ Case Reports*, vol. 13, no. 9, Article ID e237616, 2020.

[16] B. Valente-Acosta, F. Moreno-Sanchez, O. Fueyo-Rodriguez, and A. Palomar-Lever, "Rhabdomyolysis as an initial presentation in a patient diagnosed with COVID-19," *BMJ Case Reports*, vol. 13, no. 6, Article ID e236719, 2020.

[17] B. Singh, P. Kaur, and R. Reid, "Case reports: rhabdomyolysis associated with COVID-19 [Letter to the editor]," *American Family Physician*, vol. 102, no. 11, pp. 645–648, 2020, https://www.aafp.org/afp/2020/1201/p645a.html.

[18] R. Husain, I. Corcuera-Solano, E. Dayan, A. H. Jacobi, and M. Huang, "Rhabdomyolysis as a manifestation of a severe

case of COVID-19: a case report," *Radiology Case Reports*, vol. 15, no. 9, pp. 1633–1637, 2020.

[19] N. R. Chedid, S. Udit, Z. Solhjou, M. Y. Patanwala, A. M. Sheridan, and E. Barkoudah, "COVID-19 and rhabdomyolysis," *Journal Of General Internal Medicine*, vol. 35, no. 10, pp. 3087–3090, 2020.

[20] B. Singh, P. Kaur, A. Mechineni, and M. Maroules, "Rhabdomyolysis in COVID-19: report of four cases," *Cureus*, vol. 12, 2020.

[21] M.-M. Alejandro, A. W. Maham, D. J. Kenar, and R.-M. Geurys, "COVID-19 related rhabdomyolysis," *Journal Of Clinical Nephrology*, vol. 4, pp. 65–69, 2020.

[22] J. R. Pellegrini, S. Parnia, E. Q. Harris, J. Varney, Jaswinder, and Singh, "An atypical case of COVID-19 induced rhabdomyolysis and acute kidney injury," *JASN*, vol. 32, 2020.

[23] W. H. Chong and B. Saha, "Severe acute respiratory syndrome coronavirus 2 (SARS-CoV-2) associated with rhabdomyolysis and acute kidney injury (AKI)," *The American Journal Of The Medical Sciences*, vol. 360, no. 6, pp. 738-739, 2020.

[24] K. H. Chan, I. Farouji, A. Abu Hanoud, and J. Slim, "Weakness and elevated creatinine kinase as the initial presentation of coronavirus disease 2019 (COVID-19)," *The American Journal Of Emergency Medicine*, vol. 38, no. 7, 2020.

[25] E. Ahmadian, S. M. Hosseiniyan Khatibi, S. Razi Soofiyani et al., "Covid-19 and kidney injury: pathophysiology and molecular mechanisms," *Reviews In Medical Virology*, vol. 31, no. 3, 2020.

[26] Y. Cheng, R. Luo, K. Wang et al., "Kidney disease is associated with in-hospital death of patients with COVID-19," *Kidney International*, vol. 97, no. 5, pp. 829–838, 2020.

[27] S. Richardson, J. S. Hirsch, M. Narasimhan et al., "Presenting characteristics, comorbidities, and outcomes among 5700 patients hospitalized with COVID-19 in the New York city area," *JAMA*, vol. 323, no. 20, p. 2052, 2020.

[28] J. Thakkar, S. Chand, M. S. Aboodi et al., "Characteristics, outcomes and 60-day hospital mortality of ICU patients with COVID-19 and acute kidney injury," *Kidney360*, vol. 1, no. 12, pp. 1339–1344, 2020.

[29] M. R. Rudnick and R. Hilburg, "Acute kidney injury in COVID-19: another challenge for nephrology," *American Journal Of Nephrology*, vol. 51, no. 10, pp. 761–763, 2020.

[30] M. Jin and Q. Tong, "Rhabdomyolysis as potential late complication associated with COVID-19," *Emerging Infectious Diseases*, vol. 26, no. 7, pp. 1618–1620, 2020.

[31] L. O. Chavez, M. Leon, S. Einav, and J. Varon, "Beyond muscle destruction: a systematic review of rhabdomyolysis for clinical practice," *Critical Care*, vol. 20, no. 1, 2016.

[32] N. Petejova and A. Martinek, "Acute kidney injury due to rhabdomyolysis and renal replacement therapy: a critical review," *Critical Care*, vol. 18, no. 3, p. 224, 2014.

[33] J. Michelsen, J. Cordtz, L. Liboriussen et al., "Prevention of rhabdomyolysis-induced acute kidney injury - a DASAIM/DSIT clinical practice guideline," *Acta Anaesthesiologica Scandinavica*, vol. 63, no. 5, pp. 576–586, 2019.

[34] D. J. Graham, J. Staffa, D. Shatin et al., "Incidence of hospitalized rhabdomyolysis in patients treated with lipid-lowering drugs," *JAMA*, vol. 292, no. 21, pp. 2585–2590, 2004.

[35] C. M. Ballantyne, A. Corsini, M. H. Davidson et al., "Risk for myopathy with statin therapy in high-risk patients," *Archives Of Internal Medicine*, vol. 163, no. 5, p. 553, 2003.

[36] K. E. Hansen, J. P. Hildebrand, E. E. Ferguson, and J. H. Stein, "Outcomes in 45 patients with statin-associated myopathy," *Archives Of Internal Medicine*, vol. 165, no. 22, p. 2671, 2005.

[37] R. Slim, C. B. Salem, M. Zamy, and M. Biour, "Pioglitazone-induced acute rhabdomyolysis," *Diabetes Care*, vol. 32, no. 7, p. e84, 2009.

A Case of Systemic Lupus Erythematosu Antineutrophil Cytoplasmic Antibody-Associated Vasculitis Overlap Syndrome with Dissociated Pathological and Immunological Findings

Kazuhiko Kato,[1] **Tetsuya Kawamura**,[2] **Risa Terashima**,[1] **Yukiko Tsuchiya**,[1] **Yasuhito Takahashi**,[1] **Kenji Kasai**,[1] **and Takashi Yokoo**[2]

[1]*Department of Internal Medicine, Fuji City General Hospital, Takashima-cho 50, Fuji-shi, Shizuoka, Japan*
[2]*Division of Nephrology and Hypertension, Department of Internal Medicine, The Jikei University School of Medicine, Tokyo, Japan*

Correspondence should be addressed to Kazuhiko Kato; kazu.j429@gmail.com

Academic Editor: Kouichi Hirayama; k-hira@tokyo-med.ac.jp

Systemic lupus erythematosus/antineutrophil cytoplasmic antibody-associated vasculitis overlap syndrome (SLE/AAV OS) describes a pathological condition that presents with overlapping features of two diseases. There have been few reports of SLE/AAV OS and none from Japan. We present the case of a 59-year-old woman admitted with chief complaints of fever and decreased renal function. SLE was suspected due to the identification of four items from the diagnostic criteria of the American College of Rheumatology, including positivity for anti-ds-DNA and antinuclear antibodies. However, pathological findings from the kidney biopsy suggested pauci-immune crescentic glomerulonephritis. She was also diagnosed with AAV according to the Chapel Hill Consensus Conference (CHCC) 2012 definitions and the classification algorithm of AAV. SLE/AAV OS was suspected, we started immunosuppressant therapy, and subsequently her renal function improved. In previous reports, initial immunological and pathological findings generally concur. In cases where clinical and pathological features appear to conflict, as in the present case, a treatment strategy decision should be based on pathological and immunological findings to improve the prognosis of OS.

1. Introduction

Systemic lupus erythematosus/antineutrophil cytoplasmic antibody-associated vasculitis overlap syndrome (SLE/AAV OS) is a disease entity proposed by Nasr et al. in 2008 [1]. This condition presents with overlapping features of two diseases in terms of physical, laboratory, and pathological findings. Previously reported cases [1–5] have described women with a mean age of 40 years who presented with symptoms characteristic of two diseases: arthritis, including cytopenia, rhinitis, pulmonary hemorrhage, and interstitial pneumonia, and kidney changes, including hematuria and proteinuria, often exhibiting rapid progression to glomerulonephritis. SLE/AAV OS exhibits features of both SLE and AAV but, in many cases, the features of one of the two diseases are more evident; in addition, the pathological and immunological findings of the more evident disease, including various autoantibodies, are predominant. No treatment has been established for SLE/AAV OS, and disease management decisions must be based on the more prominent features of either SLE or AAV. In past reports [1–5], the initial immunological and pathological findings often agreed; however, they were inconsistent in the present case.

2. Case Presentation

A 59-year-old woman with no family history of kidney disease was receiving treatment for hypertension and dyslipidemia. The patient was taking oral olmesartan medoxomil (20 mg once daily), oral amlodipinebesylate (10 mg once daily), and oral rosuvastatin calcium (2.5 mg once daily). She had been experiencing symptoms of a common cold for approximately one month and developed a night fever 14 days before admission. Oral antipyretics and similar drugs did not improve her symptoms. Her serum creatinine level reached 2.4 mg/dL 14 days before admission and increased to 3.6 mg/dL on the day of admission, which was the day when she was referred to our hospital for an investigation of her worsening renal function. Findings on her arrival were as follows: body height, 160 cm; body weight, 60 kg; blood pressure, 138/80 mmHg; pulse, 80 beats/min; body temperature, 37.3°C; no anemia in the palpebral conjunctiva; breathing sounds were clear/no secondary noises; no heart murmurs; no edema in the legs; no joint pain or eruption; and no oral enanthem.

Blood test results on admission were as follows: white blood cell count, 12,900 cells/μL; lymphocytes, 800 cells/μL; monocytes, 11,000 cells/μL; neutrocytes, 10,800 cells/μL; eosinophils, 100 cells/μL; basophils, 0 cells/μL; red blood cell count, 3.57×10^6 cells/μL; hemoglobin, 10.9 g/dL; hematocrit, 31.7%; platelets, 350×10^3 cells/μL; aspartate transaminase, 62 IU/L; alanine transaminase, 119 IU/L; lactate dehydrogenase, 289 IU/L; total protein, 6.3 g/dL; albumin, 2.3 g/dL; urea nitrogen, 35 mg/dL; creatinine, 3.73 mg/dL; sodium, 136 mmol/L; potassium, 3.8 mmol/L; calcium, 8.0 mg/dL; phosphate, 4.8 mg/dL; C-reactive protein, 14.25 mg/dL; immunoglobulin G, 1,169 mg/dL; immunoglobulin A, 413 mg/dL; immunoglobulin M, 98 mg/dL; complement component, 3 132 mg/dL; complement component, 4 30.3 mg/dL; and 50% hemolytic complement, 98.8 U/mL. Furthermore, serine proteinase 3 antineutrophil cytoplasmic antibody, <0.51 IU/mL; myeloperoxidase antineutrophil cytoplasmic antibody (MPO-ANCA), 8.2 IU/mL; anti-double-strand (ds)-DNA antibody IgG, 54.9 IU/mL; anti-Smith antibody, negative; anticardiolipin immunoglobulin, 1 U/mL; and lupus anticoagulant, negative. Antinuclear antibody homogeneous pattern 160-fold and nucleolar pattern 80-fold were identified.

Urine testing revealed proteinuria (2081 mg/day) and hematuria (red blood cells ≥ 100/high-power field (poikilocytes 0–10%)). Plain thoracoabdominal computed tomography indicated reticular shadows in both inferior lobes. Renal size was preserved.

We suspected SLE because four items from the diagnostic criteria of the American College of Rheumatology (ACR) were satisfied: presence of antinuclear antibodies, positivity for anti-ds-DNA antibody, serum lymphocytopenia, and urine protein of 2.0 g/day. Treatment with mycophenolate mofetil (MMF) (1000 mg/day, orally) and prednisolone (PSL) (40 mg/day, orally) was started for SLE/lupus nephritis. On the 32nd hospital day, results of the renal biopsy that was taken on the 7th hospital day were confirmed. The disease course after admission is shown in Figure 1.

Global sclerosis was observed in two of a total 17 glomeruli. Cellular crescents and fibrinoid necrosis with rupture of Bowman capsule were observed in 14 of the remaining 15 glomeruli (Figure 2).

The degree of tubulointerstitial injury was 85%. Immunofluorescence showed pauci-immune type crescentic glomerulonephritis (1+ deposition in a granular manner in the mesangial area of C3 only) (Figure 3).

She was diagnosed as AAV according to the Chapel Hill Consensus Conference (CHCC) 2012 definitions [6] and the classification algorithm of AAV by Watts et al. [7]. She was suspected of SLE/AAV OS with serological features of SLE, and the treatment was changed to PSL monotherapy on day 8. Thereafter, the dosage of PSL was gradually decreased, and serum creatinine levels improved from a maximum of 7.06 mg/dL to 3.39 mg/dL on day 56.

3. Discussion

SLE is an autoimmune disease caused by the deposition of autoantibodies, including antinuclear antibodies [8]. Various clinical symptoms are associated with SLE, and 30–60% of patients present with lupus nephritis (LN) [9, 10].

The diagnostic criteria of the ACR are widely used for the diagnosis of SLE. The application of these criteria for the diagnosis of Japanese patients has been reported to have a sensitivity of 97% and specificity of 89% [11]. Double-stranded-DNA antibodies are specific to SLE, and the specificity of this approach is reportedly 97.4% [12].

LN is characterized by immune-complex deposition in the glomeruli [13]; specifically, pathological findings show deposition in the glomerular basement membrane [14]. Thus, the renal biopsy and assessment of pathological findings from a renal lesion are useful for diagnosing LN/SLE.

The autoimmune disease AAV targets small- and medium-sized blood vessels and is characterized by ANCA-positive laboratory results [15]. This disease has three possible patterns: granulomatosis with polyangiitis, microscopic polyangiitis, or eosinophilic granulomatosis with polyangiitis [16]. Renal pathological findings include the absence of immune-complex deposition in the glomeruli, and the condition is characterized by pauci-immune necrotizing crescentic glomerulonephritis [17]. Our patient was also diagnosed as AAV according to the Chapel Hill Consensus Conference (CHCC) 2012 definitions [6] and the classification algorithm of AAV by Watts et al. [7].

A positive result for ANCA is not representative of a classic presentation of SLE; however, approximately 20% of cases are reportedly positive for ANCA [18–20]. It has been reported that antinuclear antibodies produce p-ANCA-like fluorescence during indirect immunofluorescence screening [21]; results of enzyme-linked immunosorbent assay

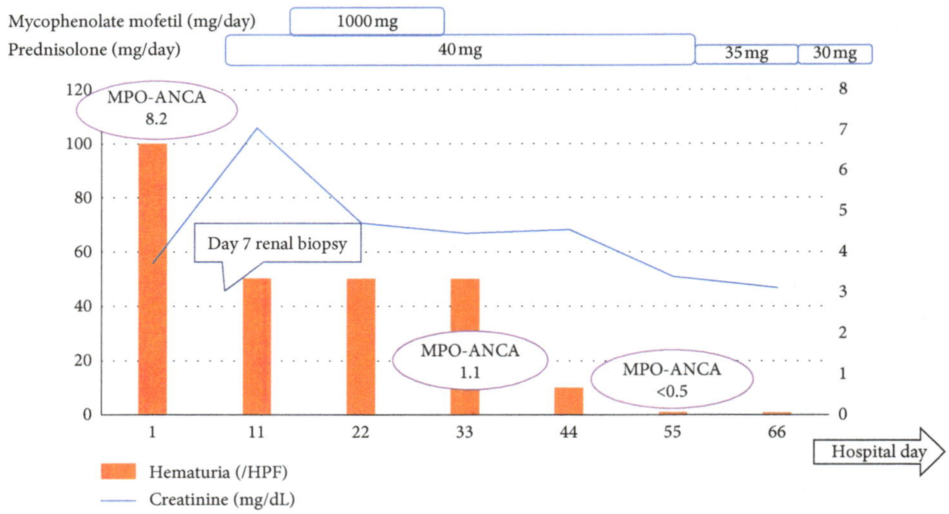

FIGURE 1: Disease course after admission. The patient was suspected of SLE/AAV OS with serological features of SLE, and the treatment was changed to PSL monotherapy on day 8. Thereafter, the dosage of PSL was gradually decreased, and serum creatinine levels improved from a maximum of 7.06 mg/dL to 3.39 mg/dL on day 56.

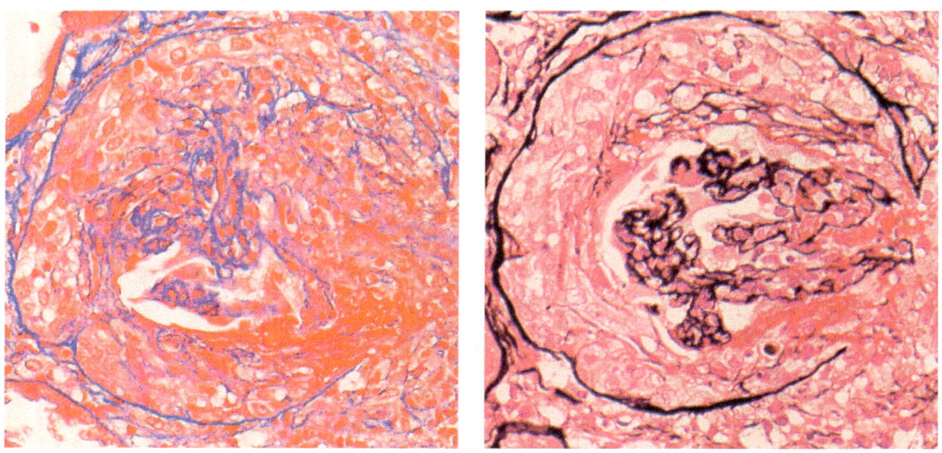

(a) (b)

FIGURE 2: Global sclerosis was observed in two of a total 17 glomeruli. Cellular crescents and fibrinoid necrosis with rupture of Bowman capsule were observed in 14 of the remaining 15 glomeruli. (a) Masson's trichrome stain and (b) PAM stain showed cellular crescents and fibrinoid necrosis, with Bowman's capsule rupture.

(ELISA) are also thought to be affected by a cross-reaction with coexisting autoantibodies. Therefore, a positive ANCA status is of little clinical significance for SLE, and it is thought that overlap of the pathology of AAV with ANCA-positive status in SLE patients is very rare [22]. Crescentic nephritis is a feature of ANCA vasculitis, which is frequently observed in severe LN [2]. In particular, LN patients with focal and segmental glomerular inflammation and necrosis that lack immune deposits, similar to AAV, have been described [23]. From reports of patients with symptoms of SLE, positive ANCA status, and AAV-like renal pathological findings, it was concluded that a condition exists in which the two diseases overlap. In 2008, SLE/AAV overlap syndrome was proposed as a disease concept.

In the present case, we identified four items from the ACR diagnostic criteria, including strong positivity for ds-DNA and presence of antinuclear antibodies. The patient was suspected of SLE and was treated with PSL and MMF. Results from the renal biopsy confirmed pauci-immune crescentic glomerulonephritis. Electron microscopy had not detected immune-complex deposition, and the formation of crescents was observed. Immunostaining was positive for C3 only, but some reports of immunofluorescence and electron microscopy in the context of AAV have shown complement deposition in the glomeruli [24]; this is believed to be consistent with the pauci-immune type. The patient was diagnosed as AAV according to the Chapel Hill Consensus

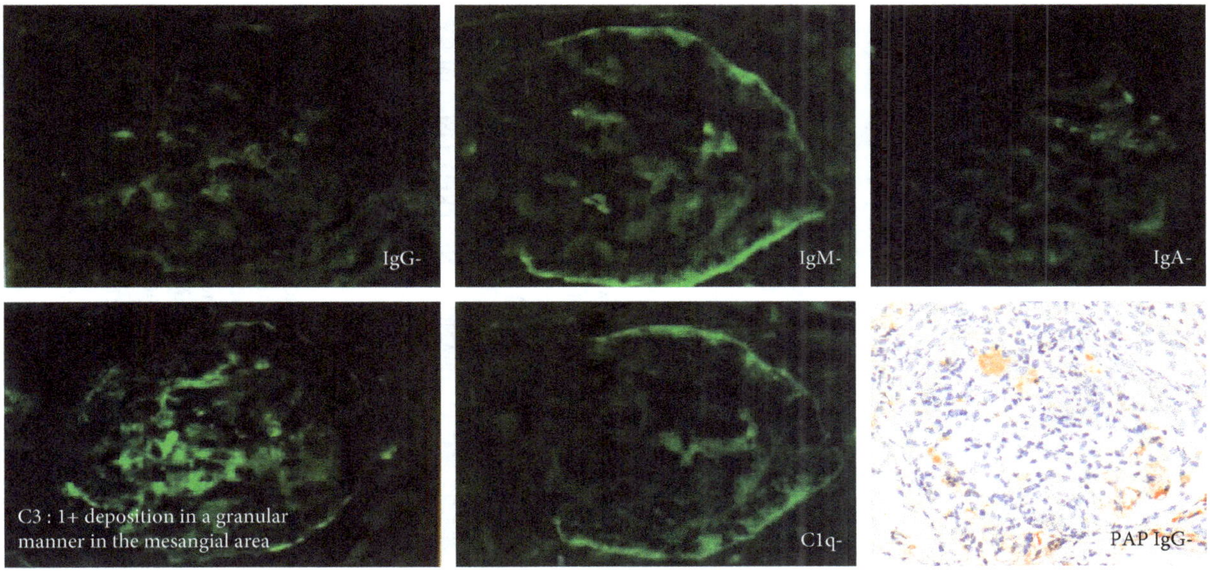

FIGURE 3: Immunofluorescence showed pauci-immune type crescentic glomerulonephritis (1+ deposition in a granular manner in the mesangial area of C3 only). Peroxidase antiperoxidase (PAP) method showed no deposition of IgG in the glomerular tuft free of crescent.

Conference (CHCC) 2012 definitions [6] and the classification algorithm of AAV by Watts et al. [7]. Given the above criteria, the patient was diagnosed with AAV.

We could not definitively diagnose SLE because this case did not meet four items from the diagnostic criteria of ACR. However, we suspected SLE/AAV OS with features of SLE. The patient's treatment was changed to PSL monotherapy.

There are only a few case reports [1–5] describing SLE/AAV OS in detail, and no cases of SLE/AAV OS have been reported in Japan. To date, 10 cases of SLE/AAV OS have been reported by Nasr et al. in 2008 [1], four cases by Hervier et al. in 2012 [2], and eight cases by Jarrot et al. in 2016 [3]. Recently, there has been one case reported in 2018 [4] and one in 2019 [5]. Of note, most of these cases had glomerular deposition of immunoglobulin, and only three cases showed pauci-immune glomerulonephritis similar to the present case. In this regard, the present case was rare among patients with SLE/AAV OS.

Many of these cases involved women with a mean age of 40 years. SLE/AAV OS presents with symptoms characteristic of the two diseases; Table 1 lists the serological and pathological features of the 21 reported cases described above (case 4 of [2] was excluded because no renal biopsy was reported). SLE/AAV OS has characteristics of both diseases, but it does not necessarily meet all the diagnostic criteria for both diseases. Likewise, the features of either SLE or AAV are generally more evident, and the pathological and immunological findings, including various autoantibodies, often agree. While many cases are positive for both antinuclear antibodies and ANCA, few are positive for both ANCA and ds-DNA, as was observed in the present case. Cases 5 and 8 of [3] were strongly positive for both ds-DNA antibodies and ANCA, but the renal pathological findings were LN, and the SLE elements appeared to be stronger than those of the present case.

Serological examination of our patient revealed clinical features classified as SLE, and the patient was strongly positive for ds-DNA. Elevation of ANCA was mild, and the pathological conditions were assumed to be SLE. However, renal biopsy findings showed pauci-immune crescentic glomerulonephritis, which revealed inconsistency between the clinical and pathological features. After PSL monotherapy, renal function improved, which brought serum creatinine levels to 3 mg/dL at discharge.

Many past studies [1–5] have reported treatment plans for SLE/AAV OS based on corticosteroids and cyclophosphamide, but outcomes have varied from significant improvement in general condition/renal function to death. Although there are established treatment protocols for SLE and AAV, no treatment method has been established for SLE/AAV OS. When immunosuppressants such as PSL are used, the therapeutic approach must be based on an evaluation of whether elements of SLE or AAV are more prominent. In past reports [1–5], serological and pathological features often align, but there have been some cases published where findings dissociate, as observed in the present case. In this context, it is difficult to assess patients by serological examination alone. The presentation of OS often reflects the pathology of microscopic polyangiitis, and many cases are characterized by renal involvement in which pathological diagnosis is only possible with a kidney biopsy. With SLE/AAV OS, performing a renal biopsy and planning treatment strategies based on pathological findings may improve the outcomes of SLE/AAV OS.

Though a rare disease, SLE/AAV OS causes damage to all organs of the body, including the kidneys. Further investigation is needed to elucidate the underlying pathological mechanisms and to establish methods of treatment that may

TABLE 1: Serological and pathological features of the 21 reported cases described above (case 4 of [2] was excluded because no renal biopsy was reported).

	Age	Sex	Hematuria	Proteinuria (g/day)	Serum creatinine (mg/dL)	ANA	Anti-dsDNA (UL/mL)	Low C3/C4	ANCA specificity	Renal biopsy	Positive immunenoreactanats	Diagnosis	Treatment
Case 1 of [1]	22	Female	Yes	1.5	2.7	Positive (1:1286)	Negative	Not determined	MPO-ANCA		IgG 3+ IgM 2+ IgA+ C3 3+ C1q 2+	LN IV-S (A/C)/ANCA GN	Intavenous CY, PSL, MMF
Case 2 of [1]	37	Female	Yes	5.9	10	Positive (1:80)	Positive	Not determined	MPO-ANCA		IgG 3+ C3 3+ C1q 1+	LN V/ ANCA GN	IntravenousCY.PSL, azathioprine
Case 3 of [1]	62	Female	Yes	2	4.7	Positive (1:848)	Positive	Not determined	Negative		IgG+ IgM+ C3 2+	LN III (A/C)/ANCA GN	IntravenousCY, PSL
Case 4 of [1]	80	Female	Yes	4	4.5	Positive (1:2560)	Negative	Not determined	Negative		IgG+ IgM+	LN II/ ANCA GN	Hydralazine, oral CY, PSL, PLX
Case 5 of [1]	19	Male	Yes	4	9.6	Positive (1:160)	Positive	Not determined	Negative		IgG 3+ IgA+ C3 2+ C1q 2+	LN IV G (A)/ANCA vasculitis	M-PRED, intavenous CY, oral CY, PSL
Case 6 of [1]	50	Female	Yes	3.2	4.4	Positive (1:160)	Negative	Not determined	MPO-ANCA		IgG3+ IgA+ C3 2+ C1q 2+	LN III (A)/ ANCA GN	M-PRED, intravenous CY, PSL
Case 7 of [1]	55	Male	Yes	3	21	Positive (1:160)	Positive	Not determined	Negative		IgG 2+ C3 2+	LN V /ANCA GN	PSL,intravenous CY
Case 8 of [1]	37	Female	Yes	6.4	1.1	Positive (1:40)	Negative	Not determined	MPO-ANCA		IgG 3+ C3 2+	LN V /ANCA GN	IntravenousCY, PSL
Case 9 of [1]	44	Female	Yes	1.7	8.8	Positive (1:320)	Positive	Not determined	Negative		IgG 2+ IgM 1+ IgA 1+ C3 2+	LN III (A/C)/ANCA GN	IntravenousCY, PSL,MMF, HC
Case 10 of [1]	78	Female	Yes	3	4.5	Positive (1:640)	Negative	Not determined	MPO-ANCA,PR-3 ANCA		IgG 2+ C3 2+	LN III(A/C)/ ANCA GN	Hydralazine, M-PRED, OSL, oral CY
[4]	40	Female	Not determined	Not determined	8.7	Positive (1:640)	Negative	Not determined	MPO-ANCA		Not determined	Pauci-immune GN	PSL, rituximab, HC, CY
[5]	48	Female	Yes	0.6	Not determined	Positive (1:40)	Negative	No/no	PR3-ANCA		IgG+ C3+	LN V	PSL, intravenous CY
Case 1 of [3]	23	Female	Yes	0.8	1.02	Positive (1:800)	23	No/yes	Negative		C3+	Pauci-immune GN	Not determined
Case 2 of [3]	43	Female	Yes	3.2	7.11	Positive (1:1280)	Negative	No/no	MPO-ANCA		IgG+ IgM+ C3+	Pauci-immune GN	Not determined
Case 3 of [3]	57	Female	Yes	3.6	5.63	Positive (1:1280)	Negative	No/no	MPO-ANCA		Pauci-immune	Pauci-immune GN	Not determined
Case 4 of [3]	29	Female	Yes	0.3	1.01	Positive (1:640)	20	No/no	MPO-ANCA		IgG 3+ IgM 2+ C1q 2+	LN II-G	Not determined
Case 5 of [3]	41	Female	Yes	4	1.53	Positive (1:2560)	50	Yes/yes	MPO-ANCA		IgG 2+ IgA 2+ C3 3+ C1q 2+	LN IV-G	Not determined
Case 6 of [3]	53	Female	Yes	6	1.62	Positive (1:600)	Negative	Yes/yes	MPO-ANCA		Negative	Pauci-immune GN	Not determined

Table 1: Continued.

	Age	Sex	Hematuria	Proteinuria (g/day)	Serum creatinine (mg/dL)	ANA	Anti-dsDNA (UL/mL)	Low C3/C4	ANCA specificity	Renal biopsy	Positive immunenoreactanats	Diagnosis	Treatment
Case 7 of [3]	27	Female	Yes	0.8	3.93	Positive (1:200)	22	No/yes	MPO-ANCA		IgG+ C3+	Pauci-immune GN	Not determined
Case 8 of [3]	74	Female	Yes	1	3.31	Positive (1:5240)	50	No/no	MPO-ANCA		IgG 2+ C3 2+	LN IV-G	Not determined
Case 1 of [4]	74	Female	Yes	0.6	4.1	Positive (1:5120)	Positive	No/yes	MPO-ANCA		IgG+ IgM+ C3+	Not determined	Not determined
Case 2 of [4]	35	Female	Yes	> 6	3.4	Positive (1:620)	Positive	No/no	MPO-ANCA		IgG+	Not determined	PSL, CY
Case 3 of [4]	21	Female	Yes	2.5	3.8	Positive (1:2560)	Positive	No/no	MPO-ANCA		IgG+ IgM+ C3+ C1q+	Not determined	PSL, oral CY, intravenous CY

ANA: antinuclear antibody, ANCA: antineutrophil cytoplasmic antibodies, LN: lupus nephritis, GN: glomerulonephritis, CY: cyclophosphamide, MMF: mycophenolate mofetil, PSL: prednisolone, M-PRED: pulse methylprednisolone, PLX: plasmapheresis, and HC: hydroxychloroquine.

mitigate the potentially serious consequences of this disease. Here, we presented a rare case where renal biopsy enabled the diagnosis of SLE/AAV OS. Renal biopsy should be considered an important tool for diagnosing SLE/AAV OS and planning treatment strategies.

References

[1] S. H. Nasr, V. D. D'Agati, H.-R. Park et al., "Necrotizing and crescentic lupus nephritis with antineutrophil cytoplasmic antibody seropositivity," *Clinical Journal of the American Society of Nephrology*, vol. 3, no. 3, pp. 682–690, 2008.

[2] B. Hervier, M. Hamidou, J. Haroche, C. Durant, A. Mathian, and Z. Amoura, "Systemic lupus erythematosus associated with ANCA-associated vasculitis: an overlapping syndrome?" *Rheumatology International*, vol. 32, no. 10, pp. 3285–3290, 2012.

[3] P. A. Jarrot, L. Chiche, B. Hervier et al., "Systemic lupus erythematosus and antineutrophil cytoplasmic antibody-associated vasculitis overlap syndrome in patients with biopsy-proven glomerulonephritis," *Medicine (Baltimore)*, vol. 95, no. 22, p. e3748, 2016.

[4] P. Curtiss, T. Liebman, C. Khorolsky, N. Brinster, J. Beasley, and K. Lo Sicco, "Systemic lupus erythematosus and antineutrophil cytoplasmic antibody-associated vasculitis: an emerging overlap syndrome with cutaneous manifestations," *JAAD Case Reports*, vol. 4, no. 5, pp. 493–496, 2018.

[5] S. Itikyala, D. Pattanaik, and S. Raza, "Systemic lupus erythematosus (SLE) and antineutrophil cytoplasmic antibody-associated vasculitis (AAV) overlap syndrome: case report and review of the literature," *Case Reports in Rheumatology*, vol. 2019, Article ID 5013904, 5 pages, 2019.

[6] C. Sunderkötter, P. Lamprecht, A. Mahr, D. Metze, and B. Zelger, "Nomenklatur der kutanen Vaskulitiden - deutschsprachige Definitionen des Dermatologischen Anhanges zur Chapel Hill Consensus Conference," *Journal der Deutschen Dermatologischen Gesellschaft*, vol. 16, no. 12, pp. 1425–1433, 2018.

[7] R. Watts, S. Lane, T. Hanslik et al., "Development and validation of a consensus methodology for the classification of the ANCA-associated vasculitides and polyarteritis nodosa for epidemiological studies," *Annals of the Rheumatic Diseases*, vol. 66, no. 66, pp. 222–227, 2007.

[8] A. Ippolito, D. Wallace, D. Gladman et al., "Autoantibodies in systemic lupus erythematosus: comparison of historical and current assessment of seropositivity," *Lupus*, vol. 20, no. 3, pp. 250–255, 2011.

[9] R. Cervera, M. A. Khamashta, J. Font et al., "Morbidity and mortality in systemic lupus erythematosus during a 10-year period," *Medicine*, vol. 82, no. 5, pp. 299–308, 2003.

[10] N. Maroz and M. S. Segal, "Lupus nephritis and end-stage kidney disease," *The American Journal of the Medical Sciences*, vol. 346, no. 4, pp. 319–323, 2013.

[11] R. Yokohari and T. Tsunematsu, "Application, to Japanese patients, of the 1982 American Rheumatism Association revised criteria for the classification of systemic lupus erythematosus," *Arthritis & Rheumatism*, vol. 28, no. 6, pp. 693–698, 1985.

[12] A. F. Kavanaugh and D. H. Solomon, "Guidelines for immunologic laboratory testing in the rheumatic diseases: anti-DNA antibody tests," *Arthritis & Rheumatism*, vol. 47, no. 5, pp. 546–555, 2002.

[13] M. Fava, C. H. Mallinckrodt, M. J. Detke, J. G. Watkin, and M. M. Wohlreich, "The effect of duloxetine on painful physical symptoms in depressed patients," *The Journal of Clinical Psychiatry*, vol. 65, no. 4, pp. 521–530, 2004.

[14] J. C. Jennette and D. B. Thomas, "Crescentic glomerulonephritis," *Nephrology Dialysis Transplantation*, vol. 16, no. 6, pp. 80–82, 2001.

[15] E. Csernok, "Anti-neutrophil cytoplasmic antibodies and pathogenesis of small vessel vasculitides," *Autoimmunity Reviews*, vol. 2, no. 3, pp. 158–164, 2003.

[16] J. C. Jennette, R. J. Falk, P. A. Bacon et al., "2012 revised international Chapel Hill consensus conference nomenclature of vasculitides," *Arthritis & Rheumatism*, vol. 65, no. 1, pp. 1–11, 2013.

[17] J. C. Jennette, A. S. Wilkman, and R. J. Falk, "Diagnostic predictive value of ANCA serology," *Kidney International*, vol. 53, no. 3, pp. 796–798, 1998.

[18] M. Chen, M.-H. Zhao, Y. Zhang, and H. Wang, "Anti-neutrophil autoantibodies and their target antigens in systemic lupus erythematosus," *Lupus*, vol. 13, no. 8, pp. 584–589, 2004.

[19] G. M1, G. Morozzi, G. D. Sebastiani et al., "Anti-neutrophil cytoplasmic antibodies in 566 European patients with systemic lupus erythematosus: prevalence, clinical associations and correlation with other autoantibodies. European Concerted Action on the Immunogenetics of SLE," *Clin Exp Rheumatol*, vol. 16, no. 5, pp. 541–546, 1998.

[20] I. Manolova, M. Dancheva, and K. Halacheva, "Anti-neutrophil cytoplasmic antibodies in patients with systemic lupus erythematosus: prevalence, antigen specificity, and clinical associations," *Rheumatology International*, vol. 20, no. 5, pp. 197–204, 2001.

[21] S. S. Lee, J. W. Lawton, and W. Chak, "Distinction between antinuclear antibody and P-ANCA," *Journal of Clinical Pathology*, vol. 44, no. 11, pp. 962-963, 1991.

[22] D. Sen and D. A. Isenberg, "Antineutrophil cytoplasmic autoantibodies in systemic lupus erythematosus," *Lupus*, vol. 12, no. 9, pp. 651–658, 2003.

[23] C. C. Najafi, S. M. Korbet, E. J. Lewis, M. M. Schwartz, M. Reichlin, and J. Evans, "Significance of histologic patterns of glomerular injury upon long-term prognosis in severe lupus glomerulonephritis," *Kidney International*, vol. 59, no. 6, pp. 2156–2163, 2001.

[24] M. Haas and J. A. Eustace, "Immune complex deposits in ANCA-associated crescentic glomerulonephritis: a study of 126 cases," *Kidney International*, vol. 65, no. 6, pp. 2145–2152, 2004.

Fibrillary Glomerulopathy with a High Level of Myeloperoxidase-ANCA: A Case Report

Tomohiko Asakawa,[1] Mea Asou,[1] Shigeo Hara,[2] Takashi Ehara,[3] and Makoto Araki[1]

[1]*Department of Internal Medicine, Suwa Central Hospital, Chino, Nagano 391-8503, Japan*
[2]*Department of Diagnostic Pathology, Kobe City Medical Center General Hospital, 2-1-1, Minatojima Minamimachi, Chuo-ku, Kobe 650-0047, Japan*
[3]*Graduate School of Health Sciences, Matsumoto University, 2095-1 Niimura, Matsumoto 390-1241, Japan*

Correspondence should be addressed to Makoto Araki; makoto.araki@gmail.com

Academic Editor: Kouichi Hirayama

An elderly woman was admitted with the chief complaint of gross hematuria. Laboratory values indicated a high myeloperoxidase-ANCA level. In renal histological examination, 40% of the glomeruli showed crescent formation, but immunofluorescence staining showed positivity for IgG, C3, and C1q. Furthermore, the deposition of fibrils in the glomerulus was noted on electron microscopy, and immunohistochemical staining showed strong positivity for DNA-J heat shock protein family member B9 (DNAJB9). Crescent formation is a common feature of fibrillary glomerulonephritis (FGN). Thus, in ANCA-positive crescentic glomerulonephritis, immunohistochemical assessments for immunoglobulins and DNAJB9, as well as electron microscopy, are important to correctly diagnose FGN.

1. Introduction

Gross hematuria with renal dysfunction suggests the possibility of rapidly progressive glomerulonephritis (RPGN) and requires urgent attention. Anti-neutrophil cytoplasmic antibody- (ANCA-) associated vasculitis (AAV) represents RPGN and is characterized by elevated serum ANCA levels and pauci-immune crescentic glomerulonephritis. But it is well known that the presence of ANCA is not highly specific for the diagnosis of vasculitis.

Fibrillary glomerulonephritis (FGN) is a rare glomerular disease characterized by noncongophilic amyloid-like fibrillary glomerular deposits. The histological type of FGN is the mesangial proliferating glomerulonephritis pattern, but it is often accompanied by crescents. FGN has a poor prognosis and often results in relatively rapid deterioration of renal function, like RPGN. The diagnosis could be made only by electron microscopy. But recently a simple immunostaining method has been established. Thus, the number of cases may increase in the future.

RPGN due to AAV is known as pauci-immune crescent glomerulonephritis, but in fact, immunoglobulin deposition is observed in many cases [1–3]. There may be cases of FGN with crescents among them. But, if electron microscopy is not performed in such cases, differentiation between the two is impossible.

2. Case Presentation

A 71-year-old woman was admitted with the chief complaint of gross hematuria. Her laboratory values indicated a creatinine (Cr) level of 1.72 mg/dl and massive proteinuria of 5.1 g/gCr. There was no fever, and her white blood cells were within the normal range. Further examination revealed a high myeloperoxidase (MPO)-ANCA level (125 U/ml, normal < 3.5), no monoclonal proteins, and normal complement protein levels (Table 1). Thus, a renal biopsy was performed; it showed mesangial proliferation in all 13 glomeruli and crescent formation in 5 glomeruli. Immunofluorescence staining showed positivity for

Table 1: Laboratory findings on admission.

		Unit
WBC	3910	/μL
Hb	7.7	g/dL
Plt	32.2	10^4/μL
TP	6	g/dL
Alb	2.6	g/dL
GOT	17	IU/L
GPT	8	IU/L
LDH	224	IU/L
T-Bil	0.35	mg/dL
ALP	174	IU/L
r-GTP	11	IU/L
HbA1C	5.8	%
BUN	23.3	mg/dL
Cr	1.72	mg/dL
Na	139.3	mEq/L
K	3.6	mEq/L
Cl	106	mEq/L
CRP	0.59	mg/dL
HBs-Ag		(−)
HCV-Ab		(−)
C3	115	mg/dL
C4	33	mg/dL
CH50	30.5	U/ml
ANA	×40	
PR3-ANCA	<1.0	U/mL
MPO-ANCA	125	IU/mL
Serum immunofixation electrophoresis	M protein (−)	
Urine immunofixation electrophoresis	M protein (−)	
FLC (κ/λ ratio)	0.97	
Uric protein	(3+)	
Uric protein	5.1	g/gCr
Uric blood	(3+)	
Urine red blood cells	55~99	/HPF
Oval fat body	(+)	
Granular cast	1~10	/WF
Waxy cast	1~10	/WF

FLC; free light chain, HPF; high power field, WF; whole field.

immunoglobulin G (IgG), C3, and C1q (Figure 1). The deposition of fibrils was noted in the glomerulus on electron microscopy (Figure 2). Additional staining showed negativity for Congo red, and there was no kappa/lambda (κ/λ) imbalance. In addition, immunohistochemical staining for DNA-J heat shock protein family member B9 (DNAJB9, Anti-DNAJB9 primary antibody was purchased from Proteintech (rabbit polyclonal antibody; catalog no. 13157-1-AP)) showed strong positivity in the glomerulus (Figure 3). These results indicated FGN.

The optimal treatment modalities were unclear based on the results primarily owing to the fact that it still remained to be determined whether the patient had FGN alone or FGN accompanied by AAV. Since there is no treatment specifically recommended for FGN, induction therapy for AAV was initiated with high-dose oral prednisone (PSL) 1 mg/kg/day and intravenous cyclophosphamide pulse therapy (IVCY, 7.5 mg/kg/day, biweekly). After 1 month, IVCY was switched to azathioprine (AZA) as renal function improved with a Cr level of 1.05 mg/dl and urinary protein of 3.0 g/gCr, and inflammatory response was negative. Two months later, she developed manic depression. Thus, AZA was discontinued and PSL was reduced to 5 mg/day because of suspected side effects of the drugs.

One and a half years later, renal function had not deteriorated; the Cr level was 0.84 mg/dl and urinary protein was 0.6 g/gCr. The titer of ANCA also remained at a low level of 10.7 IU/ml, and the patient's mental condition was stable with the administration of valproic acid.

3. Discussion

We encountered a case of elevated serum MPO-ANCA level and anti-DNAJB9 positive staining indicating glomerulonephritis with crescent formation. FGN is a rare glomerular disease noted in 0.6–1% of all kidney biopsies. The clinical features of FGN, usually present in older adults and include proteinuria, hematuria, and hypertension [4–6], which are similar to those of AAV. In renal biopsy, AAV is characterized by crescent formation, but about 25% of cases of FGN also show crescents. The hallmark of renal damage caused by AAV is pauci-immune, which is very difficult to determine by immunostaining when FGN is in the background. To our knowledge, FGN with serum MPO-ANCA positivity, like in our case, is very rare.

Although the etiology of FGN is still unknown, diagnostic criteria based on morphological features have been proposed. This case fulfilled the following previously-established diagnostic criteria [7, 8]: glomerular deposition of fibrils that were (i) randomly oriented, (ii) lacked hollow centers at magnification of <30,000, (iii) were Congo-red negative, and (iv) stained positively with antisera to immunoglobulins on immunofluorescence staining. DNAJB9 was identified as a biomarker of FGN in 2017 [6–9]. DNAJB9 is found in the endoplasmic reticulum (ER) and functions as a co-chaperone for heat shock protein 70 (Hsp 70). Its role appears to be ensuring proper folding of proteins. DNAJB9 is ubiquitously expressed. Immunohistochemically, DNAJB9 shows weak granular expression in the cytoplasm of tubular epithelial cells, glomerular cells, and vascular smooth muscle cells in normal renal tissues. In FGN, there is prominent staining for DNAJB9 outside the cell of the glomerulus, making it easy to distinguish from its expression pattern in normal tissues. In fact, in this case, there were apparent staining differences between the renal tubules and the mesangial region. DNAJB9 immunostaining is known to be positive in 98–100% of FGN cases [6, 8] and is expected to be a new diagnostic tool to replace electron microscopy in such cases.

FGN can present morphologically with varying patterns of glomerular injury, including crescent formation. In FGN, the mesangial proliferative glomerulonephritis pattern is seen in as many as 70% of the cases [10], and the endocapillary proliferative glomerulonephritis, segmental membranous nephropathy, and diffuse sclerosing glomerulonephritis patterns are also recognized. Crescent formation is common and has been observed in 17–31% of patients [4, 7, 11]. Glomerular damage due to FGN including crescent formation is thought to be caused by an immune complex-type renal disorder. FGN shows immunofluorescence staining for deposition of C3 (92%), C1q (36%), as well as IgG (100%,

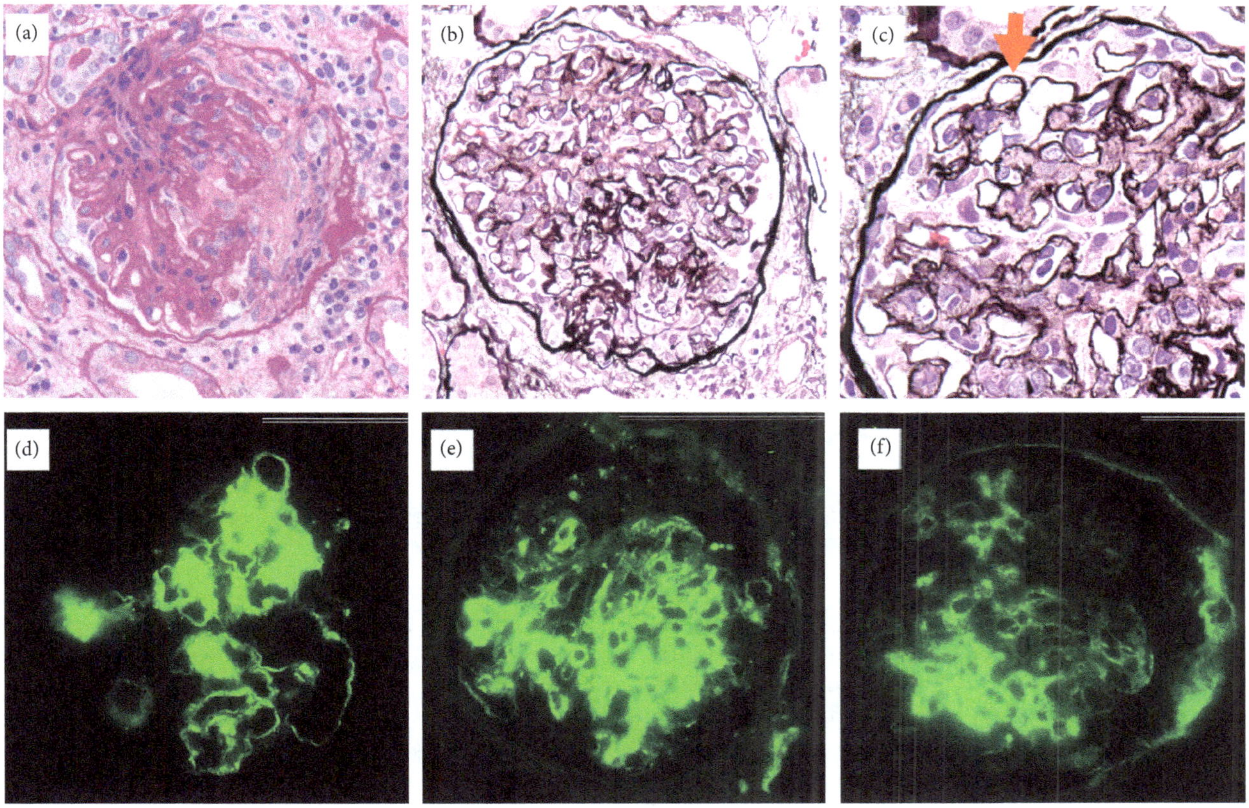

FIGURE 1: Light microscopic appearance. Periodic acid–Schiff (PAS) staining showed crescents formation (a) (×200). Periodic acid methenamine silver (PAM) staining showed mesangium expansion (b) (×200) and segmental duplication of glomerular basement membrane (c) (×200 arrow). Positive immunofluorescent staining of IgG (d), C3 (e), and C1q (f). IgM and IgA were negative.

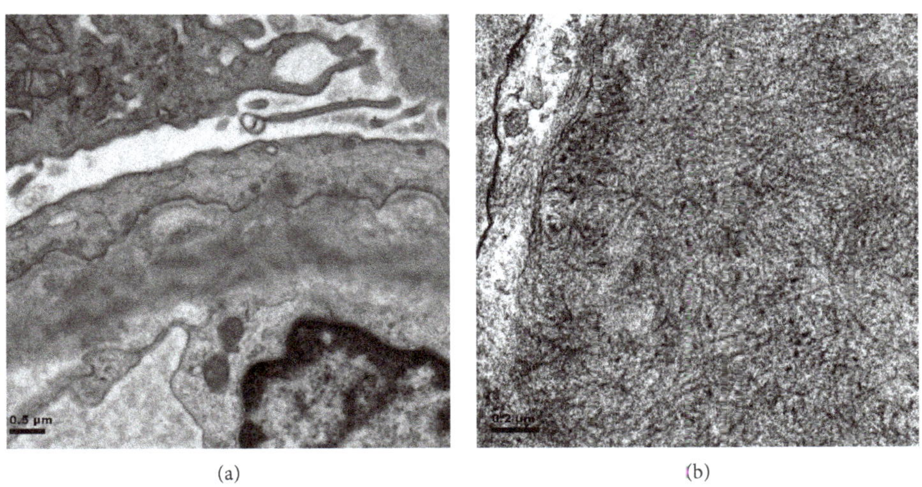

FIGURE 2: Electron micrographs of a glomerular tuft. (a) Electron microscopic showed the presence of electron-dense deposits in the glomerular mesangium and capillary walls. (b) Higher magnification reveled deposits as random arrangement of nonbranching fibrils (×7,000 and ×20,000).

significant for IgG1 and IgG4) [8]. Although FGN may be classified as one of the monoclonal gammopathies of renal significance (MGRS), only approximately 11% of cases show κ or λ light-chain restriction [4]; that is, most FGN cases are characterized by polyclonal IgG deposits, as this case. Furthermore, only 2% of the patients have hypocomplementemia. Despite fibrils and IgG coexist, whether fibrils are composed of IgG remains unclear, and there is a possibility that the fibril deposition is secondary to an immune response [12].

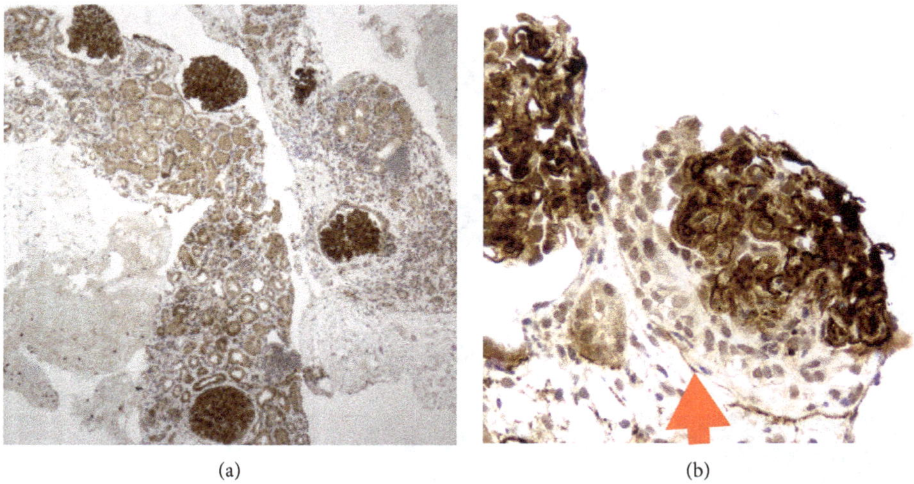

FIGURE 3: Immunohistochemistry of DNAJB9. (a) Glomeruli are strongly stained (×40). (b) In contrast to the glomerulus, crescent (arrow) is not stained (×400).

A small number (2/34) of p-ANCA-positive FGN cases with crescents have been reported [7]. However, because diseases other than AAV are sometimes positive for ANCA [13], the interpretation of its staining is difficult except in typical vasculitis. In addition, systemic diseases such as autoimmune diseases, malignant tumors, and chronic infections are known to be associated with 1/3rd of FGN cases [14]. The pathogenicity of ANCA is thought to be due to differences in its epitopes [15]; however, there is no ideal way to distinguish between them. Furthermore, AAV with immune complex deposition is often experienced [1–3]. If ANCA is elevated serologically and crescents are present, FGN may be missed because electron microscopic examination is infrequent. Since FGN can be diagnosed by immunohistochemical staining with the advent of DNAJB9, it is possible to increase the number of reports that the ANCA-associated glomerulonephritis associated with immune complex deposition was actually FGN. The etiology of FGN is not yet known, but it is hypothesized to be an ER stress/misfolding-related disease. Although immune responses and inflammation are known to be associated with ER stress, the relationship between ANCA and FGN remains unclear [16].

FGN is difficult to treat, and half of the patients progress to end-stage renal disease within 4 years of diagnosis [4, 5, 17, 18]. However, some cases of spontaneous cure have been reported [19]. The standard treatment of FGN has not been established; nonspecific immunosuppressive therapy targeting immune-complexes is being attempted, and there is much overlap between treatment modalities for AAV and FGN. Specific therapies for FGN are expected to be developed in the future based on its association with DNAJB9.

4. Conclusion

Based on the histological findings, it was considered that the patient's renal dysfunction was caused by either FGN alone or from concomitant AAV and FGN. There is no ideal way to know if ANCA has pathological significance, and no conclusion could be reached based on this case. Altogether, in cases of ANCA-positive crescentic glomerulonephritis, if immunostaining reveals immunoglobulin deposition, the diagnosis of FGN may be missed if electron microscopy or DNAJB9 staining is not performed.

References

[1] R. Morizane, K. Konishi, A. Hashiguchi et al., "MPO-ANCA associated crescentic glomerulonephritis with numerous immune complexes: case report," *BMC Nephrology*, vol. 13, p. 32, 2012.

[2] O. Hirose, M. Itabashi, T. Takei, K. Honda, and K. Nitta, "Antineutrophil cytoplasmic antibody-associated glomerulonephritis with immunoglobulin deposition," *Clinical and Experimental Nephrology*, vol. 21, no. 4, pp. 643–650, 2017.

[3] M. Haas and J. A. Eustace, "Immune complex deposits in ANCA-associated crescentic glomerulonephritis: a study of 126 cases," *Kidney International*, vol. 65, no. 6, pp. 2145–2152, 2004.

[4] J. L. Rosenstock, G. S. Markowitz, A. M. Valeri, G. Sacchi, G. B. Appel, and V. D. D'Agati, "Fibrillary and immunotactoid glomerulonephritis: distinct entities with different clinical and pathologic features," *Kidney International*, vol. 63, no. 4, pp. 1450–1461, 2003.

[5] A. Fogo, N. Qureshi, and R. G. Horn, "Morphologic and clinical features of fibrillary glomerulonephritis versus immunotactoid glomerulopathy," *American Journal of Kidney Diseases*, vol. 22, no. 3, pp. 367–377, 1993.

[6] N. K. Andeen, H.-Y. Yang, D.-F. Dai, M. J. MacCoss, and K. D. Smith, "DnaJ homolog subfamily B member 9 is a putative autoantigen in fibrillary GN," *Journal of the American Society of Nephrology*, vol. 29, no. 1, pp. 231–239, 2018.

[7] S. H. Nasr, A. M. Valeri, L. D. Cornell et al., "Fibrillary glomerulonephritis: a report of 66 cases from a single institution," *Clinical Journal of the American Society of Nephrology*, vol. 6, no. 4, pp. 775–784, 2011.

[8] S. H. Nasr, J. A. Vrana, S. Dasari et al., "DNAJB9 is a specific immunohistochemical marker for fibrillary glomerulone-

phritis," *Kidney International Reports*, vol. 3, no. 1, pp. 56–64, 2018.

[9] S. Dasari, M. P. Alexander, J. A. Vrana et al., "DnaJ heat shock protein family B member 9 is a novel biomarker for fibrillary GN," *Journal of the American Society of Nephrology*, vol. 29, no. 1, pp. 51–56, 2018.

[10] N. Leung, M. E. Drosou, and S. H. Nasr, "Dysproteinemias and glomerular disease," *Clinical Journal of the American Society of Nephrology*, vol. 13, no. 1, pp. 128–139, 2018.

[11] S. S. Iskandar, R. J. Falk, and J. C. Jennette, "Clinical and pathologic features of fibrillary glomerulonephritis," *Kidney International*, vol. 42, no. 6, pp. 1401–1407, 1992.

[12] C. E. Alpers and J. Kowalewska, "Fibrillary glomerulonephritis and immunotactoid glomerulopathy," *Journal of the American Society of Nephrology*, vol. 19, no. 1, pp. 34–37, 2008.

[13] C. G. M. Kallenberg, "Usefulness of antineutrophil cytoplasmic autoantibodies in diagnosing and managing systemic vasculitis," *Current Opinion in Rheumatology*, vol. 28, no. 1, pp. 8–14, 2016.

[14] F. Payan Schober, M. A. Jobson, C. J. Poulton et al., "Clinical features and outcomes of a racially diverse population with fibrillary glomerulonephritis," *American Journal of Nephrology*, vol. 45, no. 3, pp. 248–256, 2017.

[15] A. J. Roth, J. D. Ooi, J. J. Hess et al., "Epitope specificity determines pathogenicity and detectability in ANCA-associated vasculitis," *Journal of Clinical Investigation*, vol. 123, no. 4, pp. 1773–1783, 2013.

[16] J. S. So, "Roles of endoplasmic reticulum stress in immune responses," *Molecules and Cells*, vol. 41, no. 8, pp. 705–716, 2018.

[17] S. A. Kalbermatter, C. Marone, D. Casartelli et al., "Outcome of fibrillary glomerulonephritis," *Swiss Medical Weekly*, vol. 142, p. w13578, 2012.

[18] N. K. Andeen, M. L. Troxell, M. Riazy et al., "Fibrillary glomerulonephritis," *Clinical Journal of the American Society of Nephrology*, vol. 14, no. 12, pp. 1741–1750, 2019.

[19] M. Sekulic, S. H. Nasr, J. P. Grande, and L. D. Cornell, "Histologic regression of fibrillary glomerulonephritis: the first report of biopsy-proven spontaneous resolution of disease," *Clinical Kidney Journal*, vol. 10, no. 6, pp. 738–741, 2017.

Monoclonal Gammopathy of Renal Significance with Deposits of Peculiar Morphology and Injuries of Secondary Thrombotic Microangiopathy: A Case Report and Review of the Literature

José C. De La Flor,[1] Marina Alonso,[2] Edna Sandoval,[3] Alexander Marschall,[4] and Miguel Rodeles[1]

[1]*Department of Nephrology, Hospital Central Defense Gomez Ulla, Madrid, Spain*
[2]*Department of Anatomic Pathology, Hospital 12 de Octubre, Madrid, Spain*
[3]*Department of Hematology, Hospital Central Defense Gomez Ulla, Madrid, Spain*
[4]*Department of Cardiology, Hospital Central Defense Gomez Ulla, Madrid, Spain*

Correspondence should be addressed to José C. De La Flor; josedelaflor81@yahoo.com

Academic Editor: Hern N. Trimarchi

We present the case of an 82-year-old woman diagnosed with monoclonal gammopathy of renal significance (MGRS) with the presence of different and peculiar kidney lesions, who began treatment with bortezomib and dexamethasone, presenting during her evolution a relapse. Although the bone marrow biopsy in this case showed plasma cells as pathologic clone and there was also a reduction after chemotherapeutic treatment, rituximab was proposed as a second line. We suspected that the relapse was possibly due to another precursor as B-cell or lymphoplasmacytic cell clone. We review the literature and suggest that the treatment for MGRS should be patient-tailored, preferably by consulting a multidisciplinary team. Future research is needed to better understand the disease course and establish the efficacy and safety of the therapeutic approach for the relapse of MGRS.

1. Introduction

The monoclonal gammopathy of renal significance (MGRS) is pathogenically characterized by the proliferation of B lymphocyte clones or plasma cell clones that synthesize and secrete a monoclonal immunoglobulin (Ig) or its components (light or heavy chains), with the ability to cause damage at the tubular, glomerular, vascular, and interstitial compartments through direct (deposition) or indirect (alterations of the alternative complement pathway) mechanisms, constituting a heterogeneous group of entities. It is unusual to find more than two forms of monoclonal immunoglobulin lesions as well as different injury mechanisms in the same biopsy, as in the case of our patient.

Proliferative glomerulonephritis with monoclonal immunoglobulin deposits (PGNMID) is a form of MGRS-associated lesions where M-protein is deposited in the glomerulus. According to the classification scheme proposed by the International Kidney and Monoclonal Gammopathy Research Group (IKMG) [1], it belongs to the lesions caused by nonorganized monoclonal immunoglobulin deposits, often leading to chronic or end-stage kidney disease (ESKD) [2, 3].

On the other hand, thrombotic microangiopathy (TMA) is a syndrome physiologically characterized by endothelial injury. TMA may be hereditary or acquired, including a variety of disorders, such as complement-mediated TMA (also known as atypical hemolytic uremic syndrome (aHUS)) and other associated conditions [4]. TMA, according to a consensus report of the IKMG in 2019 [5], belongs to the lesions without deposits. Its pathophysiology is not fully understood, but it might be related to the monoclonal Ig acting as an autoantibody against a complement regulatory protein, which could trigger the development of aHUS and other forms of TMA [6].

The optimal treatment for most subtypes of MGRS is not known, but there is recent consensus among experts that treatment should be specific for the underlying clone [7]. This is probably due to the low detection rate of circulating paraproteins and pathogenic clones in PGNMID, highlighting the need for better diagnostic tools [8]. We report a case of MGRS with lesions of PGNMID, glomerular TMA, and deposits of peculiar morphology with torpid evolution despite chemotherapeutic treatment adapted to the nature of the cell clone.

2. Case Presentation

Our patient was an 82-year-old female with a past medical history of arterial hypertension (AHT) and dyslipidemia. Her medication included angiotensin II receptor blockers (ARBs) and statin. The patient presented with asthenia, fatigue, and uncontrolled AHT for a one-month duration. On admission, physical examination revealed a blood pressure of 250/130 mmHg, a respiratory rate of 24 breaths/min, an oxygen saturation of 90% while breathing room air, pulmonary rales, and peripheral edema. Furthermore, the patient presented with fever and low level of consciousness. Her laboratory values indicated a creatinine (Cr) level of 1.93 mg/dl, hypoalbuminemia without hypercholesterolemia, a massive proteinuria of 4.9 g/gCr, and blood smear with schistocytes <1%. Other laboratory test results are shown in Table 1.

Thus, a kidney biopsy was performed; 14 glomeruli could be analyzed. Three of the glomeruli were globally sclerotic. Under light microscopy, all of the remaining 11 glomeruli showed mesangial proliferation and endocapillary hypercellularity without crescent formation. 60% of the glomeruli had mesangial expansion and basement membrane duplication (Jones methenamine silver stain). Congo red and thioflavin staining were negative. One glomerulus showed mesangiolysis and a thrombus at the vascular pole (silver methenamine-stained section) with capillary wall remodeling, multiple layering, and double-contour formation in the section stained with periodic acid-Schiff- (PAS-) positive. The arteries and arterioles showed intimal fibrosis that decreased the light by approximately 25%. In only one of the arterioles, a luminal thrombus with phenomena of hematic extravasation and fragmentation of red blood cells could be seen. Immunohistochemical staining for CD61 was positive in the arteriole described histologically, as well as in some of the glomeruli. There were mild tubular atrophy and interstitial fibrosis as estimated at 15–20% (as shown in Figure 1). Routine frozen tissue immunofluorescence (IF-F) showed four glomeruli with unspecific deposits of C1q and IgM, without the presence of deposits for the rest of the antisera used (IgA, IgG, C4, fibrinogen, kappa, and lambda). On the other hand, the IF on pronase-digested paraffin-embedded (IF-P) sections showed subendothelial deposits of IgG and kappa light chain (++/+++) with negative staining for C3 and lambda light chain (as shown in Figure 2). There was no light chain staining in IF-F nor in IF-P in the tubule and renal interstitium. Detection of IgG subclasses was not performed. Electron microscopy (EM) showed electron-dense nonorganized subendothelial deposits; on this amorphous background, there were some fibrils with parallel arrangement and a diameter ranging from 10 to 15 nm. These fibrils did not correspond to typical amyloid deposits, nor could they be identified as the ones seen in fibrillary glomerulopathy (FGN). The immunohistochemistry technique for DNAJB9 was negative, which ruled out FG (as shown in Figure 3).

Bone marrow (BM) biopsy revealed <3% plasma cells, with negative Congo red staining. The immunophenotypic study showed that 2.1% of the total cellularity were plasma cells and, of these, 97% had an abnormal phenotype with monoclonality for the kappa light chain. IdentiClone assay was not performed. A PET/CT (positron emission tomography-computed tomography) scan revealed the absence of data on lymphoproliferative syndrome, solitary plasmacytoma, and other extramedullary affectations.

Given the diagnosis of MGRS with lesions of PGNMID (IgG-kappa), glomerular TMA, and light-chain deposits of peculiar morphology (DNAJB9 negative) seen in EM, treatment with cycles of bortezomib and dexamethasone (BordD) chemotherapy was initiated and well tolerated. After receiving three cycles, a partial renal response (renal function improved with serum creatinine decreasing to 1 mg/dL and proteinuria >50% to 1.2 g protein/day) and a partial hematological response (reduction >50% of kappa light chain) were achieved. Nevertheless, after the sixth cycle, the patient presented a worsening of kidney function with creatinine increasing to 2.4 mg/dl, proteinuria to 2.7 g/day, and kappa light chain (26.6 mg/d) in an immunophenotypic study that showed a slight decrease in abnormal cellularity (2% of the total cellularity were plasma cells and, of these, 75% had an abnormal phenotype of the kappa light chain).

For this reason, and given the evidence of relapse, different therapeutic options were evaluated (according to the first response, toxicity, general status, and renal function). Treatment with intravenous rituximab (two infusions, 1000 mg each, administered 14 days apart) and prednisone (0.8 mg/kg/day) tapered to 10 mg/d over 3–6 weeks followed by a gradual discontinuation after 3 months, was initiated. Four months later, our patient presented improvement in renal function with a Cr of 1.7 mg/dl and a proteinuria of 1.43 g/day. The following controls were delayed due to the onset of the COVID-19 pandemic and the patient died 3 months later of COVID-19 pneumonia.

3. Discussion

The spectrum of renal involvement in MGRS is wide. Most of the cases are due to M-protein deposits, while in other occasions it occurs indirectly through the dysregulation of the alternative complement pathway that leads to C3 glomerulopathy (GNC3) or more rarely to an aHUS [1, 5]. The most accepted classification for renal involvement by deposits is based on the configuration of its structure, dividing the disorder into organized and unorganized, whose ultrastructural measurement is the key to guide the diagnosis and to be able to discern the type of fiber or immunoglobulin deposited [5]. Although in clinical practice it is not

Table 1: Laboratory findings on admission.

		Reference range/unit
WBC	3978	U/L
Hemoglobin (Hb)	11.3	12–16 g/dL
Platelet count (PLt)	168	$10^3/\mu L$
Reticulocyte count	2.77	2–4%
Haptoglobin	93	30–200 mg/dL
Lactate dehydrogenase (LDH)	385	135–214 IU/L
ADAMTS 13 activity	15	<10%
Coombs test	Negative	NA
Total bilirubin	0.3	0.1–1 mg/dL
Total protein (TP)	5.9	6.4–8.7 g/dL
Serum albumin (Alb)	2.6	3–5.5 g/dL
GOT	29	5–32 IU/L
GPT	21	5–33 IU/L
Urea	83	17–60 mg/dL
Creatinine	1.93	0.6–1.2 mg/dL
Na	141	135–145 mmol/L
K	4.2	3.5–5.5 mmol/L
Cl	101	95–110 mmol/L
CRP	2.51	0.1–0.5 mg/dL
HbsAg	Negative	NA
HCV-Ab	Negative	NA
HIV	Negative	NA
CH50	45	40–90 U/ml
CFH	250	225–760 μg/mL
Autoantibodies CFH	Negative	<18 AU/L
C3 nephritic factor (C3NF)	Negative	Ratio > 1.022
C3	60	90–180 mg/dL
C4	13.3	10–40 mg/dL
RF	Negative	<15 IU/ml
ANA, anti-ds-DNA, ANCA, and cryoglobulin	Negative	NA
Anti-GBM	Negative	<1 AI
Anti-PLA2R Ab (ELISA)	Negative	NA
IgG	1060	800–1600 mg/dL
IgA	100	70–400 mg/dL
IgM	127	90–180 mg/dL
Urine protein	4.9	<0.03 g/gCr
Urine red blood cells	25–35	/HPF
Protein excretion	>300	mg/dl
SPEP M-protein concentration	3.83	Negative g/L
SIF	IgG κ	NA
Urine immunofixation electrophoresis: IgG κ	43.1	NA mg/dL
FLC κ	26.6	0.33–1.54 mg/dL
FLC λ	28.6	0.57–2.63 mg/dL
FLC κ/λ	0.93	0.26–1.65

AI: activity index, AU: arbitrary units, NA: not applicable, CFH: complement factor H, ANA: antinuclear antibody, anti-ds-DNA: anti-double-stranded DNA antibody, ANCA: antineutrophil cytoplasmic autoantibody, anti-GBM: antiglomerular basement membrane, RF: rheumatoid factor, anti-PLA2R Ab: antiphospholipase A2 receptor antibody, ELISA: enzyme-linked immunosorbent assay, SPEP: serum protein electrophoresis, SIF: serum immunofixation, FLC: free light chain, and HPF: high-power field.

uncommon for more than one entity to show an overlap of the damage mechanisms in the MGRS biopsy [9], it is rare to have more than three concurrent monoclonal immunoglobulin-related lesions of different mechanisms of injury in the kidney, which makes it more difficult to classify it [10].

Klomjit et al. [11] recently published the first study to evaluate the rate and clinical predictors of finding an MGRS lesion in a kidney biopsy specimen. They identified 6300 patients who had monoclonal gammopathy (MG) from Mayo Clinic medical records from 2013 to 2018. 160 (2.5%) had undergone a kidney biopsy. Of the 160 patients, 64 (40%) had an MGRS lesion; amyloid light-chain amyloidosis was the most common finding ($n = 28$, 43.8%); PGNMID was the second most common lesion ($n = 12$, 18.8%), followed by light-chain proximal tubulopathy (LCPT) ($n = 6$, 9.4%), light-chain deposition disease ($n = 5$, 7.8%), and type I cryoglobulinemic GN ($n = 5$, 7.8%). 96 patients (60%) had a kidney lesion that was unrelated to the monoclonal protein (non-MGRS group). The authors identified the following clinical predictors for the increase of odds of finding an MGRS lesion: proteinuria ≥1.6 g/d, hematuria, low serum C3 levels, abnormal FLC, and abnormal bone marrow biopsy

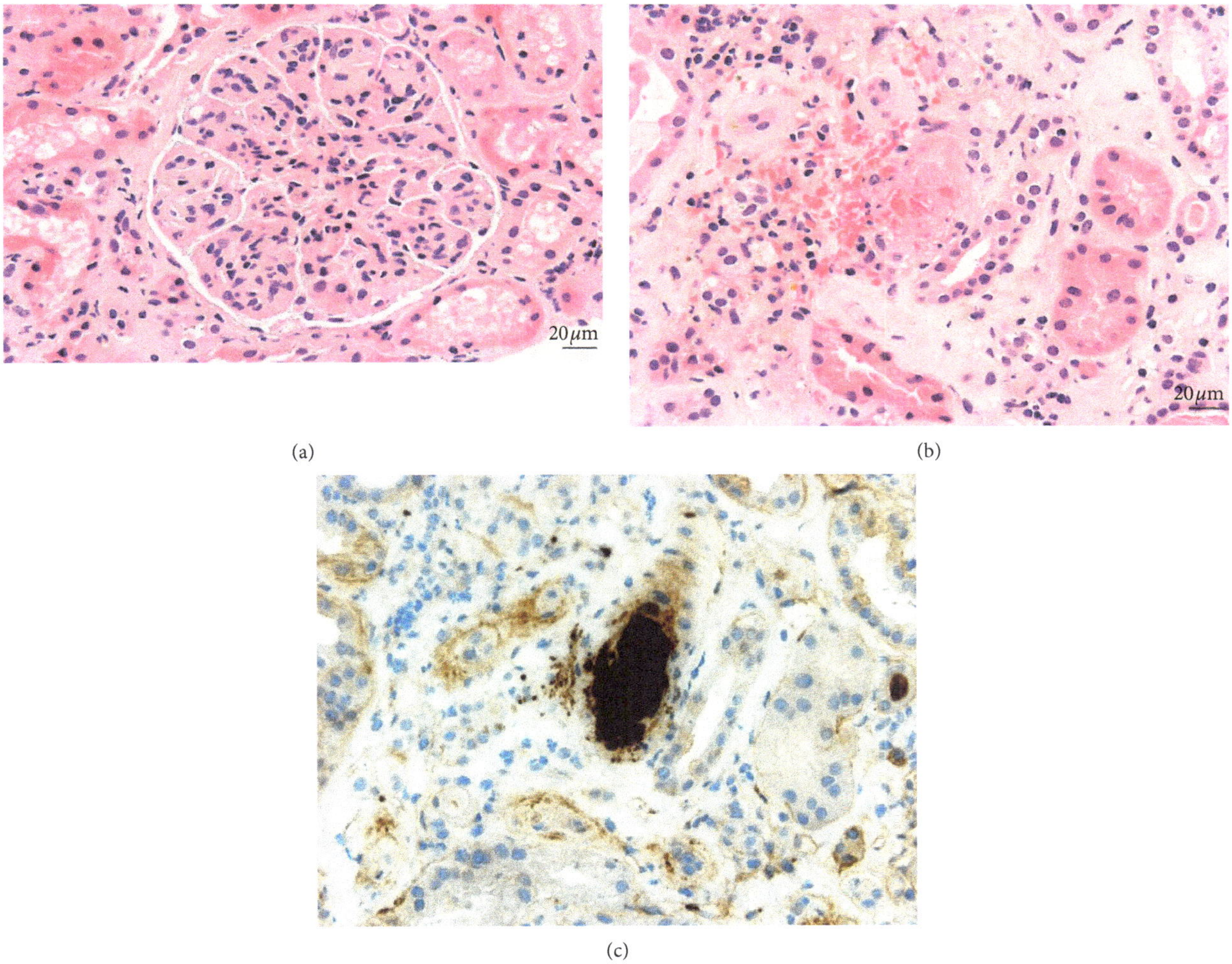

FIGURE 1: All the glomeruli displayed membranoproliferative features, with increased cellularity and a lobular pattern (a) (H-E, 400x). A single arteriole showed a luminal thrombus, composed of fibrin and platelets, together with blood extravasation and karyorrhectic debris (b) (H-E, 400x). CD61 immunostaining was performed (400x), which demonstrated platelet content (c).

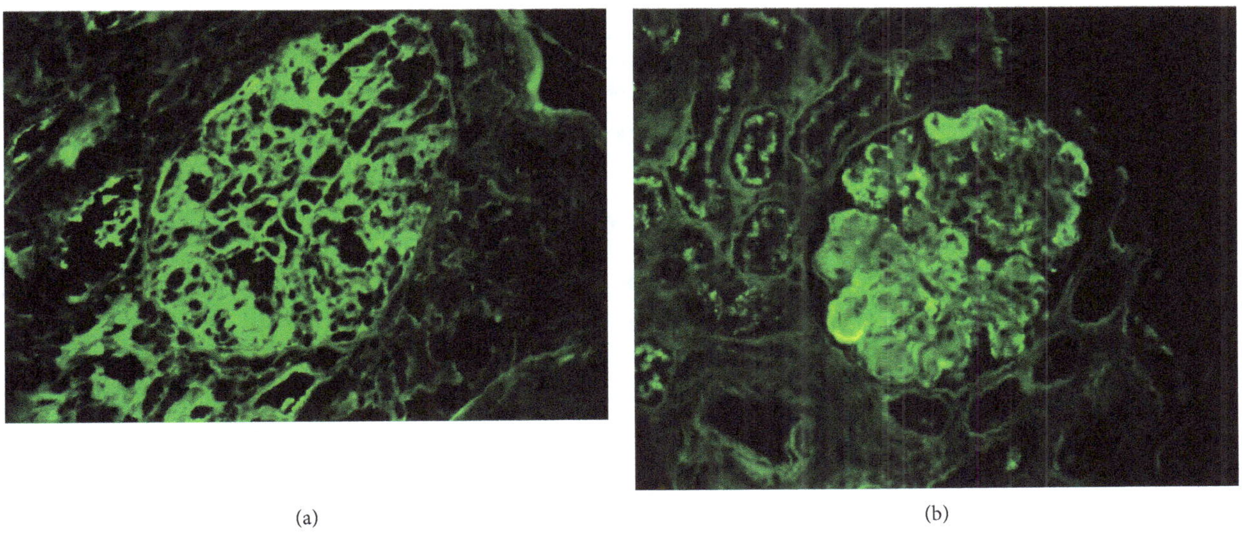

FIGURE 2: Direct immunofluorescence on fresh frozen tissue was performed; no evidence of deposits was observed (a) (IgG, 400x). Direct immunofluorescence on paraffin-embedded, pronase-digested sections was carried out; in contrast to routine IF, there were deposits of IgG and kappa light chains in the capillary walls (b) (kappa, 400x).

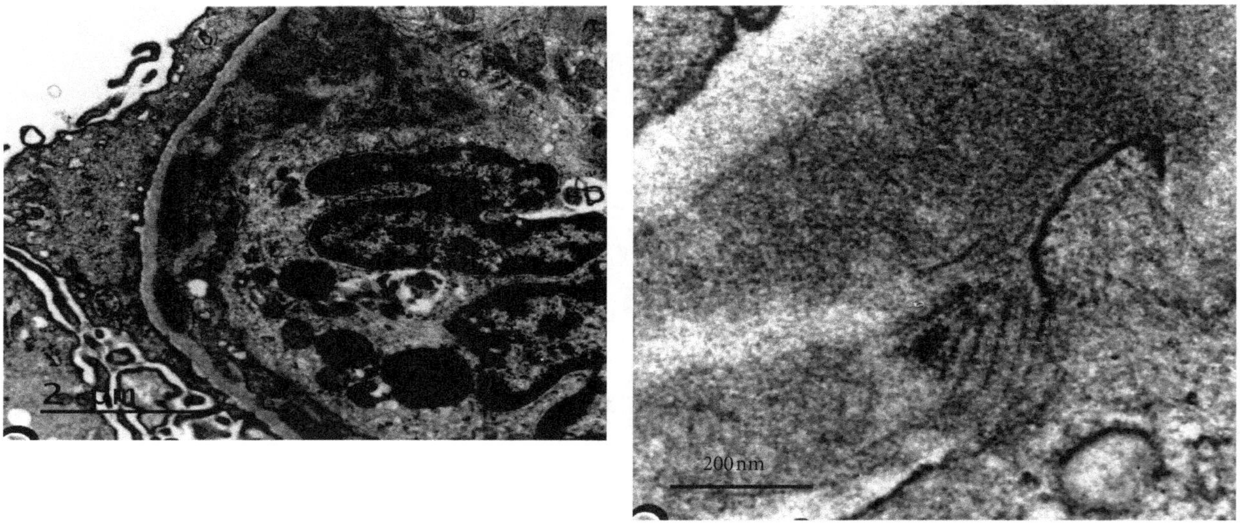

(a) (b)

Figure 3: Electron microscopy showed subendothelial and mesangial deposits (a) (10000x); for the most part, these were nonorganized; however, there were some fibrillary deposits with parallel arrangement measuring approximately 10–15 nm (b) (30000x).

specimen. Our case presented 4 of the 5 parameters described according to the study of the Mayo Clinic group.

In our case, the renal biopsy showed an MPGN pattern of glomerular injury by light microscopy. In routine IF, it presented a false-negative staining for monoclonal immunoglobulins, which was unmasked by performing IF-P. These paraffin rescue techniques are used when a valid kidney tissue is not available in IF-F. It has a high probability of success for the immunohistochemical detection of light chains [12]. Furthermore, this technique unmasks glomerular monoclonal deposits, and it helped us to establish the diagnosis of PGNMID IgG-kappa. Larsen et al. [13] reported twenty-six patients with a known monoclonal gammopathy who had a kidney biopsy showing C3 only or glomerulonephritis (GN) with negative glomerular staining for IgG, IgM, IgA, kappa, lambda, and C3 by routine IF. However, 21 samples had a residual paraffin tissue to undergo paraffin IF, including 11 cases of C3 GN, 6 dense deposit disease (DDD), and 4 unclassified MPGN/cryoglobulinemic GN cases. Paraffin IF identified 7 (33%) cases (4 of 11 C3 GN cases and 3 of the 4 unclassified MPGN/cryoglobulinemic GN cases) with positive staining for Ig. The authors strongly recommend performing paraffin IF in all patients with clinical evidence of MG in whom kidney biopsy shows C3 GN or MPGN with negative IF findings and when routine IF does not match either the clinical scenario or electron microscopic findings. Masked deposits are a rare phenomenon, and paraffin IF is certainly not warranted in most cases.

The lesions of glomerular TMA associated with MG were also observed in our patient, without presence in the clinical setting of microangiopathic hemolytic anemia (MAHA) and thrombocytopenia, and with normal levels of factor H autoantibody, the diagnosis of aHUS (complement-mediated TMA) was ruled out. Ravindran et al. [6] observed a high prevalence of MG in complement-mediated glomerulonephritis (C3 GN). Monoclonal Ig can cause dysregulation of the alternative pathway of complement by multiple mechanisms. One of these mechanisms is to act as an autoantibody to the complement factor H and interfering with its complement regulating function, and the other is its function as an autoantibody to the complement factor B that is a component of C3 convertase [14, 15]. The authors hypothesized that monoclonal Ig may facilitate the development of TMA directly or indirectly. The M-protein may injure the endothelial cells directly or interfere with the fibrin structure or indirectly via functional inhibition of proteins that regulate thrombosis. Finally, they conclude that all patients with TMA should undergo evaluation for MG. In our patient, the pathophysiological explanation of this disorder is not clear because TMA was not associated with C3 GN. Moreover, the other lesions in this category are glomerular microangiopathy associated with polyneuropathy, organomegaly, endocrinopathy, monoclonal gammopathy, and skin changes (POEMS) syndrome [16, 17]. In these cases, the lesion is a subacute to chronic glomerular thrombotic microangiopathy and is not associated with MAHA. Our patient had a similar injury, but she did not meet the criteria for this syndrome.

The most striking finding was the presence of electron-dense deposits with fibrils of 10–15 nm in the EM. These images are not typically observed in FGN or amyloidosis (fibrils < 20 nm with random orientation in mesangial cells and capillaries). Therefore, these images could correspond to a special way of crystallizing light-chain deposits or are unique features of this biopsy, demonstrating the unusual appearances that abnormal light chains can display. The fibrillar deposits are easy to confuse with each other since we only have the diameter, structure, and organization to differentiate them in EM. For this reason, it is necessary to perform amyloid stains and DNJB9 immunostaining for their better classification. In our case, the immunohistochemistry technique for DNAJB9 was negative. This is in line with a recent study published by Said et al. [18] although monotypic FGN is currently classified as a MGRS. The authors of this study performed IF-P on 35 cases of FGN that showed apparent light-chain restriction on IF-F and correlated the IF-P findings, IgG subtype staining, and SPEP/SIF. Only one of 11 cases had a detectable circulating monoclonal protein on SPEP/SIF. Said et al. conclude that DNAJB9-positive monotypic FGN (confirmed by IF-P and IgG subclass staining) is very rare and is not associated with MGRS in most patients.

MGRS treatment strategies are based on chemotherapy that must be adapted to the nature of the cell clone, both lymphocytic or plasma, renal function, and the presence or absence of extrarenal involvement. The evaluation of hematological response is crucial because the reduction of monoclonal Ig components is associated with the best renal outcomes. However, renal response is not contingent on the resolution of the M-protein in PGNMID [19]. Recently, Van Kruijsdijk et al. [20] reported 2 cases of PGNMID and raised the question if clone-directed therapy is always necessary, given the probability that the M-protein can disappear spontaneously without treatment, in cases when the quantification is only 0.4%. The authors detect incongruities probably because of a small sample size and the risk for confounding by indications that can be made with the results of 65 patients with PGNMID of three observational studies [2, 8, 19]. 73% of the patients who received clone-directed therapy had complete or partial renal response, but also 54% of the patients who received no clone-directed therapy (steroids, mycophenolate mofetil, and/or cyclosporine) and 29% of the patients who received no treatment or renin-angiotensin system blockade alone achieved complete or partial renal response.

In our case, the flow cytometric immunophenotyping of bone marrow showed the presence of plasma cells with abnormal kappa. Therefore, treatment with cycles of BordD chemotherapy was initiated, with good outcomes at the beginning. However, at the end of the sixth cycle, both renal and hematological relapse was evident, despite observing a 26.8% reduction in plasma cells with an abnormal phenotype for kappa. Given the heterogeneity of multiple kidney lesions associated with MGRS, and even more so in cases of relapse, to date, there is little experience regarding the optimal treatment of these complex forms [8, 19]. Different regimens including cyclophosphamide, bortezomib, melphalan, lenalidomide, rituximab, and daratumumab have been used according to the degree of glomerular filtration and proteinuria, with limited results [10]. In our case, rituximab treatment was proposed as a second line. Rituximab is a treatment option for cases of MGRS associated with IgM lambda deposits with identification of the B lymphocyte clone [2]. Despite the fact that the bone marrow biopsy showed plasma cells as pathologic clone and there was also a reduction after chemotherapeutic treatment, we suspected that the relapse of the disease occurred because the detected M-protein could not have been properly produced by this clone, if by another precursor as the B-lymphocyte clone.

New diagnostic tools need to be investigated in cases where the M-protein is little or not detected since clonal identification is even more difficult [7]. Despite the initial improvement with rituximab, we were unable to monitor the response to our treatment because the patient died of COVID-19 at the beginning of the pandemic in Spain.

In conclusion, we recommend that the treatment for MGRS should be patient-tailored, preferably by consulting a multidisciplinary team Future larger, prospective, and multicenter studies on pathophysiology are needed to better understand the disease course and to establish the efficacy and safety of therapy in the relapse of MGRS.

Consent

The patient has given her written informed consent to publish her case (including publication of images).

References

[1] F. Bridoux, N. Leung, C. A. Hutchison et al., "Diagnosis of monoclonal gammopathy of renal significance," *Kidney International*, vol. 87, no. 4, pp. 698–711, 2015.

[2] S. H. Nasr, A. Satoskar, G. S. Markowitz et al., "Proliferative glomerulonephritis with monoclonal IgG deposits," *Journal of the American Society of Nephrology*, vol. 20, no. 9, pp. 2055–2064, 2009.

[3] M. A. Lusco, A. B. Fogo, B. Najafian, and C. E. Alpers, "AJKD atlas of renal pathology: proliferative glomerulonephritis with monoclonal immunoglobulin deposits," *American Journal of Kidney Diseases*, vol. 67, no. 3, pp. e13–e15, 2016.

[4] T. Barbour, S. Johnson, S. Cohney, and P. Hughes, "Thrombotic microangiopathy and associated renal disorders," *Nephrology Dialysis Transplantation*, vol. 27, no. 7, pp. 2673–2685, 2012.

[5] N. Leung, F. Bridoux, V. Batuman et al., "The evaluation of monoclonal gammopathy of renal significance: a consensus report of the international kidney and monoclonal gammopathy research group," *Nature Reviews Nephrology*, vol. 15, no. 1, pp. 45–59, 2019.

[6] A. Ravindran, R. S. Go, F. C. Fervenza, and S. Sethi, "Thrombotic microangiopathy associated with monoclonal gammopathy," *Kidney International*, vol. 91, no. 3, pp. 691–698, 2017.

[7] J.-P. Fermand, F. Bridoux, R. A. Kyle et al., "How I treat monoclonal gammopathy of renal significance (MGRS)," *Blood*, vol. 122, no. 22, pp. 3583–3590, 2013.

[8] A. Kousios, N. Duncan, F. W. K. Tam et al., "Proliferative glomerulonephritis with monoclonal Ig deposits (PGNMID): diagnostic and treatment challenges for the nephrologist!" *Kidney International*, vol. 95, no. 2, pp. 467-468, 2019.

[9] S. Adapa, V. M. Konala, S. Naramala, and C. C. Nast, "Multiple morphological phenotypes of monoclonal immunoglobulin disease on renal biopsy: significance of treatment," *Clinical Nephrology—Case Studies*, vol. 8, no. 1, pp. 17–24, 2020.

[10] F. Caravaca-Fontán, E. Gutiérrez, R. Delgado Lillo, and M. Praga, "Gammapatías monoclonales de significado renal," *Nefrología*, vol. 37, no. 5, pp. 465–477, 2017.

[11] N. Klomjit, N. Leung, F. Fervenza, S. Sethi, and L. Zand, "Rate and predictors of finding monoclonal gammopathy of renal significance (MGRS) lesions on kidney biopsy in patients with

monoclonal gammopathy," *Journal of the American Society of Nephrology*, vol. 31, no. 10, pp. 2400–2411, 2020.
[12] S. H. Nasr, S. J. Galgano, G. S. Markowitz, M. B. Stokes, and V. D. D'Agati, "Immunofluorescence on pronase-digested paraffin sections: a valuable salvage technique for renal biopsies," *Kidney International*, vol. 70, no. 12, pp. 2148–2151, 2006.
[13] C. P. Larsen, N. C. Messias, P. D. Walker et al., "Membranoproliferative glomerulonephritis with masked monotypic immunoglobulin deposits," *Kidney International*, vol. 88, no. 4, pp. 867–873, 2015.
[14] S. Meri, V. Koistinen, A. Miettinen, T. Törnroth, and R. Seppäilä, "Activation of the alternative pathway of complement by monoclonal lambda light chains in membranoproliferative glomerulonephritis," *Journal of Experimental Medicine*, vol. 175, no. 4, pp. 939–950, 1992.
[15] T. S. Jokiranta, A. Solomon, M. K. Pangburn, P. F. Zipfel, and S. Meri, "Nephritogenic lambda light chain dimer: a unique human miniautoantibody against complement factor H," *Journal of Immunology*, vol. 163, no. 8, pp. 4590–4596, 1999, http://www.ncbi.nlm.nih.gov/pubmed/10510403.
[16] Y. Nakamoto, H. Imai, T. Yasuda, H. Wakui, and A. B. Miura, "A spectrum of clinicopathological features of nephropathy associated with POEMS syndrome," *Nephrology, Dialysis, Transplantation*, vol. 14, no. 10, pp. 2370–2378, 1999.
[17] Y. Nakamura, M. Nishimura, T. Terano et al., "A patient with POEMS syndrome: the pathology of glomerular microangiopathy," *The Tohoku Journal of Experimental Medicine*, vol. 231, no. 3, pp. 229–234, 2013.
[18] S. M. Said, N. Leung, M. P. Alexander et al., "DNAJB9-positive monotypic fibrillary glomerulonephritis is not associated with monoclonal gammopathy in the vast majority of patients," *Kidney International*, vol. 98, no. 2, pp. 498–504, 2020.
[19] R. Gumber, J. B. Cohen, M. B. Palmer et al., "A clone-directed approach may improve diagnosis and treatment of proliferative glomerulonephritis with monoclonal immunoglobulin deposits," *Kidney International*, vol. 94, no. 1, pp. 199–205, 2018.
[20] R. C. M. Van Kruijsdijk, A. C. Abrahams, T. Q. Nguyen, M. C. Minnema, J. F. M. Jacobs, and M. Limper, "Clone-directed therapy for proliferative glomerulonephritis with monoclonal immunoglobulin depositions: is it always necessary?" *Journal of Nephrology*, vol. 33, no. 3, pp. 611–617, 2020.

Acute Renal Failure in a Patient with Rivaroxaban-Induced Hypersensitivity Syndrome: A Case Report with a Review of the Literature and of Pharmacovigilance Registries

Gisela Marcelino, Ould Maouloud Hemett, and Eric Descombes

Service of Nephrology, HFR Cantonal Hospital Fribourg, 1708 Fribourg, Switzerland

Correspondence should be addressed to Gisela Marcelino; giselamarcelino1988@hotmail.com

Academic Editor: Sophia Lionaki

Direct oral anticoagulants (DOACs) are among the most commonly prescribed medications, and DOAC-associated kidney dysfunction may be a problem that is underrecognized by clinicians. We report on the case of an 82-year-old patient who, two weeks after the prescription of rivaroxaban for atrial fibrillation, was hospitalized for a drug-induced hypersensitivity syndrome whose main clinical manifestations were low-grade fever with a petechial rash in the legs and acute renal failure (ARF). Within one week after rivaroxaban withdrawal, the patient's clinical condition improved and the renal function normalized. In a review of the literature, we only found five case reports of rivaroxaban-related ARF: two patients had tubulo-interstitial nephritis (TIN), two had anticoagulant-related nephropathy (ARN), and the last one had IgA nephropathy. As some recent publications suggest that kidney injury due to anticoagulation drugs may be largely underdiagnosed, we also analyzed the data from the VigiAccess database, the World Health Organization pharmacovigilance program that collects drug-related adverse events from 134 national registries worldwide. Among all the rivaroxaban-associated adverse events reported in VigiAccess since 2006, 4,323 (3.5%) were renal side effects, of which 2,351 (54.3%) were due to unspecified ARF, 363 (8.4%) were due to renal hemorrhage (characteristically associated with ARN), and 24 (0.6%) were due to TIN. We also compared these results with those reported in VigiAccess for other DOACs and vitamin K antagonists. This analysis suggests that the frequency of renal adverse events associated with rivaroxaban and other DOACs may be appreciably higher than what one might currently consider based only on the small number of fully published cases.

1. Introduction

Since the introduction of direct oral anticoagulants (DOACs) into the market at the beginning of the century, they have rapidly risen to become one of the most commonly prescribed medications by clinicians [1]. Their utility in the prevention of systemic embolization and stroke in atrial fibrillation or in the treatment of venous thromboembolism, or even their simpler use in comparison to warfarin, has led medical doctors to prefer DOACs as their molecule of choice, to the detriment of the well-known vitamin K antagonist [1].

However, since the introduction of DOACs in clinical practice, some authors have highlighted the risk of renal dysfunction associated with the use of DOACs [2–10]. Warfarin has also been associated with acute and chronic renal failure (often in the setting of overanticoagulation, i.e. INR >3), but this has been considered an uncommon complication up to now [8, 11–17]. In the literature, two types of kidney injury induced by DOACs are reported. The first is immune-mediated (namely, tubulointerstitial nephritis) and associated with different immuno-allergic mechanisms [18–20]. The second, first described by Brodsky et al. in 2009 and known as anticoagulant-related nephropathy (previously called warfarin-related nephropathy), is due to tubular obstruction by red blood cell casts, secondary to glomerular injury [11]. Anticoagulant-related nephropathy is hypothesized to be associated with the lack of an endothelial trophic factor (that can be caused either by DOACs or warfarin), which leads to the disruption of the glomerular barrier and causes glomerular hemorrhage and an inflammatory response, further aggravating renal injury [8, 11, 12]. In an animal model, Brodsky and colleagues showed that warfarin and dabigatran can cause renal dysfunction and progressive hematuria in a dose-dependent manner [15–17]. It should be noted, however, that the general underlying physiopathological mechanisms of anticoagulant-related nephropathy are not yet fully understood and that further research is required in this area.

So, the aim of the present work is to present the case of a patient who developed rivaroxaban-induced hypersensitivity syndrome with reversible acute renal failure (ARF), to review the cases associating rivaroxaban with renal dysfunction that have already been reported in the literature and to search the pharmacovigilance data to establish if there is, indeed, an increased risk of renal injury associated with rivaroxaban and other DOACs, when compared to antivitamin K.

2. Case Report

An 82-year-old Caucasian woman with a known history of metabolic syndrome (hypertension, dyslipidemia, type II diabetes, and hyperuricemia) developed atrial fibrillation 15 days before admission to our hospital and received 20 mg of rivaroxaban once a day, in addition to the usual treatment that she had regularly been undergoing for a long time and that remained unchanged, namely, moxonidine 0.2 mg/day, metoprolol 200 mg/day, losartan 100 mg/day, spironolactone 50 mg/day, furosemide 20 mg/day, simvastatin 40 mg/day, ezetimibe 10 mg/day, allopurinol 100 mg/day, 500 mg of calcium, and 400 UI of cholecalciferol/day.

Three days before admission, she noticed petechial lesions in the legs and developed progressive bilateral pitting edema in the lower limbs, associated with a weight gain of 4–5 kg, which made her fall twice at home. At admission, the clinical examination was remarkable for a petechial rash of the legs and the massively swollen lower limbs with pitting edema. The patient had low-grade fever with a temperature of 38.0°C. The blood pressure was 132/70 mmHg, heart rate was regular at 92/min, and oxygen saturation was 94%. The remainder of the exam was unremarkable. Diuresis was conserved at a rate of 0.55–0.60 ml/kg/hour. Table 1 summarizes the results of the laboratory analysis performed at admission. There was marked acute renal dysfunction (serum creatinine = 215 μmol/l) with a moderate inflammatory response (C-reactive protein = 129 mg/l), a mild hepatic dysfunction, and a marked lymphopenia at 0.11 G/l (normal >1.0 G/l) but no eosinophilia. The urine exam showed massive leucocyturia (without eosinophils), no hematuria, and a mild tubular proteinuria of 0.72 g/day (25% albumin). The renal ultrasound and the posteroanterior and the lateral chest X-ray were normal. The echocardiography showed a normal ejection fraction (60%) without signs of diastolic dysfunction. As the patient had fallen before admission, a native cerebral CT scan was also performed and showed two small asymptomatic subdural hematomas (4 mm left-parietal and 1 mm right-parietal). The autoimmune screening was negative for antinuclear antibodies, rheumatoid factor, antineutrophil cytoplasmic antibodies, antiglomerular basement membrane antibodies, and cryoglobulins. C3 and C4 were within the normal range. The serologies for human immunodeficiency virus, hepatitis B, and hepatitis C were negative. The urine and blood cultures were sterile.

At admission, rivaroxaban was immediately stopped. In the first 48 hours of the hospitalization, the diuretics were stopped, and the patient received cautious intravenous hydration with vitamin K supplementation. Over the following days, we observed a rapid clinical and biological improvement. The petechial lesions in the lower limbs improved, while the edema affecting the legs rapidly diminished under low-dose diuretics (5 mg/day of torasemide), with a weight loss of 4.3 kg in five days. At the same time, the blood analysis showed a rapid and spontaneous improvement in the renal and hepatic dysfunction, as well as in the inflammatory syndrome (see Table 1 and Figure 1). As the renal function rapidly and spontaneously improved, neither a renal biopsy was performed nor were steroids prescribed.

3. Discussion

The patient we report presented with features of a drug-induced hypersensitivity syndrome fulfilling the RegiSCAR diagnostic criteria for DRESS [21], including reaction suspected to be drug-related occurring two weeks after the prescription of a new medications, hospitalization, pethechial rash in the legs, low-grade fever, renal and hepatic dysfunction, and severe lymphopenia. From a nephrological point of view, the renal findings were consistent with an acute tubulointerstitial nephritis (ARF with sterile leucocyturia and tubular proteinuria) [18]. As the renal function rapidly improved after rivaroxaban was stopped, a kidney biopsy was finally not performed in accordance with the algorithm for management of drug-induced acute interstitial nephritis of the Yale University [19]. It should also be noted that a rechallenge with rivaroxaban to confirm the relation between the prescription of rivaroxaban and the hypersensitivity syndrome [22] was not performed for ethical reasons.

Over the recent years, some publications have pointed out that there may be an increased risk of renal dysfunction in patients receiving DOACs. However, we found only five fully published case reports reporting an association between rivaroxaban and ARF in our review of the literature [2–6]. The main features of these five cases are summarized in Table 2. Overall, when taking into account all these case reports, including the one presented here, four of the cases involved men, with a median age of 76 years; two had preexisting chronic kidney disease, and five out of six cases exhibited several cardiovascular risk factors. In fact, older people and those with cardiovascular risk factors are the people who are most at the risk for ARF induced by DOACs [7, 9]. ARF developed within two days to two months after the prescription of rivaroxaban in all these cases, with one exception. Renal histology showed tubulointerstitial

TABLE 1: Laboratory results of the patient at admission and at discharge from our hospital.

Blood analysis (reference ranges)	At admission	At discharge
Hemoglobin (120–160 g/l)	105 g/l	109 g/l
Leucocytes (4.0–10.0 G/l)	7.2 G/l	5.8 G/l
Eosinophils (0–0.7 G/l)	0.36 G/l	—
Lymphocytes (1.0–4.0 G/l)	0.11 G/l	—
Platelets (150–300 G/l)	156 G/l	317 G/l
Urea (2.8–7.0 mmol/)	23.2 mmol/l	9.7 mmol/l
Creatinine (50–95 μmol/l)	215 μmol/l	86 μmol/l
Sodium (136–146 mmol/l)	133 mmol/l	139 mmol/l
Potassium (3.7–5.0 mmol/l)	4.1 mmol/l	4.2 mmol/l
Albumin (37–51 g/l)	30.2 g/l	—
Aspartate transaminase (<44 U/l)	77 U/l	48 U/l
Alanine aminotransferase (<44 U/l)	70 U/l	58 U/l
Alkaline phosphatase (35–105 U/l)	107 U/l	75 U/l
Gamma-glutamyl transferase (<40 U/l)	54 U/l	40 U/l
Total bilirubin (3.1–18.8 μmol/l)	25.7 μmol/l	14.3 μmol/l
Direct bilirubin (<3.4 μmol/l)	19.6 μmol/l	9.7 μmol/l
Prothrombin time % (75–100%)	34%	69%
Partial thromboplastin time (26–36 sec)	58 sec	—
Factor VII (70–120%)	66%	—
Creatinine kinase (<170 U/l)	210 U/l	—
C-reactive protein (<5 mg/l)	129 mg/l	24 mg/l

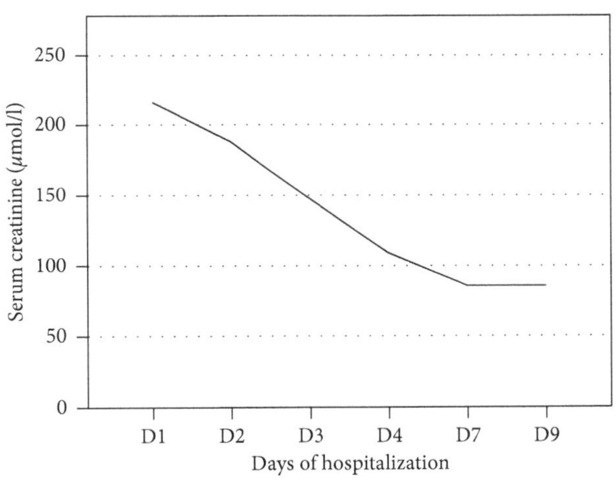

FIGURE 1: Time course of creatinine after stopping rivaroxaban from admission up to day 9, the day of discharge from our hospital.

nephritis (TIN) in two patients, anticoagulant-related nephropathy in two others, and IgA nephropathy in the last one. From a prognostic point of view, among these five cases, renal function improved in two (who had TIN at renal biopsy and who had received low-dose corticotherapy), while two of the three others had to undergo chronic dialysis (see Table 2).

In the process of carrying out the abovementioned review, we were surprised by the small number of cases that could be retrieved from the literature, which is in contrast to the alarming tone of some recent articles associating anticoagulation with ARF [7–17]. So, we questioned whether renal injury associated with anticoagulants, including rivaroxaban, might be greatly underdiagnosed and/or underreported, as has already been suggested by some authors [10, 12, 13]. Therefore, we consulted VigiAccess, which is an international pharmacovigilance database that collects data from 134 countries that are members of the World Health Organization Program for International Drug Monitoring [23]. The data we retrieved from the VigiAccess database concerning rivaroxaban are reported in Table 3. It is interesting to note that, from 2006 (when the first case was reported) to the end of April 2019, 121,038 adverse drug events associated with the prescription of rivaroxaban have been reported in VigiAccess. Among them, 4,323 (3.5%) were kidney-related adverse events. Renal side effects were the 8th most frequent type of adverse drug reaction reported for rivaroxaban; the side effects were equally distributed among genders and were more frequent in patients older than 65 years. According to the VigiAccess database, dabigatran and rivaroxaban are the drugs for which the proportion of kidney-related adverse events is higher: 4.6% and 3.5%, respectively, compared to only 2.0% for apixaban and 1.7% for edoxaban [23]. Table 3 shows that the clinical presentation was ARF (54.3%) in the majority of the cases reported for rivaroxaban, with only a small number developing CKD or ESRD (2.1%). Also, these data suggest that the mechanism of renal injury most frequently associated with rivaroxaban seems to be anticoagulant-related nephropathy (as it is characteristically associated with renal hemorrhage, which occurred in 363 cases), rather than tubulointerstitial nephritis with only 24 cases reported.

Therefore, even though we are aware of the limitations of the accuracy of the data obtained from registries, renal side effects associated with rivaroxaban and other DOACs seem to be more frequent than one might consider based only on the small number of published cases. In a recent paper, Glassock suggested that warfarin-/anticoagulation-related nephropathy were "the real McCoy" but that they are "rather uncommon but likely underdiagnosed clinicopathologic entities" [13]. Therefore, we also analyzed the renal adverse

TABLE 2: Clinical characteristics of the full-published case reports of rivaroxaban-associated acute renal failure.

Country	Age (y)	Sex	Comorbidities	Nephrological signs	Time to appearance	Renal biopsy	Treatment	Evolution
France (2017) [2]	87	M	Hypertension	ARF with conserved diuresis	2 days	TIN	Steroids (0.5 mg/kg for 1 month followed by a taper schedule)	Partial recovery
			Dyslipidemia	Proteinuria 1 g/l				
			Heart failure	Microscopic hematuria				
			Atrial fibrillation Stroke in the past Carotid artery stenosis Arteriopathy of the lower limbs	Leucocyturia				
Netherlands (2017) [3]	82	M	Hypertension	ARF with decreased diuresis	3 weeks	TIN	Steroids (40 mg prednisone for 2 weeks followed by a taper schedule of 5 mg/week)	Full recovery
			Pacemaker for a third-degree atrioventricular block	Proteinuria 0.3 g /24 h				
			Atrial fibrillation	Microscopic hematuria				
			CKD (eGFR 39 ml/ min/1.73 m2)	Leucocyturia but concomitant urinary infection				
Portugal (2017) [4]	82	F	CKD (eGFR 52.4 ml/min/ 1.73 m2)	ARF with conserved diuresis Macroscopic hematuria Proteinuria 0.56 g/24 h	2 months	Anticoagulant-related nephropathy	N-Acetylcystein 600 mg/day	Chronic hemodialysis
Australia (2018) [5]	45	M	Asthma	ARF with conserved diuresis Nephrotic range proteinuria Microscopic hematuria RBC casts	7 days	IgA nephropathy	Ramipril	CKD
Japan (2019) [6]	75	M	Hypertension	ARF	3 years	Anticoagulant-related nephropathy	No specific treatment was initiated	Chronic hemodialysis
			Diabetes mellitus	Nephrotic range proteinuria				
			Atrial fibrillation	Macroscopic hematuria				
			Stroke in the past	RBC and granular casts				
			IgA vasculitis					

F, female; M, male; ARF, acute renal failure; CKD, chronic kidney disease; TIN, tubulointerstitial nephritis; RBC, red blood cells.

events associated with anticoagulation reported in the VigiAccess database, not only for the four abovementioned DOACs but also those reported for antivitamin K drugs (warfarin, acenocoumarol, and phenprocoumanone). This analysis is reported in Table 4 and shows that the reported annual rate of renal adverse events is almost ten-fold higher for NOACs (7,725 cases in 15 years) than that reported for antivitamin K drugs (2,145 cases reported in 50 years). Of course, this difference may be related, to some extent, to bias in diagnosing and/or reporting the side effects for these

TABLE 3: Number and type of renal side effects reported for rivaroxaban (until 27 April 2019) retrieved from the VigiAccess database of the WHO Program for International Drug Monitoring (available at http://www.vigiaccess.org/).

	Rivaroxaban
First case reported	**2006**
Total number of side effects	**121,038**
Sex, *n* (%)	
Female	54,116 (45)
Male	54,865 (45)
Age, *n* (%)	
<65 years	23,295 (19)
≥65 years	62,105 (52)
Renal side effects, *n* (%)	**4,323 (3.5)**
Acute renal failure	2,351 (54.3)
Renal hemorrhage	363 (8.4)
Chronic kidney disease	84 (1.9)
Tubulointerstitial nephritis	24 (0.6)
Nephritic and nephrotic syndromes	16 (0.4)
End-stage renal disease	10 (0.2)

Results are presented as number of subjects (valid percentage).

TABLE 4: Number and type of renal side effects for DOACs and antivitamin K retrieved (until 27th April 2019) from VigiAccess database of the WHO Program for International Drug Monitoring (available at http://www.vigiaccess.org/).

	DOACs	AVKs
Total number of reported side effects	$n = 235{,}457$	$n = 117{,}015$
First case reported	2003	1968
Renal side effects, *n* (%)	7,725 (3.3)	2,145 (1.8)
Acute kidney injury	3,796 (49.1)	904 (42.1)
Renal failure unspecified	2,802 (36.3)	704 (32.8)
Renal hemorrhage	553 (7.2)	147 (6.9)
Chronic kidney disease	209 (2.7)	75 (3.5)
Tubulointerstitial nephritis	55 (0.7)	36 (1.7)

Results are presented as number of subjects (valid percentage). DOACs, direct oral anticoagulants; AVKs, antivitamin K. All DOACs include rivaroxaban, apixaban, edoxaban, and dabigatran. Acenocoumarol, warfarin, and phenprocoumone were regrouped as AVKs.

different classes of anticoagulants. Nevertheless, the data from the pharmacovigilance registries reported above may suggest that anticoagulation-related nephropathy, although probably sometimes underdiagnosed, was probably a rare complication in the era of antivitamin K drugs, but that this may no longer be the case in the DOACs era.

This statement is at odds with the conclusions of some recent studies, suggesting that the risk of DOAC-associated renal dysfunction may be lower than for warfarin [7, 24–29]. However, it should be emphasized that several of these retrospective cohort studies have methodological flaws with respect, for example, to the doses of the anticoagulant prescribed or the degree of chronic renal dysfunction already present points that are critical to the correct interpretation of the results. This fact has been well-established in a recent meta-analysis conducted by de Aquino Moura et al. [30] who concluded that studies concerning anticoagulant-related nephropathy are "scarce and heterogeneous and present significant methodological limitations". For example, the majority of the participants in the two studies carried out by Chan et al. [7, 24] received low doses of DOACs (61% for apixaban, 89% for dabigatran, and 93% for rivaroxaban), and this was the case for 22.6% of the patients reported on by Hernandez et al. [25], an element that can clearly reduce the risk of complications as, according to an animal model, the risk of renal dysfunction is dose-dependent [15–17]. It is, therefore, clear that only further well-planned prospective studies will be able to satisfactorily clarify this question.

In summary, although we found only a few case reports of rivaroxaban-associated renal dysfunction reported in the literature, the data from the international pharmacovigilance register, VigiAccess, suggest that the frequency of renal adverse events associated with the prescription of rivaroxaban and other DOACs may be appreciably higher than that presently considered by clinicians. According to the reported data, the mechanism of renal injury most frequently involved in rivaroxaban-associated ARF seems to be anticoagulant-related nephropathy, rather than tubulointerstitial nephritis. From a practical point of view, it is, therefore, important that clinicians are aware of the risks of renal dysfunction in patients receiving DOACs and anticoagulant drugs in general. As already proposed by Wheeler et al. [31], we agree that systematic screening of the renal function is required in patients taking DOACs and that regular monitoring of renal function should be performed in all patients receiving therapeutic anticoagulation.

Abbreviations

ARF: Acute renal failure
CKD: Chronic kidney disease
ESRD: End-stage renal disease
DOACs: Direct oral anticoagulants
TIN: Tubulointerstitial nephritis.

Authors' Contributions

All authors contributed to the writing of the paper and to the interpretation and analysis of the data. GM was responsible for the literature review and for retrieving the data from VigiAccess. All authors read and approved the final manuscript.

References

[1] G. Lippi, C. Mattiuzzi, G. Cervellin, and E. J. Favaloro, "Direct oral anticoagulants: analysis of worldwide use and popularity using google trends," *Annals of Translational Medicine*, vol. 5, no. 16, p. 322, 2017.

[2] A. Dantec, J.-S. Virot, A. Filancia, R. Angonin, and H. Nefti, "Néphrite tubulo-interstitielle au rivaroxaban (Xarelto)," *La Presse Médicale*, vol. 46, no. 5, pp. 541-542, 2017.

[3] R. C. Monahan, M. M. Suttorp, and B. A. T. F. Gabreëls, "A case of rivaroxaban-associated acute tubulointerstitial

nephritis," *Netherland Journal of Medicine*, vol. 75, pp. 169–171, 2017.

[4] M. Oliveira, C. Lima, M. Góis, H. Viana, F. Carvalho, and S. Lemos, "Rivaroxaban-related nephropathy," *Portuguese Journal of Nephrology and Hypertension*, vol. 31, pp. 212–216, 2017.

[5] E. Y. Chung, J. Chen, and S. Roxburgh, "A case report of henoch-schonlein purpura and IgA nephropathy associated with rivaroxaban," *Nephrology*, vol. 23, no. 3, pp. 289-290, 2018.

[6] Y. Fujino, C. Takahashi, K. Mitsumoto, and T. Uzu, "Rivaroxaban-related acute kidney injury in a patient with IgA vasculitis," *BMJ Case Reports*, vol. 12, no. 1, Article ID e227756, 2019.

[7] Y.-H. Chan, Y.-H. Yeh, M.-Y. Hsieh et al., "The risk of acute kidney injury in Asians treated with apixaban, rivaroxaban, dabigatran, or warfarin for non-valvular atrial fibrillation: a nationwide cohort study in Taiwan," *International Journal of Cardiology*, vol. 265, pp. 83–89, 2018.

[8] S. Brodsky, J. Eikelboom, and L. A. Hebert, "Anticoagulant-related nephropathy," *Journal of the American Society of Nephrology*, vol. 29, no. 12, pp. 2787–2793, 2018.

[9] Z. Hijazi, S. H. Hohnloser, U. Andersson et al., "Efficacy and safety of apixaban compared with warfarin in patients with atrial fibrillation in relation to renal function over time," *JAMA Cardiology*, vol. 1, no. 4, pp. 451–460, 2016.

[10] T. Oliver, L. A. Salman, B. Ciaudelli, and D. A. Cohen, "Anticoagulation-related nephropathy: the most common diagnosis you've never heard of," *The American Journal of Medicine*, vol. 132, no. 8, pp. e631–e633, 2019.

[11] S. V. Brodsky, A. Satoskar, J. Chen et al., "Acute kidney injury during warfarin therapy associated with obstructive tubular red blood cell casts: a report of 9 cases," *American Journal of Kidney Diseases*, vol. 54, no. 6, pp. 1121–1126, 2009.

[12] S. V. Brodsky, T. Nadasdy, B. H. Rovin et al., "Warfarin-related nephropathy occurs in patients with and without chronic kidney disease and is associated with an increased mortality rate," *Kidney International*, vol. 80, no. 2, pp. 181–189, 2011.

[13] R. J. Glassock, "Anticoagulant-related nephropathy," *Clinical Journal of the American Society of Nephrology*, vol. 14, no. 6, pp. 935–937, 2019.

[14] L. Golbin, C. Vigneau, G. Touchard et al., "Warfarin-related nephropathy induced by three different vitamin K antagonists: analysis of 13 biopsy-proven cases," *Clinical Kidney Journal*, vol. 10, no. 3, pp. 381–388, 2017.

[15] M. Ryan, K. Ware, Z. Qamri et al., "Warfarin-related nephropathy is the tip of the iceberg: direct thrombin inhibitor dabigatran induces glomerular hemorrhage with acute kidney injury in rats," *Nephrology Dialysis Transplantation*, vol. 29, no. 12, pp. 2228–2234, 2014.

[16] A. Ozcan, K. Ware, E. Calomeni et al., "5/6 nephrectomy as a validated rat model mimicking human warfarin-related nephropathy," *American Journal of Nephrology*, vol. 35, no. 4, pp. 356–364, 2012.

[17] S. V. Brodsky, "Anticoagulants and acute kidney injury: clinical and pathology considerations," *Kidney Research and Clinical Practice*, vol. 33, no. 4, pp. 174–180, 2014.

[18] M. Praga and E. González, "Acute interstitial nephritis," *Kidney International*, vol. 77, no. 11, pp. 956–961, 2010.

[19] D. G. Moledina and M. A. Perazella, "Drug-induced acute interstitial nephritis," *Clinical Journal of the American Society of Nephrology*, vol. 12, no. 12, pp. 2046–2049, 2017.

[20] R. Raghavan and S. Shawar, "Mechanisms of drug-induced interstitial nephritis," *Advances in Chronic Kidney Disease*, vol. 24, no. 2, pp. 64–71, 2017.

[21] T. Shiohara and Y. Mizukawa, "Drug-induced hypersensitivity syndrome (DiHS)/drug reaction with eosinophilia and systemic symptoms (DRESS): an update in 2019," *Allergology International*, vol. 68, no. 3, pp. 301–308, 2019.

[22] C. Bailey, D. Peddie, M. E. Wickham et al., "Adverse drug event reporting systems: a systematic review," *British Journal of Clinical Pharmacology*, vol. 82, no. 1, pp. 17–29, 2016.

[23] Uppsala Monitoring Centre, "VigiAccess data base from WHO program for international drug monitoring," 2019, http://www.vigiaccess.org/.

[24] Y.-H. Chan, Y.-H. Yeh, L.-C. See et al., "Acute kidney injury in asians with atrial fibrillation treated with dabigatran or warfarin," *Journal of the American College of Cardiology*, vol. 68, no. 21, pp. 2272–2283, 2016.

[25] A. V. Hernandez, G. Bradley, M. Khan et al., "Rivaroxaban versus warfarin and renal outcomes in non-valvular atrial fibrillation patients with diabetes," *European Heart Journal Quality of Care and Clinical Outcomes*, 2019.

[26] C. I. Coleman, R. Kreutz, N. Sood et al., "Rivaroxaban's impact on renal decline in patients with nonvalvular atrial fibrillation: a US MarketScan claims database analysis," *Clinical Applied Thrombosis And Hemostasis*, vol. 25, 2019.

[27] J.-I. Shin, S. Luo, G. C. Alexander et al., "Direct oral anticoagulants and risk of acute kidney injury in patients with atrial fibrillation," *Journal of the American College of Cardiology*, vol. 71, no. 2, pp. 251-252, 2018.

[28] X. Yao, N. Tangri, B. J. Gersh et al., "Renal outcomes in anticoagulated patients with atrial fibrillation," *Journal of the American College of Cardiology*, vol. 70, no. 21, pp. 2621–2632, 2017.

[29] G. Maura, C. Billionnet, J. Coste, A. Weill, A. Neumann, and A. Pariente, "Non-bleeding adverse events with the use of direct oral anticoagulants: a sequence symmetry analysis," *Drug Safety*, vol. 41, no. 9, pp. 881–897, 2018.

[30] K. B. De Aquino Moura, P. M. P. Behrens, and R. Pirolli, "Anticoagulant-related nephropathy: systematic review and meta-analysis," *Clinical Kidney Journal*, vol. 12, pp. 400–407, 2019.

[31] D. S. Wheeler, R. P. Giugliano, and J. Rangaswami, "Anti-coagulation-related nephropathy," *Journal of Thrombosis and Haemostasis*, vol. 14, no. 3, pp. 461–467, 2016.

Anterior Ischemic Optic Neuropathy in a Child Receiving Chronic Hemodialysis

Joyce Moore,[1] Jennifer Klowak,[2] Gloria Isaza,[3] Steven Arora,[4] Vladimir Belostotsky,[4] Nina Stein,[5] and Rahul Chanchlani[4]

[1]*Department of Medicine, Michael G. DeGroote School of Medicine, McMaster University, Hamilton, Ontario, Canada*
[2]*Department of Pediatrics, McMaster Children's Hospital, Hamilton, Ontario, Canada*
[3]*Department of Ophthalmology, McMaster University, Hamilton, Ontario, Canada*
[4]*Division of Nephrology, Department of Pediatrics, McMaster Children's Hospital, Hamilton, Ontario, Canada*
[5]*Department of Radiology, McMaster University, Hamilton, Ontario, Canada*

Correspondence should be addressed to Rahul Chanchlani; chanchlr@mcmaster.ca

Academic Editor: Raoul Bergner

Anterior ischemic optic neuropathy (AION) occurs due to hypoperfusion of the optic nerve and is a rare complication in patients receiving maintenance dialysis. To date, AION has only been reported in 22 children, all of whom were receiving peritoneal dialysis. We report the first case of AION in a 2-year 11-month-old child receiving chronic hemodialysis secondary to polycystic kidney disease from a phosphomannomutase 2 gene mutation. This case highlights the consideration for frequent blood pressure monitoring and ophthalmic screening in a certain cohort of children receiving chronic dialysis.

1. Background

Anterior ischemic optic neuropathy (AION) is characterized by hypoperfusion of the posterior ciliary arteries resulting in optic nerve infarction [1]. AION has been reported as a complication of hypotension secondary to chronic dialysis in adult patients, but it is much less common in children [2]. To our knowledge, only 22 cases of pediatric AION have been reported and all of them were receiving peritoneal dialysis [1, 3–5]. We present what we believe to be the first case report of AION in a child receiving chronic intermittent hemodialysis.

2. Case Report

We report a 2-year 11-month-old male on chronic hemodialysis secondary to polycystic kidney disease (PCKD) who underwent bilateral nephrectomy. He had a compound heterozygous phosphomannomutase 2 promoter and missense mutation, accounting for PCKD and congenital hyperinsulinism. His left kidney was removed in February 2017 due to respiratory insufficiency from mass effect. Seven months later, with significantly reduced kidney function, he underwent a left nephrectomy due to respiratory compromise and hypertension. Following his second nephrectomy, he began intermittent hemodialysis five days a week; decreased to four days a week after 6 months.

Prior to his second nephrectomy, he was being treated for hypertension with an angiotensin-converting enzyme inhibitor, beta-blocker, and furosemide. After the second nephrectomy, his intradialytic systolic blood pressure used to be around 68 mmHg. For this reason, he was started on 2.5 mg midodrine during hemodialysis for systolic blood pressure below 90 mmHg. His ultrafiltration was minimized to avoid further hypotensive episodes during hemodialysis. Despite that, his systolic blood pressure stayed around 60 mmHg. Other medications included diazoxide, omeprazole, levothyroxine, and darbepoetin. He was G-tube fed without salt restriction. His blood work five days prior to presentation demonstrated normocytic, mild anemia (hemoglobin 95 g/L) with a reticulocyte count of 20×10^9/L. His electrolytes were grossly normal (sodium 136 mmol/L,

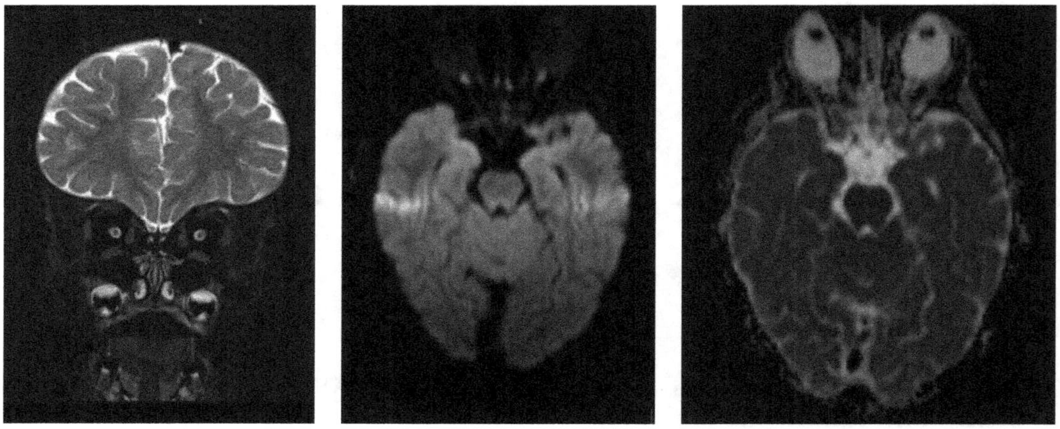

(a) (b) (c)

FIGURE 1: Brain MRI at patient's presentation. Coronal T2 turbo spin echo with fat saturation of the orbits showing normal thickness and T2 signal of the optic nerves. No asymmetry noted (a). Diffusion weighted imaging B1000 (b) and apparent diffusion coefficient map (c). The visualization of the optic nerves is distorted by the presence of artifacts, and allowing for this limitation, no restricted diffusion was observed on the apparent diffusion coefficient map.

potassium 3.8 mmol/L, chloride 91 mmol/L, and calcium 2.77 mmol/L) and his albumin was low at 30 g/L. Creatinine was elevated at 421 μmol/L. His echocardiogram showed normal biventricular function.

In June 2018, 9 months after initiating hemodialysis, he presented to the emergency department with an unsteady gait and difficulty focusing and following objects starting approximately two hours after completion of hemodialysis that day. Parents noted a pupil size change from small to large bilaterally, documented at 8 mm. On his initial neurological examination, his pupils were dilated but responsive, and he had poor visual acuity and an unsteady gait. He was otherwise alert, oriented, and comfortable. Vitally, his blood pressure was 59/33 mmHg, heart rate was 92 bpm, and he was afebrile. Laboratory findings on admission demonstrated a normocytic, mild anemia with a hemoglobin level of 101 g/L and an MCV of 92.7 fL. His sodium was found to be low at 127 mmol/L, with a potassium level of 4.4 mmol/L, and a chloride level of 98 mmol/L. Repeat blood work displayed a sodium level of 134 mmol/L, and thus, no hypertonic saline was administered. Creatinine was elevated at 166 μmol/L. Tox screen was negative, and AST, ALT, and INR were all normal. He had no history of trauma, toxin ingestion, sick contact exposure, or seizure activity.

Head CT displayed nonspecific findings of bifrontal subcortical white matter hypodensities. MRI displayed multiple foci of increased fluid-attenuated inversion recovery signal, mainly on bilateral subcortical white matter of the frontal lobes and corona radiata. Optic nerve size and signal intensity were normal (Figure 1). Ophthalmology noted decreased visual acuity to hand motion and optic disk pallor, and diagnosed optic nerve atrophy. He was treated with a five-day course of intravenous pulse methylprednisolone (15 mg/kg, 225 mg daily). Enteral midodrine was administered three times a day, and fluids were titrated for a blood pressure goal above 70/40 mmHg.

He was discharged after steroid treatment with a diagnosis of bilateral AION. Ophthalmology follow-up two months after his acute presentation revealed his vision to be 20/800 in the left eye and 20/30 in the right eye (Figure 2). He continued midodrine until his related living donor kidney transplant. He is currently stable and normotensive six months posttransplant. His vision at 10 months following his initial presentation is 20/40 in the right eye and no light perception in the left.

3. Discussion

AION results from poor perfusion of the optic nerve and is a rare but serious condition that can occur in patients on chronic dialysis [2]. The optic nerve is supplied by the posterior ciliary arteries which arise from the ophthalmic artery [3]. Compromised blood flow through these arteries may lead to ischemia of the optic nerve [3, 5]. If adequate blood flow is not promptly restored, permanent vision loss can occur [3, 5]. Many factors can contribute to hypoperfusion of the optic nerve, and the risk factors vary between adults and children [3, 5]. In adults, AION is classified as either arteritic or nonarteritic [6]. The former is commonly associated with giant cell arteritis and results due to thromboembolism in the posterior ciliary arteries [6]. The latter is more common in adults and occurs due to risk factors such as diabetes, vasospasm, nocturnal hypotension, and sleep apnea [6]. On the other hand, children do not have risk factors associated with aging, and infarction of the optic nerve is more commonly related to systemic hypotension [3]. Risk factors in children include young age at dialysis onset, chronic hypotension (often with previous hypertension), history of bilateral nephrectomy, autosomal recessive polycystic disease, and anemia [1, 2, 5].

To date, 22 cases of AION have been reported in children, all of whom were on peritoneal dialysis. Similarities of our case with the previously reported 22 cases are the

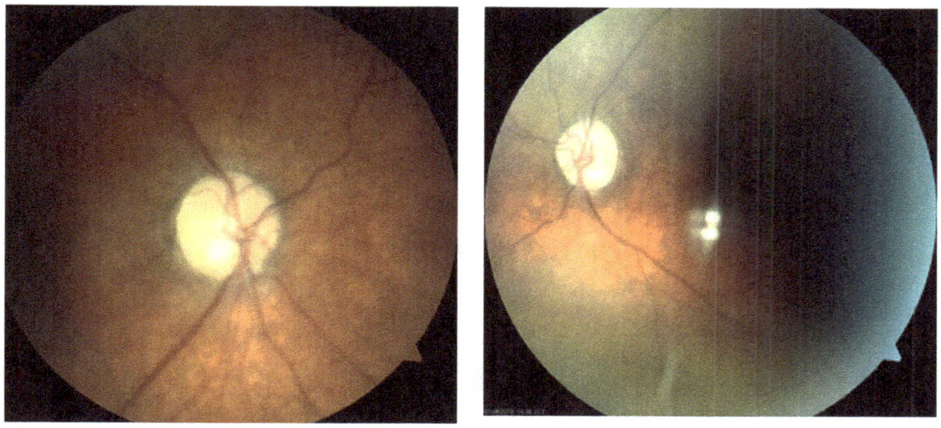

(a) (b)

FIGURE 2: Fundoscopic images of retina from two-month follow-up. The left optic nerve (a) is more pale than the right (b). Vision at this time was 20/800 in the left eye and 20/30 in the right eye.

bilateral nature of vision loss in 95% (21/22) of patients and sudden presentation in all patients [1, 3–5]. As with our case, 77% (17/22) of the cases also presented with hypotension, further supporting systemic hypotension as a risk factor for AION. The mean age of patients was 3.3 years. Of the 21 patients available for follow-up, 62% (13/21) had partial vision recovery, as did our patient, and 38% (8/21) remained blind [1, 3–5]. The optic disc pallor seen at presentation in our case has been reported previously in acute pediatric AION related to dialysis [3]. Unique features are that this is the first reported case of pediatric AION during hemodialysis and that it was bilateral, whereas adult AION following hemodialysis typically presents with monocular loss. However, AION following peritoneal dialysis in both children and adults is usually a bilateral disease [3]. This suggests that the mechanism for AION in children may be similar in both hemo- and peritoneal dialysis patients and highlights the need for better screening across all patients.

This case emphasizes the importance of blood pressure control in children receiving chronic hemo- or peritoneal dialysis. Dialysis patients have frequent contact with the health care system, providing ample opportunity for blood pressure monitoring and management. All children with risk factors for AION, such as anemia, young age, chronic hypotension, bilateral nephrectomy, and polycystic kidney disease, should be regularly screened for AION with an early involvement of ophthalmology as needed. Adequate medical management of low blood pressure and early diagnosis of AION could reduce both the incidence of AION and the associated potential for complete vision loss in patients receiving chronic dialysis.

Consent

Informed consent was obtained from the patient's parents.

Acknowledgments

The authors would like to acknowledge the patient's family for their cooperation and support. The authors would like to particularly acknowledge the co-author, Dr. Gloria Isaza, a well-respected ophthalmologist, who unfortunately passed shortly before publication.

References

[1] A. M. Chutorian, J. M. S. Winterkorn, and M. Geffner, "Anterior ischemic optic neuropathy in children: case reports and review of the literature," *Pediatric Neurology*, vol. 26, no. 5, pp. 358–364, 2002.

[2] Y.-S. Chang, S.-F. Weng, C. Chang et al., "Risk of nonarteritic anterior ischemic optic neuropathy following end-stage renal disease," *Medicine*, vol. 95, no. 12, p. e3174, 2016.

[3] G. Di Zazzo, I. Guzzo, L. De Galasso et al., "Anterior ischemic optical neuropathy in children on chronic peritoneal dialysis: report of 7 cases," *Peritoneal Dialysis International: Journal of the International Society for Peritoneal Dialysis*, vol. 35, no. 2, pp. 135–139, 2015.

[4] A. Al-Kaabi, A. Haider, M. Shafeeq, M. El-Naggari, I. El-Nour, and A. Ganesh, "Bilateral anterior ischaemic optic neuropathy in a child on continuous peritoneal dialysis: case report and literature review," *Sultan Qaboos University Medical Journal*, vol. 16, no. 4, pp. e504–507, 2016.

[5] S. Dufek, M. Feldkoetter, E. Vidal et al., "Anterior ischemic optic neuropathy in pediatric peritoneal dialysis: risk factors and therapy," *Pediatric Nephrology*, vol. 29, no. 7, pp. 1249–1257, 2014.

[6] Y. J. Liao and J. J. Hwang, "Treatment of anterior ischemic optic neuropathy: clues from the bench," *Taiwan Journal of Ophthalmology*, vol. 4, no. 1, pp. 9–16, 2014.

Tubulocystic Renal Cell Carcinoma of the Native Kidney in a Renal Transplant Recipient: A Rare Case Report

Brianna Ruch,[1] **Ashley J. Limkemann**,[1] **Paulo Garcia**,[2] **Cameron Benedict**,[3] **Gaurav Gupta**,[1] **Marlon Levy**,[1] **and Amit Sharma**[1]

[1]*Hume-Lee Transplant Center, Virginia Commonwealth University, Richmond, VA, USA*
[2]*Department of Pathology, Virginia Commonwealth University, Richmond, VA, USA*
[3]*School of Medicine, Virginia Commonwealth University, Richmond, VA 23298, USA*

Correspondence should be addressed to Amit Sharma; amit.sharma@vcuhealth.org

Academic Editor: Mahzuz Karim

Tubulocystic renal cell carcinoma (TCC) is a rare and newly recognized variant of renal cell carcinoma, which may mimic benign cystic disease of the kidney. To our knowledge, we present the first reported case of a patient who, despite standard preoperative workup, developed TCC of his native kidney soon after receiving kidney transplantation. He was appropriately treated with native nephrectomy and has had no signs of reoccurrence 7 years postoperatively. Given the significant risk of malignancy in renal transplant patients, this case emphasizes the need for close monitoring of native cystic disease before and after transplantation, with low threshold to proceed with surgical intervention.

1. Introduction

Tubulocystic renal cell carcinoma (TCC) of the kidney is a rare variant of renal cell carcinoma (RCC), and it was not recognized as a distinct entity by the World Health Organization until 2016 [1]. Literature review only yields approximately 100 reported cases, the majority of which focuses on histologic features and differentiation. There are no reported cases of TCC in transplant recipients, despite the high risk of renal cancer in this population [2]. We report a rare case of tubulocystic renal cell carcinoma occurring in the native left kidney of a renal transplant recipient.

2. Case Presentation

A 65-year-old African American male underwent a native right nephrectomy for RCC 25 years ago. Five years later, he began hemodialysis for end-stage renal disease (ESRD) secondary to hypertension and insulin-dependent diabetes. As part of a workup for renal transplant consideration, he underwent contrast-enhanced computed tomography (CT) of the abdomen in 2010 that demonstrated multiple low-attenuation cysts, too small to characterize, and a 3.1 cm × 2.6 cm nonenhancing lesion in the left renal upper pole consistent with a Bosniak class II renal cyst. Based on these findings, no further follow-up was recommended (Figure 1(a)). Subsequently, he underwent a living-related kidney transplant in 2012 with an immunosuppression regimen consisting of rabbit antithymocyte globulin (thymoglobulin; Genzyme Corp., Cambridge, MA) for induction (day 0 to day 3 at 1.5 mg/kg) and maintenance therapy of tacrolimus, mycophenolate mofetil, and a tapering dose of prednisone.

The patient presented to the clinic five months after his transplant with complaints of hematuria and left leg swelling. Abdominal CT scan revealed an enlarging, minimally enhancing hypodense 3.3 × 3.8 cm cystic mass, Bosniak class IV, in the upper pole of the native left kidney that was suspicious for RCC (Figure 1(b)). Venous duplex of the left leg demonstrated deep venous thrombosis extending from the popliteal to the left common femoral vein. Patient underwent thrombolysis, placement of the inferior vena cava filter, and systemic anticoagulation followed by an uneventful laparoscopic left radical nephrectomy. Macroscopic

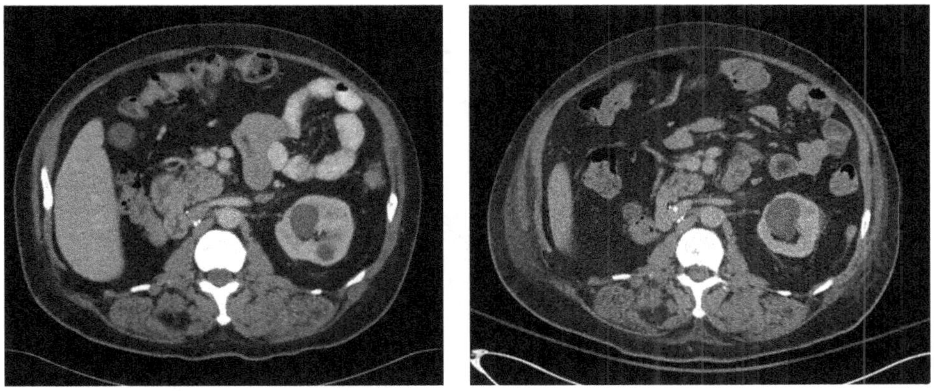

(a) (b)

Figure 1: Contrast-enhanced CT scan of the abdomen (a) two years before transplant and (b) five months after transplant. (a) Left kidney showing a 3.1 × 2.6 cm, nonenhancing, cystic lesion at the upper pole. (b) Enlarged and minimally enhancing 3.3 × 3.8 cm mass in the upper pole of the left kidney suspicious for renal cell cancer (white arrow).

evaluation of the specimen showed a 2.3 × 2.1 × 2.0 cm well encapsulated, polycystic mass in the superior pole of the left kidney abutting the pelvis but not invading the renal parenchyma. Immunohistochemical analysis of the neoplastic cyst-lining cells was positive for racemase, CD10, vimentin, and focal positive staining with CK7, as well as negative staining with EMA (Figure 2). The patient was diagnosed with tubulocystic renal cell carcinoma of the kidney, Fuhrman nuclear grade 3, confined to the kidney.

Postoperatively, our patient was followed per the 2018 National Comprehensive Cancer Network (NCCN) guidelines with abdominal imaging at one year and chest imaging annually over three years [3]. He was considered tumor-free based on his last abdominal magnetic resonance imaging in 2014, which showed no recurrent or residual disease. He continued to do well, about seven years after his renal transplant and left native nephrectomy, with a serum creatinine of 1.59 mg/dL and eGFR 49 mL/min/1.73 m^2. His current immunosuppression consists of tacrolimus 2 mg twice a day, mycophenolate mofetil 750 mg twice a day, and prednisone 10 mg daily.

3. Discussion

Cystic lesions of the kidneys may present a diagnostic dilemma in ESRD patients, especially if they are being considered for renal transplantation. Tubulocystic renal cell carcinoma (TCC) of the kidney is a rare, recently recognized entity of renal cell carcinoma (Table 1) [1, 4–7]. To our knowledge, TCC occurring within the native kidney of a renal transplant recipient has not been previously reported.

Tubulocystic renal cell carcinoma is often diagnosed incidentally. However, some patients may present with hematuria, leg swelling, or abdominal pain [8]. It occurs most frequently in the fifth or sixth decades with a strong male predominance (male : female ratio: 7 : 1), and approximately 60% occur in the left kidney [2]. The differential diagnosis of TCC includes other tumors with cystic appearance on imaging, such as multilocular cystic RCC and adult cystic nephroma [7]. It is not uncommon to have TCC described on imaging as cysts with unusual or atypical features [9] and can vary in appearance from Bosniak class II to IV [7]. Macroscopically, TCCs are well-circumscribed lesions comprising small cysts with multiple thin septa that give them a "bubble wrap" appearance. Although relatively indolent, TCC can behave aggressively, and it should be treated with partial or total nephrectomy [10]. Recurrence and/or metastasis occur in less than 10% of cases.

Renal transplant recipients have an increased risk (0.5–1.0%) of developing renal cancer when compared to those with ESRD (0.3%) and the general population (0.005%) [11–14]. The highest incidence of renal cancers occurs in the native kidney but may also occur in the renal allograft or even be transmitted from the donor [15]. This makes renal cancer the third most common solid tumor in transplant recipients and accounts for 10% of all cancer-related deaths following renal transplantation [16]. Risk factors for RCC in renal transplant recipients include the length of time on dialysis, the presence of renal cysts, male sex, and African descent [17, 18].

Most patients who have been on dialysis more than 3 years will have acquired renal cysts, of which 2% will develop RCC (11). These renal cysts may be categorized based on their radiologic characteristics (septa, cyst content, and enhancement) into Bosniak I, II, IIF, III, and IV classifications [19, 20]. The Bosniak classifications stratify malignancy risk, with a recent 2016 review finding malignancy occurring in 9% of type II cysts, 18% of type IIF, 51% of type III, and 86% of type IV [21]. Standard practice recommends no further intervention for Bosniak I and II, interval imaging follow-up for Bosniak IIF, and surgical intervention for Bosniak III and IV cysts [20].

Despite the increased frequency of renal cysts and RCC in patients with ESRD, there are no widely accepted screening protocols or lower interventional thresholds either before or following transplantation [11, 22, 23]. The lack of screening can be attributed to the relatively high mortality

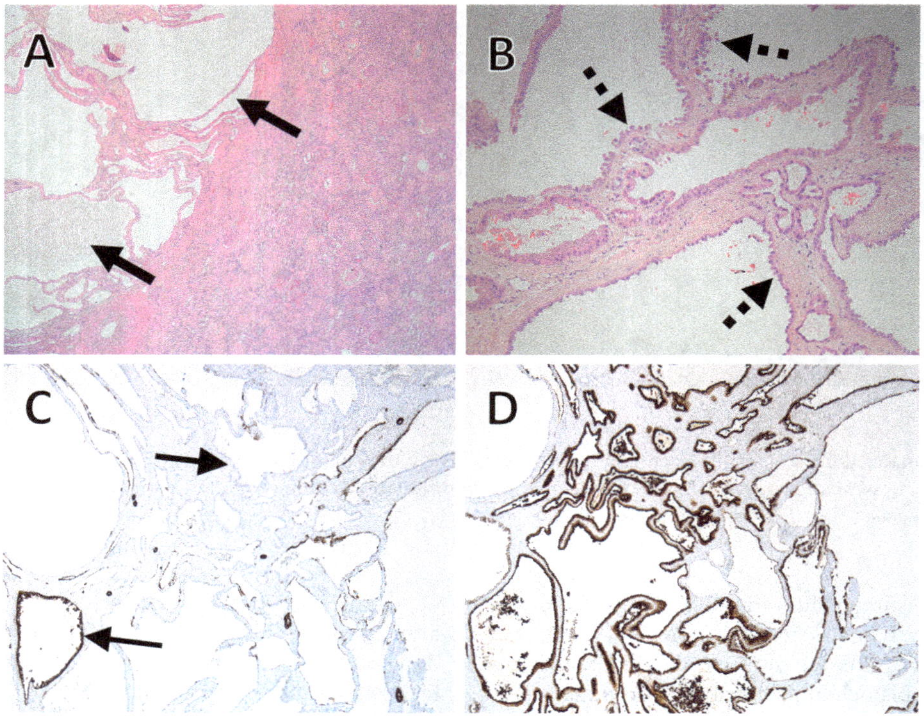

FIGURE 2: (a) Well-demarcated lesion of small- to intermediate-sized tubules admixed with cystically dilated tubules (solid thick arrows). (b) Tubules and cysts comprising a single epithelial layer of flat to hobnail-shaped cells with abundant, pink cytoplasm and large nuclei with prominent nucleoli (dashed thick arrows). The stroma was fibrotic and paucicellular, while mitotic activity was low to absent. No papillary architecture or epithelial cell clearing was observed. (c) Immunohistochemical stain for CK7 showed patchy reactivity (thin solid arrows) in the lesional areas. (d) CD10 showed strong reactivity.

TABLE 1: Common subtypes of renal cell carcinoma [3–5].

Renal cell carcinoma	Associations	Imaging	Morphologic characteristics	Behavior	Incidence
Clear cell	Patients >50 years Von Hippel–Lindau tuberous sclerosis	Hypervascular Heterogeneous (hemorrhage, necrosis, or cysts) Originates from the renal cortex	Cells with clear cytoplasm, prominent nucleoli, and extensive intricate branching vasculature, arranged in a nested architectural pattern.	Aggressive	75%
Papillary cell	Patients >50 years Hereditary papillary RCC End-stage renal	Hypovascular Homogeneous More common to be bilateral or multifocal	Neoplastic cells arranged in discrete papillary fronds with fibrovascular cores and can also be in a papillary-trabecular or papillary-solid architectural pattern.	Aggressive	10–15%
Chromophobe	Patients >50 years Birt–Hogg–Dube syndrome	Hypovascular spoke-wheel contrast enhancement Indistinguishable from oncocytomas	Smaller eosinophilic and larger pale neoplastic cells with wrinkled nuclei and perinuclear halos arranged in a predominantly solid architectural pattern.	Favorable, low mortality	5–11%
Collecting duct	Male-to-female ratio: 2 : 1 Patients: fourth and fifth decades	Heterogeneous (necrosis, hemorrhage, and calcification) infiltrative growth Originates from the medullary center	High-grade neoplastic cells with variable architectural patterns ranging from cribriform, papillary, solid, and tubular. Prominent stromal desmoplasia.	Very aggressive, 1/3 metastatic on diagnosis	1%

Table 1: Continued.

Renal cell carcinoma	Associations	Imaging	Morphologic characteristics	Behavior	Incidence
Renal medullary	Associated with sickle cell trait Male-to-female ratio: 2 : 1 Mean age: 22 years	Hypovascular Heterogeneous (hemorrhage and necrosis) Liver and lung metastasis	High-grade eosinophilic, neoplastic cells in varying architectural patterns. Cribriform pattern is the most common. Prominent desmoplastic stroma.	Very aggressive Mean survival: 15 weeks	1%
Multiloculated cystic	Mean age: 50 years Predominate in women with male-to-female ratio 1 : 4	Largely cystic lesions, <25% solid	Multiple cysts with thin septa, lined by clear cells.	Indolent, favorable prognosis	Less than 1%
Tubulocystic	Patients >50 years Male-to-female ratio: 7 : 1	Predominately cystic lesion with thin septa	Purely tubular and cystic growth pattern. Cysts lined by a single layer of neoplastic cells with hobnail appearance.	Largely indolent, rare reports of metastatic disease	Rare (less than 100 cases reported)

associated with ESRD and the fact that screening has not been shown to significantly increase life expectancy except when performed in younger patients. Currently, many dialysis centers will only perform routine renal screening on patients who are on the transplant waitlist [22]. For ESRD patients on the renal transplant waitlist (or undergoing evaluation) that have suspicious or complex cystic lesions, we suggest a nephrectomy in (a) young patients with a history of long-standing dialysis, (b) prior history of renal cell carcinoma in the contralateral kidney, and (c) those who may be expected to follow-up with their local nephrologists for long-term posttransplant care.

We conclude that tubulocystic renal cell carcinoma is a distinct entity of RCC. This rare case report highlights the elevated risk of developing renal cancer in transplant recipients, especially those with known renal cystic disease prior to transplantation. Therefore, such high-risk recipients should undergo either close postoperative monitoring, with annual surveillance ultrasound [16], or undergo a native nephrectomy prior to transplantation.

Abbreviations

TCC: Tubulocystic renal cell carcinoma
RCC: Renal cell carcinoma
ESRD: End-stage renal disease
CT: Computed tomography
CD: Cluster of differentiation
CK: Cytokeratin
EMA: Epithelial membrane antigen.

Acknowledgments

The authors thank Dr. Jinxing Yu for his assistance in reading the radiological images.

References

[1] H. Moch, A. L. Cubilla, P. A. Humphrey, V. E. Reuter, and T. M. Ulbright, "The 2016 WHO classification of tumours of the urinary system and male genital organs-part A: renal, penile, and testicular tumours," *European Urology*, vol. 70, no. 1, pp. 93–105, 2016.

[2] J. S. Bhullar, N. Varshney, A. K. Bhullar, and V. K. Mittal, "A new type of renal cancer-tubulocystic carcinoma of the kidney: a review of the literature," *International Journal of Surgical Pathology*, vol. 22, no. 4, pp. 297–302, 2014.

[3] National Comprehensive Cancer Network, *Kidney Cancer (Version 4.2018)*, National Comprehensive Cancer Network, Plymouth Meeting, PA, USA, 2018, https://www2.tri-kobe.org/nccn/guideline/urological/english/kidney.pdf.

[4] S. R. Prasad, P. A. Humphrey, J. R. Catena et al., "Common and uncommon histologic subtypes of renal cell carcinoma: imaging spectrum with pathologic correlation," *Radiographics*, vol. 26, no. 6, pp. 1795–1806, 2006.

[5] V. F. Muglia and A. Prando, "Renal cell carcinoma: histological classification and correlation with imaging findings," *Radiologia Brasileira*, vol. 48, no. 3, pp. 166–174, 2015.

[6] J. J. Hsieh, M. P. Purdue, S. Signoretti et al., "Renal cell carcinoma," *Nature Reviews. Disease Primers*, vol. 3, Article ID 17009, 2017.

[7] Y. Honda, Y. Nakamura, K. Goto et al., "Tubulocystic renal cell carcinoma: a review of literature focused on radiological findings for differential diagnosis," *Abdominal Radiology*, vol. 43, no. 7, pp. 1540–1545, 2018.

[8] I. Banerjee, S. S. Yadav, V. Tomar, S. Yadav, and S. Talreja, "Tubulocystic renal cell carcinoma: a great imitator," *Reviews in Urology*, vol. 18, no. 2, pp. 118–21, 2016.

[9] J. R. Srigley and B. Delahunt, "Uncommon and recently described renal carcinomas," *Modern Pathology*, vol. 22, no. S2, pp. S2–S23, 2009.

[10] Y. Ishibashi, T. Koie, N. Fujita et al., "Tubulocystic renal cell carcinoma in the left kidney: a case report," *Journal of Medical Case Reports*, vol. 8, p. 265, 2014.

[11] A. Chewcharat, C. Thongprayoon, T. Bathini et al., "Incidence and mortality of renal cell carcinoma after kidney transplantation: a meta-analysis," *Journal of Clinical Medicine*, vol. 8, no. 4, p. 530, 2019.

[12] S. Karami, E. L. Yanik, L. E. Moore et al., "Risk of renal cell carcinoma among kidney transplant recipients in the United States," *American Journal of Transplantation*, vol. 16, no. 12, pp. 3479–3489, 2016.

[13] B. L. Kasiske, J. J. Snyder, D. T. Gilbertson, and C. Wang, "Cancer after kidney transplantation in the United States,"

American Journal of Transplantation, vol. 4, no. 6, pp. 905–913, 2004.

[14] P. Maisonneuve, L. Agodoa, R. Gellert et al., "Cancer in patients on dialysis for end-stage renal disease: an international collaborative study," *The Lancet*, vol. 354, no. 9173, pp. 93–99, 1999.

[15] C. Morath, M. Mueller, H. Goldschmidt, V. Schwenger, G. Opelz, and M. Zeier, "Malignancy in renal transplantation," *Journal of the American Society of Nephrology*, vol. 15, no. 6, pp. 1582–1588, 2004.

[16] G. M. Frascà, S. Sandrini, L. Cosmai et al., "Renal cancer in kidney transplanted patients," *Journal of Nephrology*, vol. 28, no. 6, pp. 659–668, 2015.

[17] A. Goh and A. Vathsala, "Native renal cysts and dialysis duration are risk factors for renal cell carcinoma in renal transplant recipients," *American Journal of Transplantation*, vol. 11, no. 1, pp. 86–92, 2011.

[18] L. A. Hickman, D. Sawinski, T. Guzzo, and J. E. Locke, "Urologic malignancies in kidney transplantation," *American Journal of Transplantation*, vol. 18, no. 1, pp. 13–22, 2018.

[19] M. A. Bosniak, "The current radiological approach to renal cysts," *Radiology*, vol. 158, no. 1, pp. 1–10, 1986.

[20] R. Boissier, I. Ouzaid, F. X. Nouhaud et al., "Long-term oncological outcomes of cystic renal cell carcinoma according to the Bosniak classification," *International Urology and Nephrology*, vol. 51, no. 6, pp. 951–958, 2019.

[21] I. G. Schoots, K. Zaccai, M. G. Hunink, and P. C. M. S. Verhagen, "Bosniak classification for complex renal cysts reevaluated: a systematic review," *Journal of Urology*, vol. 198, no. 1, pp. 12–21, 2017.

[22] J. L. Holley, "Screening, diagnosis, and treatment of cancer in long-term dialysis patients," *Clinical Journal of the American Society of Nephrology*, vol. 2, no. 3, pp. 604–610, 2007.

[23] A. Schwarz, S. Vatandaslar, S. Merkel, and H. Haller, "Renal cell carcinoma in transplant recipients with acquired cystic kidney disease," *Clinical Journal of the American Society of Nephrology*, vol. 2, no. 4, pp. 750–756, 2007.

Permissions

All chapters in this book were first published by Hindawi Publishing Corporation; hereby published with permission under the Creative Commons Attribution License or equivalent. Every chapter published in this book has been scrutinized by our experts. Their significance has been extensively debated. The topics covered herein carry significant findings which will fuel the growth of the discipline. They may even be implemented as practical applications or may be referred to as a beginning point for another development.

The contributors of this book come from diverse backgrounds, making this book a truly international effort. This book will bring forth new frontiers with its revolutionizing research information and detailed analysis of the nascent developments around the world.

We would like to thank all the contributing authors for lending their expertise to make the book truly unique. They have played a crucial role in the development of this book. Without their invaluable contributions this book wouldn't have been possible. They have made vital efforts to compile up to date information on the varied aspects of this subject to make this book a valuable addition to the collection of many professionals and students.

This book was conceptualized with the vision of imparting up-to-date information and advanced data in this field. To ensure the same, a matchless editorial board was set up. Every individual on the board went through rigorous rounds of assessment to prove their worth. After which they invested a large part of their time researching and compiling the most relevant data for our readers.

The editorial board has been involved in producing this book since its inception. They have spent rigorous hours researching and exploring the diverse topics which have resulted in the successful publishing of this book. They have passed on their knowledge of decades through this book. To expedite this challenging task, the publisher supported the team at every step. A small team of assistant editors was also appointed to further simplify the editing procedure and attain best results for the readers.

Apart from the editorial board, the designing team has also invested a significant amount of their time in understanding the subject and creating the most relevant covers. They scrutinized every image to scout for the most suitable representation of the subject and create an appropriate cover for the book.

The publishing team has been an ardent support to the editorial, designing and production team. Their endless efforts to recruit the best for this project, has resulted in the accomplishment of this book. They are a veteran in the field of academics and their pool of knowledge is as vast as their experience in printing. Their expertise and guidance has proved useful at every step. Their uncompromising quality standards have made this book an exceptional effort. Their encouragement from time to time has been an inspiration for everyone.

The publisher and the editorial board hope that this book will prove to be a valuable piece of knowledge for researchers, students, practitioners and scholars across the globe.

List of Contributors

Hideaki Yamabe
Department of Nephrology, Hirosaki University Hospital, Hirosaki, Japan
Internal Medicine, EST Clinic, Hirosaki, Japan

Mitsuaki Kaizuka and Satoru Tsunoda
Internal Medicine, EST Clinic, Hirosaki, Japan

Tasuku Nagasawa
Internal Medicine, Japanese Red Cross Ishinomaki Hospital, Ishinomaki, Japan

Kazuo Nomura
Aoyama Nomura Dermatology Clinic, Hirosaki, Japan

Michiko Shimada
Department of Nephrology, Hirosaki University Hospital, Hirosaki, Japan

Norio Nakamura
Community Medicine, Hirosaki University Graduate School of Medicine, Aomori, Japan

Masamichi Nakata, Daiki Nagawa, Ikuyo Narita, Takeshi Fujita, Reiichi Murakami, Michiko Shimada and Hirofumi Tomita
Department of Cardiology and Nephrology, Hirosaki Graduate School of Medicine, Aomori, Japan

Yuta Nakamura, Kaoru Tada, Masashi Matsuta, Atsuro Murai and Hiroyuki Tsuchiya
Department of Orthopaedic Surgery, Graduate School of Medical Sciences, Kanazawa University, 13-1 Takara-machi, Kanazawa 920-8641, Japan

Jason Galo, Bianca Madrid and Warren Kupin
Jackson Memorial Hospital/University of Miami Hospital, Miami, FL, USA

Faten Aqeel
Johns Hopkins University School of Medicine, Department of Medicine, Division of Nephrology, Baltimore, MD, USA

Jennifer Del Castillo
Department of Internal Medicine, MedStar Health, Baltimore, MD, USA

Bernard G. Jaar
Johns Hopkins University School of Medicine, Department of Medicine, Division of Nephrology, Baltimore, MD, USA
Nephrology Center of Maryland, Baltimore, MD, USA
The Johns Hopkins Bloomberg School of Public Health, Department of Epidemiology, Baltimore, MD, USA
The Welch Center for Prevention, Epidemiology, and Clinical Research, Baltimore, MD, USA

Mohamad Hanouneh
Johns Hopkins University School of Medicine, Department of Medicine, Division of Nephrology, Baltimore, MD, USA
Nephrology Center of Maryland, Baltimore, MD, USA

Alexander G. Goglia
Rutgers Robert Wood Johnson Medical School, 675 Hoes Ln W, Piscataway, NJ 08854, USA

Michael Makar
Rutgers Robert Wood Johnson Medical School, Department of Internal Medicine, 125 Paterson Street, New Brunswick, NJ 08901, USA
Penn Medicine Princeton Medical Center, Department of Internal Medicine, 1 Plainsboro Rd, Plainsboro Township, NJ 08536, USA

Craig Vanuitert
Penn Medicine Princeton Medical Center, Department of Pathology, 1 Plainsboro Rd, Plainsboro Township, NJ 08536, USA

Vadim Finkelstein
Penn Medicine Princeton Medical Center, Princeton Hypertension and Nephrology, 1 Plainsboro Rd, Plainsboro Township, NJ 08536, USA

Ryo Togashi, Yoshikazu Nemoto, Kaito Waki, Michito Nagura, Shigeyuki Arai, Yoshifuru Tamura, Shunya Uchida, Shigeru Shibata and Yoshihide Fujigaki
Department of Internal Medicine, Teikyo University School of Medicine, Itabashi-ku, Tokyo, Japan

Yasutoshi Oshima and Fukuo Kondo
Department of Pathology, Teikyo University Hospital, Itabashi-ku, Tokyo, Japan

Ryuji Ohashi
Department of Diagnostic Pathology, Nippon Medical School Musashikosugi Hospital, Kasasaki-City, Kanagawa, Japan

Ibtissam Fares, Tarik Bouattar, Hadja Moussokoro Kone, Hajar Benzouina, Meryem Benbella, Naima Ouzeddoun, Rabia Bayahia and Loubna Benamar
Nephrology Dialysis and Transplantation Department, Ibn Sina Teaching Hospital, Rabat, Morocco
Faculty of Medicine and Pharmacy of Rabat, Morocco

Sarah L. Tan, Rachel Y. P. Tan and Jeffrey Barbara
Department of Nephrology, Flinders Medical Centre, Flinders Drive, Bedford Park, South Australia 5042, Australia
College of Medicine and Public Health, Flinders University, Sturt Road, Bedford Park, South Australia 5042, Australia

Gabrielle Cehic
Department of Nuclear Medicine, Flinders Medical Centre, Flinders Drive, Bedford Park, South Australia 5042, Australia
Centre for Translational Cancer Research, University of South Australia (Cancer Research Institute), 101 Currie Street, Adelaide, South Australia 5001, Australia

Michael Wu
Department of Surgery and School of Clinical Sciences, Monash Health, 246 Clayton Road, Clayton, Victoria 3168, Australia
Monash University, Wellington Road, Clayton, Victoria 3800, Australia

John Kanellis
Department of Nephrology, Monash Health, 246 Clayton Road, Clayton, Victoria 3168, Australia
Centre for In2ammatory Diseases and Department of Medicine, Monash University, Wellington Road, Clayton, Victoria 3800, Australia

Ruhin Yuridullah, Vinod Kumar, Sushant Nanavati, Monisha Singhal and Chandra Chandran
Saint Joseph's University Medical Center, USA

Sasmit Roy
Department of Medicine, Centra Health, Lynchburg, VA 24501, USA

Sumit Patel
Department of Internal Medicine, Adventist Health Community Care, Hanford, CA 93230, USA

Hardhik Kummamuru
University of Texas, Arlington, TX 76019, USA

Amarinder Singh Garcha and Sreedhar Adapa
Kaweah Delta Health Care District, Visalia, CA 93291, USA

Rohan Gupta
Community Regional Medical Center, Fresno, CA 93721, USA

Erasmia Sampani, Chrysostomos Dimitriadis, Efstratios Kasimatis, Evangelos Memmos and Aikaterini Papagianni
Department of Nephrology, School of Medicine, Aristotle University of Thessaloniki, General Hospital "Hippokratio", Thessaloniki, Greece

Kuang-Yu Jen
Department of Pathology and Laboratory Medicine, University of California, Davis School of Medicine, Sacramento, CA, USA

Ari Auron
Department of Pediatric Nephrology, !e Permanente Medical Group, Roseville, CA, USA

Thuan V. Nguyen, Nada M. Bader, Harpreet Sidhu, Caprice Cadacio, Susana M. Mendoza and Phuong Chi T. Pham
Olive View-UCLA Medical Center, Division of Nephrology and Hypertension, Los Angeles, CA 91342, USA

Phuong Thu T. Pham
David Geffen School of Medicine at UCLA, Kidney Transplant, Los Angeles, CA 90095, USA

Jessica Cruz-Whitley and Nolan Giehl
Department of Internal Medicine, University of California at Davis, Sacramento, CA, USA

Kuang-Yu Jen
Department of Pathology, University of California at Davis, Sacramento, CA, USA

Brian Young
Department of Internal Medicine, Division of Nephrology, University of California at Davis, Sacramento, CA, USA

Joseph McAllister, Pradeep Nagisetty and Kay Tyerman
Paediatric Nephrology, Leeds Childrens Hospital, Leeds LS2 9NS, West Yorkshire, UK

Samantha Bateman
Central and Northern Adelaide Renal and Transplantation Service (CNARTS), Royal Adelaide Hospital, Adelaide, Australia

Maleeka Ladhani
Central and Northern Adelaide Renal and Transplantation Service (CNARTS), Royal Adelaide Hospital, Adelaide, Australia
Sydney School of Public Health, University of Sydney, Australia

Shilpanjali Jesudason
School of Medicine, University of Adelaide, South Australia, Australia

P. Ventura-Aguiar, F. Diekmann and M. J. Ricart
Department of Nephrology and Renal Transplant, Hospital Clínic, Barcelona, Spain

M. T. Cibeira, M. Aymerich and J. Blade
Department of Hematology, Hospital Clínic, Barcelona, Spain

A.Martinez and M. Cuatrecasas
Department of Pathology, Hospital Clínic, Barcelona, Spain

J. Ferrer
Department of Hepatobiliopancreatic Surgery, Hospital Clínic, Barcelona, Spain

F. Touzani and A. Pozdzik
Department of Nephrology and Dialysis, Centre Hospitalier Universitaire, Hospital Brugmann, Brussels, Belgium
Faculty of Medicine, Université Libre de Bruxelles (ULB), Brussels, Belgium

C. Geers
Department of Pathology, Centre Hospitalier Universitaire, Hospital Brugmann, Brussels, Belgium

Latif A. Salam, Khabbab Amin, Regina Cheng and Noriyuki Murakami
Department of Internal Medicine, Section of Hospital Medicine, State University of New York (SUNY) Downstate Health Sciences University, 450 Clarkson Avenue, Brooklyn, NY 11203, USA

Clinton Brown
Brooklyn Health Disparities Center, Division of Nephrology, State University of New York (SUNY) Downstate Health Sciences University, 450 Clarkson Avenue, Brooklyn, NY 11203, USA

Lawrence Kwon
Department of Internal Medicine, Division of Nephrology, State University of New York (SUNY) Downstate Health Sciences University, 450 Clarkson Avenue, Brooklyn, NY 11203, USA

Ravinder D. Bhanot
Division of Pulmonary and Critical Care, St. Mary's of Michigan Medical Center, Saginaw, MI, USA
Department of Internal Medicine, Wayne State University, Detroit, MI, USA

Jasleen Kaur
Department of Internal Medicine, Wayne State University, Detroit, MI, USA

Zeenat Bhat
Division of Nephrology, Department of Internal Medicine, Wayne State University, Detroit, MI, USA

Ilya Seleznev, Dinara Jumadilova and Francesca Cainelli
Department of Medicine, Nazarbayev University School of Medicine, Nur-Sultan, Kazakhstan

Assiya Naushabayeva and Kairat Kabulbayev
Research Institute of Cardiology and Medicine, Almaty, Kazakhstan

Gulaiym Karashasheva
National Scientific Center for Oncology and Transplantation, Nur-Sultan, Kazakhstan

Rabin Nepali and Dibya Singh Shah
Department of Nephrology and Transplant Medicine, Tribhuvan University Teaching Hospital, Kathmandu, Nepal

Shreya Shrivastav
Department of Pathology, Tribhuvan University Teaching Hospital, Kathmandu, Nepal

Kamel El-Reshaid
Department of Medicine, Faculty of Medicine, Kuwait University, Kuwait City, Kuwait

Shaikha Al-Bader and Hossameldin Sallam
Department of Medicine, Nephrology Unit, Al-Amiri Hospital, Ministry of Health, Kuwait City, Kuwait

Daniele Sforza, Matteo Ciancio Manuelli, Linda De Luca, Simona Grande and Massimo Villa
Department of Emergency, Policlinico Tor Vergata Hospital, Rome, Italy

Leandro Siragusa, Bruno Sensi and Michele Grande
Department of Surgery, Tor Vergata University of Rome, Rome, Italy

Renato Argirò and Marco Nezzo
Department of Diagnostic Imaging and Interventional Radiology, Tor Vergata University of Rome, Rome, Italy

Carolina Ormonde and Raquel Cabral
Nephrology Department, Hospital do Divino Esp´ırito Santo, Ponta Delgada, Portugal

Sara Serpa
Radiology Department, Hospital do Divino Esp´ırito Santo, Ponta Delgada, Portugal

Sasmit Roy
Lynchburg Nephrology Physicians, 2091 Langhorne Road, Lynchburg, VA 24501, USA

Srikanth Kunaparaju
Richmond Nephrology Associates, 671 Hioaks Road, Suite B, Richmond, VA 23225, USA

Narayana Murty Koduri
Great Plains Health, 601 W Leota St, North Platte, NE 69101, USA

Vikram Sangani and Mytri Pokal
Quantum HC, Department of Internal Medicine, Navicent Health, 777 Hemlock Street, Macon, GA 31201, USA

Venu Madhav Konala
Precision Cancer Center, 122 St Christopher Dr, Ashland, KY 41101, USA

Mamtha Balla
Promedica Toledo Hospital, 2142 N Cove Blvd, Toledo, OH 43606, USA

Sreedhar Adapa
Adventist Medical Center, 115 Mall Drive, Hanford, CA 93230, USA

Gordon Audley
Division of General Medicine, Department of Medicine, Faculty of Health Sciences, University of Cape Town and Groote Schuur Hospital, Cape Town, South Africa

Bianca Davidson, Erika Jones, Brian Rayner, Nicola Wearne and Zibya Barday
Division of Nephrology and Hypertension, Department of Medicine, Faculty of Health Sciences, University of Cape Town and Groote Schuur Hospital, Cape Town, South Africa

Brendon Price
Division of Anatomical Pathology, Department of Pathology, Faculty of Health Sciences, University of Cape Town/National Health Laboratory Services, Groote Schuur Hospital, Cape Town, South Africa

Vasiliki Zoi, Dimitra Bacharaki, Aggeliki Sardeli, Minas Karagiannis and Sophia Lionaki
Department of Nephrology, National and Kapodistrian University of Athens, Attikon Hospital, Athens, Greece

Roberto Rivera and Salvador Vila
Department of Medicine, University of Puerto Rico School of Medicine, Guillermo Arbona Building Room A824A, San Juan, PR 00936-5067, USA

D. O. Beraldo and A. A. Teixeira
Hospital Renascentista, Pouso Alegre, MG, Brazil
Escola Paulista de Medicina—UNIFESP, São Paulo, Brazil

S. B. C. P. Duarte and R. A. Teixeira
Hospital Renascentista, Pouso Alegre, MG, Brazil
Instituto do Coração—FMUSP, São Paulo, Brazil

R. B. Santos, C. G. Mendes, M. P. Silveira, A. S. Neto, M. M. Silva, L. G. Oliveira and A. V. Bonfim
Hospital Renascentista, Pouso Alegre, MG, Brazil

Harshad Chaudhari, Nityasree Srialluri and Smita Mahendrakar
Rutgers University Department of Nephrology and Hypertension, Newark, NJ, USA

Jennine Michaud, Christine Granz and Michael Yudd
Department of Veterans Affairs, Renal Section, East Orange, NJ, USA

Thavathurai Priyanthan
Department of Nephrology, Odense University Hospital, Odense, Denmark

Anne Pernille Hermann
Department of Endocrinology, Odense University Hospital, Odense, Denmark
Department of Clinical Research, University of Southern Denmark, Odense, Denmark

Jonas Asgaard Bojsen
Department of Clinical Research, University of Southern Denmark, Odense, Denmark
Department of Radiology, Odense University Hospital, Odense, Denmark

Anne Bruun Krøigaard
Department of Pathology, Odense University Hospital, Odense, Denmark

Claus Bistrup and Erik Bo Pedersen
Department of Nephrology, Odense University Hospital, Odense, Denmark
Department of Clinical Research, University of Southern Denmark, Odense, Denmark

Daniel Guck, Andry Van de Louw and Philippe Haouzi
Division of Pulmonary and Critical Care Medicine, Department of Medicine, Pennsylvania State University, College of Medicine, Hershey, PA, USA

Reynaldo Hernandez and Steven Moore
Department of Emergency Medicine, Pennsylvania State University, College of Medicine, Hershey, PA, USA

Christian Maalouli, Arnaud Devresse and Valentine Gillion
Division of Nephrology, Cliniques Universitaires Saint-Luc, Université Catholique de Louvain, Brussels, Belgium
Division of Human Genetics, Cliniques Universitaires Saint-Luc, Université Catholique de Louvain, Brussels, Belgium

Karin Dahan
Division of Human Genetics, Cliniques Universitaires Saint-Luc, Université Catholique de Louvain, Brussels, Belgium
Center of Human Genetics, Institut de Pathologie et de Génétique, Charleroi, Belgium

Ahmad Makeen
Department of Internal Medicine, National Guard Hospital, Jeddah, Saudi Arabia

Faisal Al-Husayni
Department of Internal Medicine, National Guard Hospital, Jeddah, Saudi Arabia
King Abdullah International Medical Research Center, Jeddah, Saudi Arabia

Turki Banamah
King Abdullah International Medical Research Center, Jeddah, Saudi Arabia
Department of Nephrology, National Guard Hospital, Jeddah, Saudi Arabia
King Saud bin Abdulaziz University for Health Sciences, Jeddah, Saudi Arabia

Keiki Nagaharu
Department of Hematology and Oncology, Suzuka General Hospital, Yamanohana 1275-53, Suzuka 513-8630, Mie Prefecture, Japan
Department of Hematology and Oncology, Mie University Graduate School of Medicine, Edobashi 2-174, Tsu 514-8507, Mie Prefecture, Japan

Yuka Sugimoto
Department of Hematology and Oncology, Mie University Graduate School of Medicine, Edobashi 2-174, Tsu 514-8507, Mie Prefecture, Japan

Keiki Kawakami
Department of Hematology and Oncology, Suzuka General Hospital, Yamanohana 1275-53, Suzuka 513-8630, Mie Prefecture, Japan

Vishaka K. Chetram, Akram I. Ahmad, Saira Farid and Tanuj Sood
Department of Internal Medicine, Washington Hospital Center, Washington, DC 20010, USA

Kazuhiko Kato, Risa Terashima, Yukiko Tsuchiya, Yasuhito Takahashi and Kenji Kasai
Department of Internal Medicine, Fuji City General Hospital, Takashima-cho 50, Fuji-shi, Shizuoka, Japan

Tetsuya Kawamura and Takashi Yokoo
Division of Nephrology and Hypertension, Department of Internal Medicine, The Jikei University School of Medicine, Tokyo, Japan

Tomohiko Asakawa, Mea Asou and Makoto Araki
Department of Internal Medicine, Suwa Central Hospital, Chino, Nagano 391-8503, Japan

Shigeo Hara
Department of Diagnostic Pathology, Kobe City Medical Center General Hospital, 2-1-1, Minatojima Minamimachi, Chuo-ku, Kobe 650-0047, Japan

Takashi Ehara
Graduate School of Health Sciences, Matsumoto University, 2095-1 Niimura, Matsumoto 390-1241, Japan

José C. De La Flor and Miguel Rodeles
Department of Nephrology, Hospital Central Defense Gomez Ulla, Madrid, Spain

Marina Alonso
Department of Anatomic Pathology, Hospital 12 de Octubre, Madrid, Spain

Edna Sandoval
Department of Hematology, Hospital Central Defense Gomez Ulla, Madrid, Spain

Alexander Marschall
Department of Cardiology, Hospital Central Defense Gomez Ulla, Madrid, Spain

Gisela Marcelino, Ould Maouloud Hemett and Eric Descombes
Service of Nephrology, HFR Cantonal Hospital Fribourg, 1708 Fribourg, Switzerland

Joyce Moore
Department of Medicine, Michael G. DeGroote School of Medicine, McMaster University, Hamilton, Ontario, Canada

Jennifer Klowak
Department of Pediatrics, McMaster Children's Hospital, Hamilton, Ontario, Canada

Gloria Isaza
Department of Ophthalmology, McMaster University, Hamilton, Ontario, Canada

Steven Arora, Vladimir Belostotsky and Rahul Chanchlani
Division of Nephrology, Department of Pediatrics, McMaster Children's Hospital, Hamilton, Ontario, Canada

Nina Stein
Department of Radiology, McMaster University, Hamilton, Ontario, Canada

Paulo Garcia
Department of Pathology, Virginia Commonwealth University, Richmond, VA, USA

Cameron Benedict
School of Medicine, Virginia Commonwealth University, Richmond, VA 23298, USA

Brianna Ruch, Ashley J. Limkemann, Gaurav Gupta, Marlon Levy and Amit Sharma
Hume-Lee Transplant Center, Virginia Commonwealth University, Richmond, VA, USA

Index